THE ART OF COOKING FOR THE DIABETIC

THIRD EDITION

MARY ABBOTT HESS, L.H.D., M.S., R.D., F.A.D.A.
ASSISTED BY JANE GRANT TOUGAS

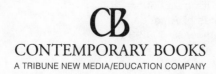

CONTEMPORARY BOOKS
A TRIBUNE NEW MEDIA/EDUCATION COMPANY

Library of Congress Cataloging-in-Publication Data

Hess, Mary Abbott.
    The art of cooking for the diabetic / Mary Abbott Hess ;
forewords by Marion J. Franz and Kathleen L. Wishner.
       p.   cm.
    Previously published: Chicago : Contemporary Books, 1988.
    Includes index.
    ISBN 0-8092-3393-2
    1. Diabetes—Diet therapy—Recipes.   I. Middleton, Katharine, d.
1987.   II. Title.
RC662.H47   1996
616.4′620654—dc20   95-21510
                                          CIP

Food Exchange Lists © 1995 American Diabetes Association and
The American Dietetic Association

Published by Contemporary Books, Inc.
Two Prudential Plaza, Chicago, Illinois 60601-6790
Manufactured in the United States of America
International Standard Book Number: 0-8092-3393-2
10   9   8   7   6   5   4   3   2   1

Contents

Foreword

If you or your family member has diabetes, you are aware of the many changes in diabetes management over the past ten years. First and foremost has been the emphasis on keeping blood glucose levels as near normal as possible. Evidence from the Diabetes Control and Complications Trial (DCCT) proved once and for all that excellent blood glucose control is important for the prevention and progression of long-term complications related to diabetes. However, evidence from the DCCT also illustrated the importance of food and nutrition in the management of diabetes. Individuals who maintained the best control of blood glucose levels reported that they followed their meal plan most of the time, treated low blood glucose levels appropriately, adjusted insulin for changes in eating that differed from their usual food pattern, and consistently ate an appropriate bedtime snack.

Besides changes in diabetes management, there have also been changes in recommendations related to food and nutrition—changes that are helping to make meal planning easier and more flexible for persons with diabetes. Among people who take insulin injections, it has been learned that those who are the most consistent in the timing of their food intake and the amount of carbohydrate they eat generally do the best with controlling their blood glucose levels. By eating consistently and monitoring blood glucose levels, you can integrate insulin regimens into your lifestyle.

For people with Type II diabetes, there are many lifestyle changes that will lead to improvement in blood glucose control: making better food choices, eating smaller portions and spreading them throughout the day, being careful of fat intake, and being more physically active. Losing ten to twenty pounds can also help. If you make these changes and still cannot control your blood glucose levels, you may need to take insulin or one of the many diabetes medications that are available today. By monitoring your blood glucose levels, you will know if the changes you are making in food and exercise are helping you achieve good control.

The good news is that there are a lot of lifestyle changes related to food and exercise that can help you better manage your diabetes. But one of the aspects of diabetes management that *hasn't* changed is the importance of planning food and meals. Another thing that hasn't changed is that—regardless of how important food and nutrition are in diabetes management—food and meals must still taste good! Information in the first section of this book can help you with diabetes management, but of more importance are the recipes in the next sections. This wonderful book can help you achieve the goal of tasty and healthful foods as well.

My wish for all of you readers and cooks is that you experience new and delightful tastes while keeping your diabetes under excellent control.

Marion J. Franz, M.S., R.D., C.D.E.
Director of Nutrition and Publications
International Diabetes Center
Minneapolis, Minnesota

Foreword

The third edition of *The Art of Cooking for the Diabetic* reflects the recent revolution in nutrition recommendations for people with diabetes. This is illustrated by the complete revision of Parts I and II, with emphasis on the flexibility of the new recommendations, including almost 300 entirely new recipes. Mary Abbott Hess has continued her tradition of preparing a book with loving care while at the same time providing accurate scientific information.

The Art of Cooking for the Diabetic is an up-to-the-minute sourcebook for anyone interested in applying the latest nutrition information to his or her daily diabetes management regimen. It highlights the American Diabetes Association's recommendation for a diabetes care team that includes a registered dietitian. It also stresses the importance of designing a meal plan that will be successful for the individual rather than attempting to follow a "diet sheet" based on outmoded, rigid guidelines that do not take lifestyle differences into consideration. In addition to the food exchange system, other methods of translating the meal plan for practical application, such as carbohydrate counting, are provided. The importance of the new food labels is demonstrated as the reader is taught how to interpret them.

The recipes in this edition reinforce the concept that a person with diabetes can enjoy gourmet dining and a wide range of food choices without having to feel guilty. In fact, the nutrition recommendations in this book should be viewed as a guide for anyone who wants to enjoy a healthy "diet."

Kathleen L. Wishner, R.D., Ph.D., M.D.
Past President (1994–95), The American Diabetes Association

Acknowledgments

Turning the science of nutrition, medical research, and new policy statements of health and professional organizations into language that the average person can understand has been a daunting task. Testing 375 wonderful and healthful recipes and calculating nutrition information in terms of grams and food exchanges has been another daunting task. These dual challenges have been met with a lot of help from many individuals who offered their time, expertise, and support.

Jane Grant Tougas worked closely with me in developing the manuscript and expanding all chapters. She also interviewed most of the registered dietitians, physicians, and other experts who generously shared their wisdom. We sincerely thank:

Barbara Barry, M.S., R.D., C.D.E.
Christine A. Beebe, M.S., R.D., C.D.E.
Brenda Broussard, R.D., M.P.H., M.B.A.
Anne Daly, M.S., R.D., C.D.E.
Deborah V. Edidin, M.D.
Joan Hill, R.D., C.D.E.
Carolyn Leontos, M.S., R.D., C.D.E.
Lindsay Leventhal, M.S., R.D., C.D.E.
Sue McLaughlin, R.D., L.D., C.D.E.
Margaret A. Powers, M.S., R.D., C.D.E.
Susan L. Thom, R.D., L.D., C.D.E.
Hope S. Warshaw, R.D., M.M.Sc., C.D.E.

Harold J. Holler, R.D., C.D.E., of the American Dietetic Association, was very helpful in providing guidance and helping to interpret the 1995 *Exchange Lists for Meal Planning*. The American Dietetic Association and American Diabetes Association granted permission to include these lists in this book.

Margaret A. Powers, M.S., R.D., C.D.E., and Susan Thom, R.D., L.D., C.D.E., reviewed the entire manuscript for technical accuracy. Each made many practical suggestions that enhanced the accuracy and usefulness of the book.

Recipes were shared by the American National CattleWomen, Marlys Bielunski and the Test Kitchens of the National Live Stock and Meat Board, Clara Coen, Karen Connit, Sharon Gourley, Barbara Grunes, Carl Jerome, Dawn Kohler, Quaker Oats, Barbara Stone, and Jeanette L. White, M.S., R.D., C.D.E.

Sharon Gourley spent almost six months working with me on every aspect of the book. She, along with my husband, Peter, colleague Karen Connit, and neighbors Linda, Claude, and Michael Garsin, taste-tested and evaluated many of the recipes. (They tasted all the rejects, too—only the best made the book.)

Lynne Hill of Hill Nutrition Associates did the computer analysis of the recipes. When we had a computer catastrophe shortly before the book deadline, North Suburban Secretarial Services entered the recipes—again. Shelly Osheff provided valuable guidance and computer consulting.

Thanks also to my literary agent, Jane Jordan Browne, attorney James Dahl, and Contemporary Books for making this book possible.

And last, but certainly not least, I thank the late Katharine S. Middleton, coauthor of the original edition of this book. She is my guardian angel, and this book is dedicated to her memory.

Introduction

According to the American Diabetes Association, almost 14 million Americans have diabetes. Nearly 90 percent of these cases are non-insulin-dependent (Type II) diabetes. More than half a million new cases of diabetes are diagnosed each year. Because Type II diabetes can develop very slowly, showing no symptoms for years, many people—perhaps as many as 7 million—are not yet aware they have the disease.

In 1994 the American Diabetes Association released its fifth edition of nutrition recommendations. Over the past 40 years, the association's recommendations have changed to reflect current scientific thinking about the role of nutrition in diabetes management. Only a decade ago, the diet prescribed for people with diabetes was rather strict and quite different from what most people ate. Following a "diabetic diet" meant avoiding sugar and using many special "diet foods" that often tasted terrible.

Now everyone is eating low-fat, sugar-free products, and many more good-tasting modified foods are available. Public health and nutrition organizations such as the United States Department of Agriculture and The American Dietetic Association are urging the general public to eat a diet based on the principles of variety, moderation, and balance. And the diet now recommended for people with diabetes is just that—a well-balanced approach to eating that is healthy for the whole family.

When all is said and done, the same healthy diet principles apply whether one has diabetes or not. The main difference is that diets planned for individuals with diabetes need greater consistency in the amounts and types of food eaten and care in the timing of meals and snacks, especially if insulin is taken. Eating suitable meals at regular mealtimes will help you avoid very high or very low blood glucose levels and long-term complications.

While moderation and portion control are still important, the philosophy of diabetes management is far more liberal than it was a few years ago. Here are some of the most dramatic changes in the American Diabetes Association's 1994 nutrition guidelines:

- An emphasis on tailoring diet plans to individual needs and lifestyles
- A new approach to sucrose (refined table sugar) as part of overall carbohydrate consumption
- A reconsideration of the role of monounsaturated fat in controlling blood glucose and fats
- An emphasis on "healthy weight," as opposed to losing weight.

People with diabetes, like everyone else, are urged to plan their meals using the federal Food Guide Pyramid, which illustrates the seven Dietary Guidelines for Americans. The 1995 Dietary Guidelines (proposed but not yet released as this book goes to press) are:

1. Eat a variety of foods.
2. Balance the food you eat with physical activity. Maintain or improve your weight.
3. Choose a diet with plenty of grain products, vegetables, and fruits.
4. Choose a diet low in fat, saturated fat, and cholesterol.
5. Choose a diet moderate in sugar.
6. Choose a diet moderate in salt and sodium.
7. If you drink alcoholic beverages, do so in moderation.

If you have diabetes, the consequences of not following a healthy eating plan can be serious. The disease requires ongoing medical and nutritional monitoring, especially as your needs change over time. The more you understand about diabetes, the more productive your appointments with your physician and your registered dietitian will be. And you will feel better because you are in control of your own health.

The Art of Cooking for the Diabetic can help you meet those challenges. Part I explains the role of the diet in diabetes management. Chapters on carbohydrates, fats, and sodium will answer many of your questions and help you make healthy choices at the supermarket and in your kitchen.

The chapters in Part II, "Living with Diabetes," give practical advice on how to deal with common situations such as eating in restaurants and at parties, traveling, and planning an exercise program. Parts I and II often mention the registered dietitian as the health professional who will counsel you about your meal plan. Although you may receive some diet information from other

Diabetes Nutrition Guidelines

What's Out	*What's In*
Primary Goal	
Weight loss as the primary goal for management of Type II diabetes	Aiming for near-normal blood glucose levels and optimal lipid levels (cholesterol, low- and high-density lipoproteins, triglycerides)
Meal Plan	
Preprinted diabetic diet plans; rigid, limited diets	Individualized food plan based on a person's food preferences, lifestyle, medication, and presence of complications
Weight	
Striving to reach an "ideal" or "desirable" weight, which may be unattainable and frustrating	Focus on reaching a "healthy" and reasonable weight that you can maintain (Even a 10- to 20-pound weight loss can improve blood glucose.)
Sugar	
The idea that simple sugars should be avoided and replaced with complex starches	Freedom to substitute some sugar, and foods that contain sugar, for other carbohydrate foods, but not simply to add them to the meal plan
Food Groups	
Six basic lists (starch/bread, meat, vegetable, fruit, milk, and fat)	Expanded lists including a new Other Carbohydrate list, a Very Low Fat Meat list, and separation of fats by saturation; advice that carbohydrate-containing foods can be used as Fruit, Starch, or Milk Exchanges

Source: Adapted from Environmental Nutrition, *June 1994.*

members of your health care team, you should rely primarily on your registered dietitian's advice.

Part III includes more than 375 delicious recipes. These recipes are not special foods for people with diabetes. They are great, healthy recipes for everyone. Each recipe has been tested, calculated, and converted to exchanges so that you can fit it into your meal plan. The exchanges match the American Diabetes Association and The American Dietetic Association's 1995 revised exchange lists. Following each recipe, a chart lists nutrition information for the specified portion size. Grams of carbohydrate are stated for those using a carbohydrate counting system. Cholesterol and fiber values are given, as well as the levels of calories, protein, fat, and sodium. If you have been told to limit your sodium intake, look for instructions at the bottom of each recipe.

Following the recipes, an appendix lists books, magazines, and many other sources of further information. A glossary gives simple definitions of terms that will help you understand information presented throughout the book.

The first edition of *The Art of Cooking for the Diabetic* was published in 1978. Much has changed since that time. For example, in the late 1970s, it was common practice to refer to someone with diabetes as a "diabetic." Today, we prefer not to label a person as a disease. Instead, we say "the person with diabetes."

Unfortunately, after almost 20 years, a copyright, and significant recognition in the marketplace, it's too late to change our title. So *The Art of Cooking for the Diabetic* it remains. Despite a "politically incorrect" title, be assured that the content of the book is very correct and up-to-date. It was developed with people like you in mind. I want to help you choose foods that fit into a healthy lifestyle. Every word has been reviewed by a superb panel of experts in diabetes care and education. They are listed in the Acknowledgments and have generously shared their experience and expertise. This edition has been prepared with the same loving care that inspired two previous editions. With it you can eat wisely—and very, very well.

Part I

Diet in Diabetes Management

When people eat, food is digested, and much of it becomes glucose—the form of sugar the body uses for fuel. The bloodstream carries the glucose to cells where it is used for energy. The cells absorb glucose with the help of the hormone insulin. People who don't have diabetes produce all the insulin they need, both for immediate energy and to store extra glucose and fat within cells for later use.

When you have diabetes, however, either your body does not make enough insulin, or it cannot properly use the insulin it does make. Without insulin, glucose can't move into the cells, and it builds up in your blood.

There are two major types of diabetes mellitus:

1. Insulin-dependent diabetes mellitus (IDDM or Type I)
2. Non-insulin-dependent diabetes mellitus (NIDDM or Type II)

Individuals with insulin-dependent diabetes do not make any or enough insulin or make very small amounts of a form that cannot be used. When the body has inadequate insulin to help use glucose for energy, it begins to burn fat. When fat is burned for energy, acid wastes called *ketones* are formed. As ketones build up in the blood, they lead to a serious condition called *ketoacidosis*. People with Type I diabetes must take insulin to avoid this life-threatening condition. Currently, insulin must be taken by injection. If it were taken as a pill, it would be digested and made inactive. However, an oral form of insulin is being developed and tested, and it may become available in the near future. That will be a wonderful breakthrough and make life easier for so many with diabetes.

People with Type II diabetes make some insulin, but either they don't make enough of it, or it does not work properly. This type of diabetes can usually be controlled by limiting the type or amount of food eaten and by increasing exercise. Oral hypoglycemic agents (diabetes pills) help some people make more insulin or use their own insulin better. The pills do not replace insulin; they only give the body a "boost" to make its own insulin. People with non-insulin-dependent diabetes sometimes require insulin injections to regulate their blood glucose levels.

The successful management of diabetes involves balancing food, physical activity, and, if needed, medication. Food raises blood glucose and blood fat levels—both of which can cause problems for people with diabetes. Activity and insulin lower blood glucose and blood fat levels. Exercise helps muscle cells use insulin better, which reduces the amount of insulin needed by the body.

Nutrition Management of Diabetes

A healthy diet provides a solid foundation for control and management of diabetes. Most cases of Type II diabetes, especially in overweight people, can be controlled by diet alone, without oral medication or insulin. This approach generally requires that meals be well-balanced, moderate in portion size, and spaced throughout the day to lessen the need for insulin production. In other words, we try to control *what to eat*, *how much to eat*, and *when to eat*. A doctor or registered dietician can also modify diets for people with diabetes to meet other individual medical needs such as sodium restriction.

Based on its 1994 guidelines, the American Diabetes Association has identified five goals for nutrition management of diabetes.

Goal 1: Keep blood glucose levels as near to normal as possible. By stabilizing your blood glucose levels, you can avoid *hyperglycemia* (high blood glucose) as well as *hypoglycemia* (low blood glucose). It is important to match the amount of food you eat with the amount of insulin in your body and your level of activity. You will feel better, and you may reduce or prevent the complications of diabetes. Blood glucose monitoring can show you the effects of foods and physical activity on your blood glucose levels. You can measure your own blood glucose using a blood glucose test meter. You will be asked to keep a monitoring record that can be evaluated by you, your doctor, dietitian, and other health care providers. The record helps identify problems related to food, exercise, and medication so that your diabetes care plan can be adjusted to meet your needs.

The Diabetes Control and Complications Trial reaffirmed the importance of controlling blood glucose levels. The results of that important study made it clear that keeping blood glucose levels as close to normal as possible dramatically reduced emergencies and long-term complications. Good blood glucose control requires frequent monitoring.

Goal 2: Achieve optimal blood fat levels. People with diabetes run triple the risk of nondiabetics to develop heart disease. That is because they often have high levels of blood fats (cholesterol and triglycerides). Chapter 5, "A New Look at Fats," discusses how to control your blood fats.

Goal 3: Maintain a reasonable weight. Eating the appropriate number of calories will help you reach and stay at a reasonable body weight. A reasonable weight is one that you and your health care team believe is achievable and maintainable over the short and long term. This weight may not be the one traditionally described as "ideal" or "desirable," but it is likely to be a healthy weight for you. Calorie needs depend on your size, age, and activity level. Your registered dietitian may change your meal plan to raise or lower calories to help you attain or maintain the weight where your body makes and/or uses insulin best.

Eating too many calories causes weight gain, which will worsen Type II diabetes and increase your risk of high blood pressure and heart disease. Children and teens with diabetes, however, must eat enough calories to grow properly. Pregnant and nursing women must eat enough calories to provide for proper development of their babies.

Physical activity also is very important. Exercise is helpful when trying to lose weight, and it helps keep your heart and blood vessels healthy, too. You can increase your activity level by walking, biking, or just taking the stairs instead of an elevator. See Chapter 9, "Exercise and Sports." If you wish to begin an intensive exercise program, check with your health care team first.

Goal 4: Prevent and treat the acute and long-term complications of diabetes. Hypoglycemia, short-term illness, and exercise-related problems can result from diabetes. Long-term complications include nephropathy (kidney disease), neuropathy (damage to nerves), hypertension (high blood pressure), retinopathy (eye disease that can lead to blindness), and cardiovascular (heart) disease.

Goal 5: Improve overall health through optimal nutrition. The Dietary Guidelines for Americans and the Food Guide Pyramid summarize nutrient needs for all Americans, including people with diabetes. It is important to eat a variety of foods that contain vitamins, minerals, carbohydrates, protein, and fat. Most foods contain a mixture of these nutrients.

Carbohydrate, which has four calories per gram, is our major source of energy. Starch and sugars in foods are carbohydrates. Starch is found in breads, pasta, cereals, and potatoes. Natural sugars are in fruits, milk, and vegetables. Added sugars are in desserts, candy, jam, and syrups. For more information, see Chapter 4, "What You Need to Know About Carbohydrates."

Protein also has four calories per gram and is needed for growth and replacement of body cells. Protein is in meats, poultry, fish, milk and other dairy products, eggs, dried beans and peas, and grain products.

Fat, the storage form of energy, is higher in calories—nine calories per gram. Fat is in margarine, butter, oils, salad dressings, nuts, seeds, milk, cheese, meat, fish, poultry, snack foods, ice cream, and desserts. For more about fat, see Chapter 5, "A New Look at Fats."

General Principles of Good Nutrition

The recipes in this book give you a head start toward achieving the American Diabetes Association goals. In addition, you should follow five general principles of good nutrition, which your registered dietitian will build into your meal plan:

Principle 1: Eat less fat. Drink skim milk and choose lean meats, poultry, and fish most of the time. Limit the portion size of fat-containing foods such as fried foods, cold cuts, pastries, gravy, salad dressing, margarine, butter, and cheese. For more information, see Chapter 5, "A New Look at Fats."

Principle 2: Choose foods high in fiber. Fiber may be beneficial in treating or preventing several gastrointestinal disorders, including colon cancer. Fiber also helps to lower blood fats. Good sources of fiber include dried beans, peas, and lentils; whole-grain breads, cereals, and crackers; and fruits and vegetables. The fiber recommendation for people with diabetes is the same as for everyone else: 20 to 35 grams of dietary fiber daily from a wide variety of food sources. More benefits of fiber are discussed in Chapter 4, "What You Need to Know About Carbohydrates."

Principle 3: Eat less sugar. Although recent studies have shown that sucrose doesn't boost blood glucose any more than other carbohydrates such as potatoes, rice, and bread, the fact remains that refined sugar has calories but no vitamins and minerals. It can cause tooth decay. Often, foods high in sugar are also high in fat, which makes them high in calories as well. For more information on the new thinking about sugar, see Chapter 4, "What You Need to Know About Carbohydrates."

Principle 4: Use less salt. The sodium in salt can cause the body to retain water. In sodium-sensitive people, it may raise blood pressure. Foods that are high in sodium, such as processed and convenience foods, are noted in the exchange lists with a special symbol: 🧂. If you are on a low-sodium diet, follow the instructions at the end of each recipe. For more on limiting your salt intake, see Chapter 6, "Cutting Down on Salt."

Principle 5: Use alcohol in moderation. The same precautions regarding alcohol use by the general population apply to people with diabetes. If your diabetes is well controlled, moderate use of alcohol will not affect your blood glucose levels. If you are using insulin, limit your alcohol use to two drinks or less per day, and always consume them with a meal. Remember that alcohol provides calories and that excess calories can cause weight gain. If you regularly drink alcohol, such as wine or beer, discuss this preference with your registered dietitian, who can build the calories into your regular meal plan. Some recent evidence suggests that one drink a day reduces risk of heart disease and increases life span. But if alcohol has not been part of your lifestyle, that doesn't necessarily mean you should add it now.

Individualizing your meal plan is the most important part of diabetes management. There is no longer a "standard diabetic diet." Your doctor and registered dietitian will help you identify your unique needs based on your cultural background, food habits, lifestyle, budget, and calorie needs. Together, you will set some goals—for blood monitoring, blood glucose and fat levels, weight, exercise, and medication. Based on your needs assessment and goals, your health care team can design a nutrition, exercise, and medication plan, tailored just for you. And they will guide you through that plan making sure you receive the education and counseling you need. Learning more about your diet, by reading this book and others, will make you more knowledgeable and confident. Periodic evaluation based on laboratory tests and monitoring records will reveal if your plan is working or needs adjustment.

1

The Meal Plan

One of your most important tools for controlling diabetes is an individual meal plan. The meal plan is a guide that indicates the number of food choices (exchanges) or the types of food you should eat at each meal or snack. Explains Barbara Barry, M.S., R.D., C.D.E., "We no longer work a meal plan into an insulin regimen. Rather, we develop the individual meal plan, then design an insulin regimen to accommodate it." Your meal plan should reflect your usual food intake and preferences, lifestyle, and the type of insulin or other medication you take.

One type of meal plan uses the food exchange lists that were revised and updated in 1995 based on the 1994 American Diabetes Association's Nutrition Guidelines. This book explains those guidelines and translates the scientific basis for them into practical information that mere mortals can understand. The new exchanges are provided and explained in detail, and all recipes have been converted to food exchanges. You and your registered dietitian may choose the exchange system or another approach such as carbohydrate counting, simplified exchanges, basic nutrition guidelines, calorie counting, fat counting, or a point system. Regardless of the approach you take, your meal plan must be tailored just for you.

For people with insulin-dependent (Type I) diabetes, the most important nutrition principle is consistency. The food you eat must balance your insulin injections and your activity. If you are not on intensive insulin therapy where you adjust your dose to food intake, you should be consistent in when you eat and the amounts of foods, particularly carbohydrate-rich foods, you eat at those times. Your plan will be developed so that you have adequate sugar in your blood at the peak time of insulin action and not too much blood sugar at other times. When your food intake and insulin are out of balance, wide swings in blood glucose can occur, causing you to suffer hypoglycemia or the symptoms of hyperglycemia.

Once you take insulin, especially the long-acting types, it will act whether or not you eat or exercise. If you are taking multiple daily injections or have an insulin pump, however, you will be able to adjust insulin times and doses on days you eat at untypical times or when you do an unusual amount of exercise.

Carbohydrate Counting

"Carbohydrate counting is a meal-planning approach for persons with diabetes that is gaining popularity across the United States," explains Anne Daly, M.S., R.D., C.D.E., who is chairman of the American Dietetic Association and American Diabetes Association Carbohydrate Counting Writing Group. "It can be simpler and more precise than food exchanges and offers greater flexibility in meal timing, food choices, and portion sizes. While it works well for some clients," she cautions, "it is not a panacea for all."

Carbohydrate counting can be used for Type I, Type II, or gestational diabetes (a form of diabetes that can occur during pregnancy). This approach is based on the fact that carbohydrates are the main influencers of blood glucose. Your meal plan indicates target goals for grams of carbohydrate to be eaten at meals and snacks. You use information from food labels, food exchange lists, and reference books to determine the amount of carbohydrate in each food you eat. You select types of foods and portion sizes to reach the set goal for total carbohydrate intake at each meal and snack.

Along with instructions on how to count carbohydrates, you receive general instructions related to amounts and types of protein and fat. Fat does not directly influence blood glucose levels. Some protein converts to blood glucose but not immediately. Modest amounts of lean protein—a 3- to 4-ounce portion of meat, for example—don't influence blood glucose levels, but a 12-ounce steak probably will.

The grams of carbohydrate to be eaten are the basis for predicting the insulin required before each meal and snack. Individuals with Type I diabetes, thus receive instructions on how much insulin to take. Eventually, the physician or dietitian will help you adjust your insulin-to-carbohydrate ratio as needed based on results of your blood glucose monitoring.

Carbohydrate counting can be easier, less time-consuming, more flexible, and more precise than a meal plan based on food exchanges. But maintaining healthy nutrition remains a challenge, especially with increased flexibility of food choices.

Carbohydrate counting is used by individuals with Type II diabetes because it is a fairly simple way to achieve good blood glucose levels. Disregarding protein and fat, however, can lead to weight gain. That can increase other health risks.

Striving for a "Healthy" Weight

Most people with non-insulin-dependent (Type II) diabetes are overweight. In fact, recent studies show that a third of all Americans—about 58 million people—are obese. Health experts now recommend that everyone start thinking in terms of healthy weight, rather than ideal weight. Studies show that even a small loss—10 to 15 pounds—can lower blood pressure, lower cholesterol and triglycerides, and boost self-esteem. For people with diabetes, a modest weight loss of 10 to 20 pounds, even if it doesn't get you near your ideal weight, usually improves blood glucose control and may be enough to prevent the need for medication. "Let's face it," says Joan Hill, R.D., C.D.E., "losing weight is very complex. Not everyone can do it. The psychosocial aspects of food are very strong. That's why *individual* plans are so important. Sometimes if you focus on controlling your blood glucose levels, weight loss follows."

For those with Type II diabetes, meal plans can address issues other than weight control. Individual plans may spread food throughout the day so that available insulin can handle controlled amounts of carbohydrate. The registered dietitian may adjust the level of fat up or down depending on the amount and type of fats in the blood. The meal plan may have more than 30 percent of calories from fat, but saturated fats are likely to be limited to less than 10 percent of calories. But don't worry about these percentages; that's the job of your dietitian, who will convert the percentages to food choices and help you to understand and use your personalized meal plan.

Many people with diabetes wonder if they can eat the same foods as the rest of their family. You do not need special foods or diet foods. Your meal plan is actually ideal for most people. Few people, however, consistently eat in such a healthy way, and it is very hard to change habits, especially those related to food.

Changing Your Meal Plan

As time goes on, your meal plan may need modification. Changes in your work schedule, school, vacation, or travel will require adjustments in the foods you eat and when you eat. Your weight may change, as might your food preferences and physical activity. These changes may affect your meal plan, too. Age also affects what you eat. More calories are needed in periods of growth, so children, teens, and pregnant women need more calories.

Results of lab tests, including periodic tests of blood fat levels, also may require that you alter your meal plan. If, for example, tests reveal the beginning of nephropathy (kidney damage), the amount or type of protein may be altered to avoid progression of the disease. By adhering to your personal meal plan, including these changes, you may be able to delay or avoid many medical complications.

Remember that your meal plan is a flexible tool that you should review regularly with your registered dietitian, who can adjust it to meet your changing needs. Regular nutrition counseling can help you make positive changes in your eating habits, provide ongoing education and support, and keep you abreast of changes in diabetes care.

Three situations require special instructions for individuals who are insulin-dependent:

1. **Plan for sick days.** Before you become ill with the flu or a cold, ask your doctor, dietitian, or diabetes nurse educator for a special sick-day plan. In general, it is important to still take your usual insulin dose. Try drinking small sips of regular soft drinks, sweetened tea, sweetened gelatin, popsicles, fruit juice, or sherbet if you can't keep solid food down. Generally, 1 cup per hour is adequate. If you can't keep any food or liquids down or if your blood glucose level is very high or very low, call your doctor immediately.

2. **Prepare for insulin reactions.** If you have symptoms of low blood glucose, test your blood. Be sure to carry glucose tablets or hard candy with you at all times to treat low blood glucose.

3. **Plan for exercise.** You may need to make some changes in your meal plan or insulin dose when you begin an exercise program. Check with your registered dietitian or doctor about it first. Be sure to carry some form of carbohydrate (such as fruit juice, dried fruit, or glucose tablets)

to treat low blood glucose. For more information, see Chapter 9, "Exercise and Sports."

Knowing what to do in advance of these situations will reduce stress; being prepared will prevent emergencies.

Portion Power

Since all meal plans are based on specific amounts of food, you will need to weigh and measure your food initially and periodically. As time goes on, you'll develop an eye for estimating portions and servings—an ability that will come in especially handy when you are eating away from home.

Portion Pointers

As you weigh and measure your food, you will eventually learn how to estimate portion sizes. Even when you are experienced at estimating, however, it's a good idea to check yourself every once in a while using a scale or measuring cup and spoons.

You can also use familiar objects to remind yourself about portion sizes. This strategy comes in handy when you are eating away from home. Here are some useful visual guides:

Portion	*Equivalent-Sized Object*
1 ounce meat	matchbox
3 ounces meat	deck of cards
medium apple or orange	tennis ball
medium potato	computer mouse
average bagel	hockey puck
1 ounce cheese	domino
1 cup fruit	baseball
1 cup broccoli	lightbulb

If you have some favorite recipes you'd like to use, ask your registered dietitian to determine their grams of carbohydrate or translate them into exchanges for you, modifying ingredients if needed. Many of the recipes you find in newspapers, magazines, and books include a nutrition analysis that states the grams of carbohydrate, protein, and fat. You can learn how to translate those numbers into exchanges. In some cases, newspaper recipes give very generous portions. You may want to prepare the recipe as printed but eat only one-half of the portion specified (and consequently only half of the nutrients, too). See Chapter 2, "Supermarket Skills," for tips on how to use nutrition labels to work foods into your meal plan.

If your meal plan doesn't follow the exchange system, ask your registered dietitian to mark this book and modify it to fit your needs. If you are counting carbohydrate, fat, or fiber, look specifically at the grams of that nutrient under every recipe. If you have dietary restrictions or specific food intolerances, this step is especially important.

2
Supermarket Skills

Do you feel as if you need a road map just to get around the *inside* of your grocery store? It's easy to get lost in today's super-sized supermarkets. So many choices! Twenty-five years ago, the average store carried about 7,800 items. Every year, more and more new products have been introduced. In 1993, more than 12,000 new products hit the supermarket shelves. Many introductions are reduced in fat, sugar, or salt. In the first three-quarters of 1994, manufacturers introduced 743 new sauces and gravies, as well as 25 entree mixes, 448 pasta products, and 135 rice dishes. These kinds of products are in response to our increasing demand for "speed-scratch" foods—prepared items we use to speed up cooking from scratch. At this rate, it's no wonder that today's superstore can carry a sometimes overwhelming choice of 30,000 products!

Planning ahead is important for everybody these days, especially for anyone with special health needs or dietary restrictions. Before you go shopping:

- Get to know the supermarket you use most often. Some stores, hospitals, and nutrition counseling firms offer store tours that teach you how to make healthy choices. Stores may also provide a printed shopping guide organized aisle by aisle—a handy checklist when you're planning your shopping trip.
- Check to see if your store has a registered dietitian or home economist on staff. She or he may be able to answer some of your questions. Your store also may have prepared a special packet on shopping for the person with diabetes.
- Before you shop, read the food section of your newspaper, and clip coupons as well as new recipes. Look through this cookbook and find recipes to try. Enjoying new foods and combinations will keep your meals interesting.
- Plan a menu for several days. Make a list from this menu, grouping together foods that you will find in the same area of the store. Keep some

options open. For example, list fresh fruit, and choose whatever looks best and is well priced. Write your grocery list on the back of an envelope that holds any coupons you have.

• Keep your list flexible so that you can take advantage of seasonal produce and suitable foods at bargain prices. For example, a sale on juice oranges might make them a better buy than the juice itself.

Try to shop soon after a meal. Studies show that we spend far more on groceries when we are hungry. Temptations jump right off the shelves into the basket! As you work the aisles, remember these tips:

• Buy as many fresh whole foods as possible. Fresh fruits, vegetables, whole grains, fish and poultry, and low-fat dairy products usually have more protective vitamins and minerals than most processed foods and are generally lower in fat, sugar, and salt. Fresh foods are usually located around the perimeter of the store.

• If you need just a little of a vegetable for a recipe, check out the salad bar. It costs more per pound, but you can buy ¼ or ½ cup of ingredients you need and will have no waste.

• If you can't find what you want, ask. The grocery business is very competitive. Consumers will be spending about half a trillion dollars in supermarkets by the year 2000. You're the customer. Don't be shy!

Healthful Staples

Stock your cupboard and freezer with these healthful basics:

A selection of vinegars, including balsamic, wine, and herb varieties

Several oils, including olive oil (choose "extra virgin" quality for salads), canola oil or corn oil for cooking, peanut oil for stir-frying

Nonstick cooking sprays—regular and perhaps olive oil and butter flavors

Various grains such as rice, couscous, barley, grits, and polenta (Many grains are available in quick-cooking or instant forms.)

An assortment of legumes, dry or canned, including a variety of peas, beans, and lentils

Several types of pasta

Canned tuna, salmon, and sardines packed in water

Baking ingredients:

• All-purpose and whole-wheat flour
• Cornstarch

- Dry bread crumbs
- Rolled oats
- Baking powder
- Baking soda
- Cream of tartar
- Unflavored gelatin
- Sugar-free gelatin dessert and pudding mixes
- Cocoa powder, unsweetened
- Semisweet chocolate chips
- Various extracts: vanilla, lemon, almond, etc.

Sweeteners:
- Granulated sugar
- Artificial sweeteners or noncaloric sweeteners—packets and/or granulated
- Honey
- Molasses
- Light (reduced-sugar) maple-flavored syrup

Seasonings:
- Salt, seasoned salt (reduced-sodium salt and seasoned salt if on a restricted-sodium plan)
- Pepper, peppercorns
- A selection of fresh spices and herbs (in pots or refrigerator) such as parsley, basil, chives
- Dried herbs—oregano, basil, Cajun seasonings; unsalted herb/vegetable blends, etc.

Canned and packaged goods:
- Tomato paste (no salt added)
- Pasta sauce
- Low-sodium canned Italian tomatoes
- Reduced-sodium canned chicken, beef, or vegetable broth
- Reduced-sodium soy sauce
- Catsup
- Salsa, tomato-based
- Fruit spreads (no sugar added)
- Peanut butter
- Light or reduced-calorie mayonnaise (fat-free mayonnaise if fat is significantly restricted)
- Several fat-free salad dressings for salads and marinades
- Canned fruit packed in juice and/or unsweetened canned fruit juice
- Dried fruits (no sugar added)

- Evaporated skimmed milk
- Nonfat dry milk
- Sugar-free cocoa mix
- Worcestershire sauce
- Mustard—Dijon, coarse-grain
- Red and white wine, to be used for cooking (not cooking wines, which may be salted)

Pantry staples:
- Onions
- Potatoes
- Fresh garlic

For the freezer:
- Frozen fruits, such as blueberries, peaches, strawberries, and/or raspberries (no sugar added)
- Fruit juice concentrates (no sugar added)
- Loaf of bread
- Soft margarine or butter (unsalted if sodium is restricted)
- Chicken breasts
- Egg substitute
- Several vegetables (no sauces added)
- Walnuts, pecans, and/or almonds

Make sure freezer items are packaged properly, labeled, and dated.

Looking at Labels

For years, consumers have been demanding more and more information about the nutritive values of the foods they eat. In answer to these demands, the Food and Drug Administration developed a standardized form of nutritional labeling in 1973. This program was strictly voluntary.

In 1990, the Nutrition Labeling and Education Act (NLEA) required that all foods regulated by the Food and Drug Administration and the U.S. Department of Agriculture bear standardized nutrition labels by May 1994. About 250,000 food products have been affected by the NLEA. Almost all packaged foods provide the information you need to make wise choices. Fresh produce and meat and on-premises cooked foods often have nutrition labeling, too.

Shoppers surveyed annually by the Food Marketing Institute (FMI) rate taste as their number-one consideration when buying food. Nutrition occupies a strong number-two slot. More than half of shoppers surveyed by FMI and

Prevention magazine say they almost always read the nutrition label on foods they buy for the first time. And 45 percent say they have changed a food-buying decision based on what they read on a nutrition label.

Nutrition Labels

Using the nutrition label should be part of your strategy for healthy eating. The nutrition label helps you compare similar foods so you can make the best choices within your daily meal plan. Remember to look at the serving size stated on the label. The nutrients listed are for that specific amount of food. For example, if you are counting carbohydrates, you may adjust the portion size up or down to meet your carbohydrate goal. If you are using the exchange system, check to see if the standard serving size is equivalent to one serving from the exchange lists. Knowing carbohydrate, fat, and calorie levels helps you translate virtually all foods into exchanges. You may want to practice translating favorite and commonly used foods into exchange list–sized portions with your registered dietitian.

Let's take a closer look at how to interpret a nutrition label. Our example is vegetable juice cocktail.

Nutrition Facts

Serving Size 8 fl. oz. (240mL)
Servings per container 4

Amount Per Serving

Calories 50	Calories from Fat 0

	% Daily Value*
Total Fat 0g	0%
Saturated Fat 0g	0%
Cholesterol 0mg	0%
Sodium 780mg	33%
Potassium 520mg	14%
Total Carbohydrate 10g	3%
Dietary Fiber 1g	4%
Sugars 7g	
Protein 2g	

Vitamin A 40% (80% as Beta Carotene)

Vitamin C 60% • Calcium 2% • Iron 4%

*Percent Daily Values are based on a 2,000 calorie diet. Your daily values may be higher or lower depending on your calorie needs.

	Calories:	2,000	2,500
Total Fat	Less than	65g	80g
Sat Fat	Less than	20g	25g
Cholesterol	Less than	300mg	300mg
Sodium	Less than	2,400mg	2,400mg
Potassium	Less than	3,500mg	3,500mg
Total Carbohydrate		300g	375g
Dietary Fiber		25g	30g

The title "Nutrition Facts" heads the label. Serving sizes, which used to vary widely, have now been standardized for 139 categories of food. The labeled serving size is not a recommended portion of that food, but an amount that is typically eaten. Sometimes label serving sizes do not exactly match the portions specified on the exchange lists used by individuals with diabetes and by dieters. In this example, 1 serving of vegetable juice at 8 fluid ounces equals 2 Vegetable Exchanges, because 1 Vegetable Exchange equals ½ cup (4 fluid ounces) of juice. All the nutrient information (grams of carbohydrate, protein, fat, milligrams of sodium, etc.) on the label is for the stated serving size.

Next comes a list of nutrients, each of which specifies the amount in grams or milligrams. To the right of these amounts is a column titled "% Daily Value." This percentage tells you how much of the recommended amount of each listed nutrient is present in one serving of that food, based on the amount of that nutrient needed in a single day. On all labels, % Daily Values are based on a 2,000-calorie diet. If you eat more than 2,000 calories a day, the food will provide a *lower* % Daily Value to your diet. If you eat less than 2,000 calories, the food will provide a *higher* % Daily Value.

Looking at the sample label, you can see that a serving contains no fat or cholesterol. But the 780 milligrams of sodium in an 8-ounce serving represent 39 percent of the total sodium someone on a 2,000-calorie diet should consume in one day. If you are on a low-sodium diet, this vegetable juice cocktail would not make a good choice. You should look for the unsalted version of vegetable juice cocktail. If this is not available, look for the nearest comparable product, perhaps unsalted tomato juice.

Note that the nutrition label distinguishes saturated fat from the total fat numbers. Manufacturers are not required to detail monounsaturated or polyunsaturated fat. (Some products high in monounsaturated fat, however, do list this number.) For the person with diabetes whose plan calls for more monounsaturated fat than usual, this lack of information can be a drawback, but you can still use the exchange lists in Chapter 3, "The Food Exchange System," or ask your dietitian to identify good sources of monounsaturated fat.

For the person with diabetes, total carbohydrate per serving is an important consideration. Total carbohydrate is the sum of all starches, sugars, and fiber. Fiber, however, does not end up as glucose in your bloodstream. We can't digest fiber, so the calories are not absorbed. Your registered dietitian will tell you how to adjust your carbohydrates if you regularly choose very high fiber cereals or muffins.

Note that there is no % Daily Value listed for sugars, although grams of sugar are listed. This omission is because the health authorities have not agreed on an appropriate Daily Value for sugar for the typical person. The grams of sugar listed include all sources of sugar—both naturally occurring and added. Sucrose, lactose (the sugar in milk), honey, corn sweeteners, high-fructose corn syrup, molasses, fruit juice concentrate, and other sugars are lumped together in the "sugars" category.

All nutrition labels must list the % Daily Value (based on a 2,000-calorie diet) for four key vitamins and minerals: A, C, calcium, and iron. If other vitamins or minerals have been added or if the product makes a claim about other vitamins or minerals, their % Daily Value must be listed, too. The label for vegetable juice cocktail shows that the juice is an excellent source of both vitamins A and C. Both of these nutrients have antioxidant properties and may protect cells from damage.

At the very bottom of the nutrition label is a footnote listing Daily Value reference numbers for a 2,000-calorie diet and a 2,500-calorie diet. This information is the same on all food labels. Foods that have only a few of the nutrients required on the standard label (such as mineral water or tea) can use a short-label format omitting this information, as can very small packages.

If your personal meal plan does not provide about 2,000 calories, you can still use % Daily Values to see which foods are good sources of key nutrients, even though the specific amounts may not apply to your diet. If fat, cholesterol, or sodium is restricted in your diet, you will want to think twice about foods that provide more than 10 percent of the Daily Value of those substances in a single serving.

Ingredient Lists

Packaged foods also must bear an ingredient list. According to an FMI/*Prevention* magazine survey, close to half of all shoppers say they almost always read the ingredient list when buying foods for the first time.

Ingredients are listed in order of weight. The ingredient list on vegetable juice cocktail puts tomato juice first, so you know there's more of that (by weight) than anything else. The ingredient list details exactly what sugars are present in the product, as well as any additives, preservatives, and colorings. We no longer advise people with diabetes to search ingredient lists for sources of sugar and to avoid sugar-containing foods. But foods with sugars listed at the beginning of the ingredient list (and recipes with a considerable amount of sugar) are likely to quickly use up exchanges on the carbohydrate lists. Similarly, these foods quickly add to grams of carbohydrate on a carbohydrate-counting regimen. Ingredient lists also enable people with food allergies or intolerances to identify and thus avoid problem ingredients.

For a handy summary of label-reading information, look for *Reading Food Labels: A Handbook for People with Diabetes*, a booklet jointly published by the American Diabetes Association, the American Heart Association, and the American Association of Diabetes Educators. Their addresses and phone numbers are listed in the Appendix, or you can look for local chapters of these organizations in your telephone book.

What Do Label Claims Really Mean?

To help you identify foods that fit into particular diets, the government now strictly regulates health claims and nutrient content claims on the front labels of packaged foods. For instance, you won't see misleading "no cholesterol" claims on foods that never had cholesterol to begin with. Health claims refer to the health benefits of foods. These are allowed in eight areas:

1. Calcium may be linked to a reduced risk of osteoporosis.
2. Fiber-containing grain products, fruits, and vegetables may be linked to a reduced risk of cancer.
3. Fruits and vegetables may be linked to a reduced risk of cancer (because of antioxidant vitamins and/or other substances).
4. Fruits, vegetables, and grain products that contain fiber may be linked to a reduced risk of coronary heart disease.
5. Reduced fat may be linked to a reduced risk of some types of cancer.
6. Reduced saturated fat and cholesterol may be linked to a reduced risk of heart disease.
7. Reduced sodium may be linked to a reduced risk of high blood pressure.
8. Sources of folic acid may be linked to a reduced risk of certain birth defects.

Nutrient content claims use terms like those listed in the following table. You can use these claims to speed your shopping by reading the front of the product label to find fat-free, light, low-fat, and low-calorie foods. Using some of these products will expand your options. When calories, fat, and sugar are reduced, you can have more of that food or can use the "saved" fat, sugar, or calories for other food choices. Remember that fresh fruits and vegetables, although not labeled with nutrient content claims, are in fact cholesterol-free and low-fat or fat-free (except for avocados and olives, which contain some fat).

COMMON NUTRIENT CONTENT CLAIMS AND THEIR MEANINGS

Claim	*Meaning*
Calorie-free	Less than 5 calories per serving
Fat-free or sugar-free	Less than ½ gram of fat or sugar per serving
Low-calorie	40 calories or less per serving
Low-fat	3 grams of fat or less per serving
Low-sodium	Less than 140 milligrams of sodium per serving of most foods (more for complete meals)
Low-cholesterol	20 milligrams or less of cholesterol and 2 grams or less of saturated fat
Reduced	Altered to contain 25 percent less of the specified nutrient or calories than in the usual product
Good source (of vitamins or minerals)	Provides at least 10% Daily Value of that vitamin or mineral per serving
High in	Provides 20% Daily Value or more of the specified nutrient per serving
High fiber	5 or more grams of fiber per serving
Light or lite	Foods altered so that they contain at least one-third fewer calories or half the fat of the usual food. A food that has most of its calories from fat must reduce fat by at least half. May also refer to color, flavor, or texture. Read labels carefully to see what "light" or "lite" really means.
Healthy	Low in fat and saturated fat and with limited sodium and cholesterol; must provide at least 10% Daily Value of vitamin A, vitamin C, iron, protein, calcium, or fiber.

Major food manufacturers are usually very careful that the nutrient information on their labels is accurate. If they do not meet federal labeling requirements, they face serious legal consequences. Unfortunately, however, some smaller manufacturers are less careful and have been known to make unsubstantiated and untrue claims about their foods. For example, an article titled "Too Good to Be True" (published in the May 1994 issue of *New York* magazine) found that the actual nutrient contents (calories, fat, and carbohydrate) of selected foods were drastically different from what the label claimed. One muffin *claimed* to have 140 calories and to be sugar-free, low-fat, and low-cholesterol but *actually had* 574 calories, 51 grams of sugar, and 21.6 grams of fat! A piece of "fat-free" cheesecake had 24.5 grams of fat. A frozen yogurt claiming to be fat-free with 47 calories really had 323 calories and 12.5 grams of fat.

Deceptive labeling is not only unfair to all customers, it is especially dangerous for those who must carefully control carbohydrate and fat in their diets. Be especially cautious with foods sold in delis, bakeries, and health food stores, and keep in mind that if something tastes "too good to be true," the label information might be erroneous. If you are concerned about a specific food, talk to your dietitian about it or call the closest regional office of the Food and Drug Administration. Their consumer affairs officers are excellent sources of information as well as fraud fighters.

3

The Food Exchange System

The exchange system is a popular way for people with diabetes to manage their food choices because it encourages moderate, consistent eating and allows you to choose from a wide variety of foods. The exchange lists and a meal plan help you know what to eat, how much to eat, and when to eat.

The food exchange system was developed in 1950 by a committee representing the American Diabetes Association, The American Dietetic Association, and the U.S. Public Health Service. The exchange lists underwent major revisions in 1976, 1986, and 1995 based on increasing knowledge about nutrition and food composition and on new approaches to the treatment of diabetes. The current exchange lists are concerned with total calorie intake based on a ratio of 10–20 percent of calories from protein to 80–90 percent of calories distributed between dietary fat and carbohydrate. Your registered dietitian will work with you to develop an individualized meal plan based on your food preferences, lifestyle, blood glucose and blood fat levels, medications, and other health needs.

If you are happy with your current meal plan and your diabetes is well controlled, you should not feel pressured to change. If, however, you think you could do better on a different type of meal plan, ask your registered dietitian to help you assess your needs and explore some new options. This chapter is intended to help you understand the latest exchange system and to ease your transition if you choose to adopt it.

What Is an Exchange?

Exchange lists group together foods that have about the same amount of carbohydrate, protein, fat, and calories. Consequently, you can exchange or trade one food on the list for another. For example, if you are tired of having ½ cup orange juice for breakfast, you might switch to a grapefruit half or a small banana. All three of these items equal one exchange on the fruit list—15 grams of carbohydrate and 60 calories.

The food exchange system is based on three main groups: carbohydrate choices, meat and meat substitute choices, and fat choices. The carbohydrate group includes starch, fruit, milk, other carbohydrate, and vegetable lists.

Placement of some foods may surprise you. For example, although corn is a vegetable, it appears on the starch list because its carbohydrate value is closer to grains and bread than to most vegetables. To give you flexibility in meal planning, several foods such as dried beans and peas, nuts, bacon, and peanut butter appear on two lists.

Each exchange list contains many foods. When you and your registered dietitian design your meal plan, you will agree on a certain number of exchanges for each meal. For example, in the morning you might plan for 2 Starch Exchanges or have a goal of 30 grams of carbohydrate. You might choose ½ cup cooked oatmeal plus one piece of toast, or one cup oatmeal, or two halves of a toasted English muffin. Each of these choices has the equivalent of 30 grams of carbohydrate, 6 grams of protein, 0 to 2 grams of fat, and 160 calories—or 2 Starch Exchanges.

It is important to eat all the food your plan calls for at each meal. It is also important to eat your meals and snacks at approximately the same time each day. Your body cannot properly use too much food at one time, especially if you are taking medication or insulin that is prescribed to help process food eaten at a specific time. (For tips on keeping mealtimes consistent when you are away from home, see Chapter 10, "Eating Out," and Chapter 11, "Traveling Safely.")

Exchange Lists

The following exchange lists (© 1995 American Diabetes Association and The American Dietetic Association) have been reprinted with permission. While designed primarily for people with diabetes and others who must follow special diets, the exchange lists are based on principles of good nutrition that apply to anyone. Each list is preceded by a brief discussion of how to use it, along with some information on the nutrients contributed by that particular food group. The use of brand names in exchange lists or in any discussion in this book is to help identify food products and is not an endorsement by the associations, publisher, or author.

Because exchange lists are based on specific portion sizes of each food listed, measuring tools are essential. You should have a set of measuring spoons, a glass measuring cup, a ruler, and a food or postage scale. (For more on kitchen equipment, see the beginning of Part III, "Recipes.")

Carbohydrate Choices

Starch Exchanges

Cereals, grains, pasta, breads, crackers, snacks, starchy vegetables, and cooked dried beans, peas, and lentils are starches. Each item on this list contains approximately 15 grams of carbohydrate, 3 grams of protein, 80 calories, and no fat.

Most starch choices are good sources of B vitamins. Dried beans, peas, and lentils are good sources of protein and fiber. They count as 1 Starch Exchange plus 1 Very Lean Meat exchange. Whole grains are also an important fiber source, averaging about 2 grams of fiber per serving.

You can choose your Starch Exchanges from any of the items on this list. If you want to eat a starch food that is not on this list, use these equivalents for 1 exchange:

- ½ cup of cereal, grain, pasta, or starchy vegetable
- 1 ounce of a bread product
- ¾–1 ounce of many snack foods (Some snack foods also have fat.)

Choose starches made with as little fat as possible. Be careful choosing bagels, rolls, and muffins. They can vary in size from 2 to 4 ounces. Each ounce of weight counts as 1 Starch Exchange. Starchy vegetables prepared with fat count as 1 Starch Exchange plus 1 Fat Exchange.

STARCH LIST

One Starch Exchange equals 15 grams carbohydrate, 3 grams protein, 0–1 gram fat, and 80 calories. Foods that contain 3 or more grams fiber per serving are identified with the symbol ⚭.

Bread

    Bagel ....½ (1 ounce)
    Bread, reduced-calorie ....2 slices (1½ ounces)

Bread, white, whole wheat,
pumpernickel, rye ....1 slice (1 ounce)

Bread sticks, crisp, 4 inches
long × ½ inch ....2 (⅔ ounce)

English muffin ....½

Frankfurter or hamburger bun ....½ (1 ounce)

Pita, 6 inches across ....½

Raisin bread, unfrosted......................1 slice (1 ounce)

Roll, plain, small ....1 (1 ounce)

Tortilla, corn, 6 inches across 1

Tortilla flour, 7–8 inches across.........1

Waffle, 4½ inches square,
reduced-fat 1

Cereals and Grains

Bran cereals ....½ cup

Bulgur (cooked) ....½ cup

Cereals (cooked)................................½ cup

Cereals, unsweetened, ready-to-eat....¾ cup

Cornmeal (dry)..................................3 tablespoons

Couscous ....⅓ cup

Flour ....3 tablespoons

Granola, low-fat ....¼ cup

Grape-Nuts ....¼ cup

Grits (cooked) ....½ cup

Kasha...½ cup

Millet ....¼ cup

Muesli ....¼ cup

Oats...½ cup

Pasta (cooked) ....½ cup

Puffed cereal ....1½ cups

Rice milk...½ cup

Rice, white or brown (cooked) ....⅓ cup

Shredded wheat ....½ cup

Sugar-frosted cereal...........................½ cup

Wheat germ ....3 tablespoons

Starchy Vegetables

Baked beans ....⅓ cup

Corn..½ cup

Corn on cob, medium........................1 (5 ounces)

Mixed vegetables with corn,
    peas, or pasta ....1 cup
Peas, green.................................½ cup
Plantain.....................................½ cup
Potato, baked or boiled...............1 small (3 ounces)
Potato, mashed ....½ cup
Squash, winter (acorn,
    butternut) ....1 cup
Yam or sweet potato, plain ....½ cup

Crackers and Snacks

Animal crackers...........................8
Graham crackers, 2½-inch
    square 3
Matzo..¾ ounce
Melba toast.................................4 slices
Oyster crackers...........................24
Popcorn (popped, no fat added or
    low-fat microwave) ....3 cups
Pretzels......................................¾ ounce
Rice cakes, 4 inches across 2
Saltine-type crackers 6
Snack chips, tortilla or potato
    (fat-free) ....15–20 (¾ ounce)
Whole-wheat crackers
    (no fat added) ....2–5 (¾ ounce)

Dried Beans, Peas, and Lentils

Count as 1 Starch Exchange plus 1 Very Lean Meat Exchange
Beans and peas—garbanzo,
    pinto, kidney, white, split,
    black-eyed (cooked).................½ cup
Lentils (cooked) ....½ cup
Lima beans (cooked) ....⅔ cup
Miso 🧂...............................3 tablespoons

Starchy Foods Prepared with Fat

Count as 1 Starch Exchange, plus 1 Fat Exchange
Biscuit, 2½ inches across 1
Chow mein noodles.....................½ cup
Corn bread, 2-inch cube..............1 (2 ounces)
Crackers, round butter type 6

Croutons...1 cup

French-fried potatoes ....16–25 (3 ounces)

Granola ....¼ cup

Muffin, small ....1 (1½ ounces)

Pancake, 4 inches across 2

Popcorn, microwave...........................3 cups

Sandwich crackers, cheese filling.......3

Sandwich crackers, peanut
    butter filling 3

Stuffing, bread (prepared) ....⅓ cup

Taco shell, 6 inches across................2

Waffle, 4½ inches square 1

Whole-wheat crackers, fat added
    (such as Triscuits).........................4–6 (1 ounce)

Planning for Cooked Starches

Some food, bought uncooked, will weigh less after you cook it. Starches, in contrast, often swell in cooking. A small amount of uncooked starch will become a much larger amount of cooked food. The following table shows some of the changes.

Food	Uncooked	Cooked
Cream of Wheat	2 tablespoons	½ cup
Dried beans	¼ cup	½ cup
Dried peas	¼ cup	½ cup
Grits	3 tablespoons	½ cup
Lentils	3 tablespoons	⅓ cup
Macaroni	¼ cup	½ cup
Noodles	⅓ cup	½ cup
Oatmeal	3 tablespoons	½ cup
Rice	2 tablespoons	⅓ cup
Spaghetti	¼ cup	½ cup

Fruit Exchanges

Fresh, frozen, and dried fruits and fruit juices are included on the Fruit Exchange list. The weights stated for fresh fruit include skin, core, seeds, and rind because that is how you buy whole fruit. Portion sizes for canned fruits are for the fruit and a small amount of juice. The average serving size for 1 Fruit Exchange equals:

- 1 small to medium fresh fruit
- ½ cup canned or fresh fruit or fruit juice
- ¼ cup dried fruit

Each item contains about 15 grams of carbohydrate, 60 calories, and about 2 grams of fiber. Fruit juices contain very little dietary fiber.

Use fresh fruits or fruits frozen or canned without added sugar most of the time. Whole fruit is more filling than fruit juice. It may be a better choice if you are trying to lose weight, and it provides a fiber bonus. The portion size for dried fruit is smaller because dried fruit is a more concentrated source of natural sugars.

Fruits, especially citrus varieties, are a good source of the antioxidant vitamin C (see discussion of antioxidants with the Vegetable Exchange list). In addition to its antioxidant properties, vitamin C is necessary for the formation of healthy connective tissue and bones. Early symptoms of vitamin C deficiency include bleeding gums and the tendency to bruise easily. Most Americans get their vitamin C at breakfast in fruits like oranges and grapefruits. Other fruits that are good sources of vitamin C include mangoes, berries, and melons. Try to have one excellent source of vitamin C each day at a meal or snack.

Fruit is also rich in the antioxidant beta-carotene, which your body converts to vitamin A. Excellent beta-carotene sources include fruits that are orange in color—mangoes, cantaloupe, papayas, and oranges.

Potassium, found in bananas, is necessary for maintaining the nervous system and fluid balance. Certain medications, particularly diuretics, can deplete the body of potassium.

Fresh fruits in season are generally the best choice for flavor and texture. If you select frozen, dried, or canned fruits, be sure to choose those labeled "unsweetened" or "no sugar added." Read Chapter 4, "What You Need to Know About Carbohydrates," for more information on sugars that may be added to fruit during processing.

Generally, fruit canned in "extra light syrup" has the same amount of carbohydrate per serving as the "no sugar added" variety or the "packed in fruit juice" variety. All canned fruits on the fruit list are based on one of these three types. If one serving of canned fruit has more than 15 grams of carbohydrate (check the nutrition label to be sure), then you will need to adjust the amount you eat.

Avoid canned fruits packed in regular syrup. Before the introduction of water- and juice-packed fruits, people with diabetes were told to use canned fruits but wash off the heavy syrup. Unfortunately, that technique did not work. A fruit that sits for months in a heavy, sugary syrup absorbs a lot of sugar. If you use fruit packed in heavy syrup and rinsed, you must cut your serving size by at least one-half or add an Other Carbohydrate Exchange to account for the extra sugar.

Fruit drinks are not included on the fruit list because they may have as little as 10 percent fruit juice and as much as 90 percent water plus added sugar. If you drink sweetened lemonade or another fruit drink, read the label and count each 15 grams of carbohydrate either toward your carbohydrate goal or as 1 Other Carbohydrate Exchange.

FRUIT LIST

One Fruit Exchange equals 15 grams carbohydrate and 60 calories. The weight for fresh fruit includes skin, core, seeds, and rind. Fruits that have 3 or more grams fiber per serving are identified with the symbol ⬬.

Fruit

Apple, unpeeled, small	1 (4 ounces)
Apples, dried	4 rings
Applesauce, unsweetened	½ cup
Apricots, fresh	4 whole (5½ ounces)
Apricots, dried	8 halves
Apricots, canned	½ cup
Banana, small	1 (4 ounces)
Blackberries	¾ cup
Blueberries	¾ cup
Cantaloupe, small	⅓ melon (11 ounces) or 1 cup cubes
Cherries, sweet, fresh	12 (3 ounces)
Cherries, sweet, canned	½ cup
Dates	3
Figs, fresh	1½ large or 2 medium (3½ ounces)
Figs, dried	1½
Fruit cocktail	½ cup
Grapefruit, large	½ (11 ounces)
Grapefruit sections, canned	¾ cup
Grapes, small	17 (3 ounces)

Honeydew melon.................................1 slice (10 ounces) or 1 cup cubes
Kiwifruit ....1 (3½ ounces)
Mandarin oranges, canned.................¾ cup
Mango, small......................................½ fruit (5½ ounces) or ½ cup
Nectarine, small ....1 (5 ounces)
Orange, small.....................................1 (6½ ounces)
Papaya ....½ fruit (8 ounces) or 1 cup cubes
Peach, medium, fresh ....1 (6 ounces)
Peaches, canned.................................½ cup
Pear, large, fresh ....½ (4 ounces)
Pears, canned.....................................½ cup
Pineapple, fresh ....¾ cup
Pineapple, canned..............................½ cup
Plums, small ....2 (5 ounces)
Plums, canned ....½ cup
Prunes 3
Raisins..2 tablespoons
Raspberries...1 cup
Strawberries.......................................1¼ cup whole berries
Tangerines, small...............................2 (8 ounces)
Watermelon ....1 slice (13½ ounces) or 1¼ cups cubes

Fruit Juice

Apple juice/cider ....½ cup
Cranberry juice cocktail ....⅓ cup
Cranberry juice cocktail,
    reduced-calorie ....1 cup
Fruit juice blends (100% juice)..........⅓ cup
Grape juice...⅓ cup
Grapefruit juice ....½ cup
Orange juice.......................................½ cup
Pineapple juice ....½ cup
Prune juice ....⅓ cup

Milk Exchanges

Each serving of milk or milk product on this list contains about 12 grams of carbohydrate and 8 grams of protein. The group does not include all dairy foods. Cheeses are on the meat list. Cream and other dairy fats are on the fat list. Look for chocolate milk, yogurt with fruit, frozen yogurt, ice milk, and ice cream on the Other Carbohydrates Exchange list. You'll find nondairy creamers on the Free Food list.

Milk and yogurt are good sources of protein and calcium. Calcium, a mineral, is needed for bone growth and repair. Everyone needs adequate calcium throughout life for strong bones and teeth. Lack of calcium is a major risk factor for osteoporosis, a crippling bone disease that affects many women in later life. Most milk sold in the United States is fortified with vitamin A (for growth, eye function, and resistance to infection) and vitamin D (for the absorption and use of calcium).

The amount of fat in milk or yogurt determines how many calories it has:

	Carbohydrate (grams)	Protein (grams)	Fat (grams)	Calories
Skim/very low fat	12	8	0–3	About 90
Low-fat	12	8	5	120
Whole	12	8	8	150

The higher the fat content of milk and yogurt, the greater the amount of saturated fat and cholesterol. Choose lower-fat varieties more often. In the store, you will find skim milk in dry, liquid, evaporated, and buttermilk forms. Very low fat milk is sometimes labeled 1% fat milk. Low-fat milk, low-fat buttermilk, and low-fat yogurt have 1½ to 2 percent fat. Whole milk has 3 to 4 percent fat. Yogurt comes in nonfat, low-fat, and regular forms. Some flavored and fruited yogurts have considerable added sugar plus added fruit. Be sure to read the nutrition label for fat, calorie, and carbohydrate content of milks and yogurts.

Most registered dietitians include milk in a meal plan because it helps so much to meet the dietary need for calcium as well as several other vitamins and minerals.

Try plain yogurt instead of some or all of the sour cream, mayonnaise, or oil in recipes and as a topping for potatoes. Explore uses for low-fat buttermilk, which adds flavor and creamy texture to many foods, including salad dressings, dips, soups, and sauces. Add fruit to milk or yogurt for a shake or dessert. Just 1 or 2 tablespoons of milk, buttermilk, or yogurt in a recipe, as a topping, or in a beverage, is 1 Free Food choice. You can also use a tablespoon of nonfat dry milk as a coffee whitener as a Free Food.

Although true allergy to food is very rare, intolerance to lactose—the sugar in milk—is quite common in adults, particularly in non-Caucasians. Lactose intolerance is caused by a diminished level or complete absence of lactase—the enzyme made by the body to convert lactose into simple sugars that can be absorbed from the digestive tract. Most lactose-intolerant adults can handle small amounts of milk (a few ounces) without much difficulty and can eat foods prepared with some milk as an ingredient. But they cannot digest larger amounts of milk. Lactose intolerance can cause bloating, abdominal pain, diarrhea, and gas.

As distressing as those symptoms are, don't give up on milk immediately. Some people who are physically intolerant of milk can eat fermented milk products such as yogurt, kefir, or cheese. Choose low-lactose dairy products, drink milk with added lactase, or take lactase in the form of tablets, liquid, or powder along with milk-based foods. If you still can't drink milk—or just don't like it—talk to your registered dietitian about increasing fruit choices so you can regularly drink calcium-fortified fruit juices. And try to eat other calcium-rich foods such as sardines and tofu, calcium-fortified muffins or breads, some green leafy vegetables, or yogurt or cheese if tolerated. Pregnant, lactating, and postmenopausal women may need to take a calcium supplement. Your registered dietitian will advise you about this and any other need for supplements.

Milk List

One Milk Exchange equals 12 grams carbohydrate and 8 grams protein.

Skim and Very Low Fat Milk

(0–3 grams fat per exchange)
Skim milk ....1 cup
½% milk...1 cup
1% milk...1 cup
Nonfat or low-fat buttermilk............1 cup
Evaporated skim milk........................½ cup
Nonfat dry milk (dry) ....⅓ cup
Plain nonfat yogurt ....¾ cup

Nonfat or low-fat fruit flavored
    yogurt, sweetened with aspartame
    or other nonnutritive sweetener.....1 cup

Low-Fat Milk

(5 grams fat per exchange)
2% milk...1 cup
Plain low-fat yogurt........................¾ cup
Sweet acidophilus milk.....................1 cup

Whole Milk

(8 grams fat per exchange)
Whole milk.......................................1 cup
Evaporated whole milk......................½ cup
Goat's milk.......................................1 cup
Kefir ....1 cup

Other Carbohydrate Exchanges

The list of other carbohydrates features foods that contain added sugar or that are mainly carbohydrates but are not starches, fruit, or milk. One exchange equals 15 grams of carbohydrate. Protein, fat, and calories vary. You can substitute food choices on this list for Starch, Fruit, or Milk Exchanges in your meal plan. Some choices will also count as one or more Fat Exchanges. Portion sizes are small because these foods are generally concentrated sources of carbohydrate and do not contain as many important vitamins and minerals as foods on the starch, fruit, and milk lists.

Foods that are high in sugar include soft drinks, candies, syrups, and sweet desserts. Foods from other lists prepared with added sugar that are in this category include sweetened yogurt, chocolate milk, and canned or frozen fruit with heavy syrup. Look at nutrition labels to determine what size portion equals 15 grams of carbohydrate. Try light jams and jellies and sugar-free or light syrups. Again, check the nutrition label for the amount that equals 15 grams of carbohydrate. For every 5 grams of fat in a serving size, count 1 Fat Exchange in addition to the carbohydrate choice. Some nonfat products made with fat replacements contain more carbohydrates, which you may need to count when you eat these foods in large amounts. Discuss this with your registered dietitian.

A new line of carbohydrate-controlled foods has recently been introduced under the brand name of Snack-15™. Each single-portion package contains 15 grams of carbohydrate, so you don't have to measure portions. The Snack-15 line includes trail mixes, spicy granola-type snacks, fruit gelatins, vegetable aspics, juice drinks, brownies, granola-type bars and cookies, and other items. A specially formulated high-glucose lemony drink is designed for use during periods of hypoglycemia.

OTHER CARBOHYDRATES

One Other Carbohydrate Exchange equals 15 grams carbohydrate, or 1 Starch, or 1 Fruit, or 1 Milk Exchange.

Food	Serving Size	Exchange(s) per Serving
Angel food cake, unfrosted	¹⁄₁₂ cake	2 Carbohydrates
Brownie, small, unfrosted	2-inch square	1 Carbohydrate, 1 Fat
Cake, unfrosted	2-inch square	1 Carbohydrate, 1 Fat
Cake, frosted	2-inch square	2 Carbohydrates, 1 Fat
Cookie, fat-free	2 small	1 Carbohydrate
Cookie	2 small	1 Carbohydrate, 1 Fat
Cookie, sandwich with cream filling	2	1 Carbohydrate, 1 Fat
Cranberry sauce, jellied	¼ cup	2 Carbohydrates
Cupcake, frosted	1 small	2 Carbohydrates, 1 Fat
Doughnut, plain cake	1 medium (1½ ounces)	1½ Carbohydrates, 2 Fats
Doughnut, glazed	3¾ inches across	2 Carbohydrates, 2 Fats
Fruit juice bars, frozen, 100% juice	1 bar (3 ounces)	1 Carbohydrate
Fruit snacks, chewy (pureed fruit concentrate)	1 roll (¾ ounce)	1 Carbohydrate
Fruit spreads, 100% fruit	1 tablespoon	1 Carbohydrate
Gelatin, regular	½ cup	1 Carbohydrate
Gingersnaps	3	1 Carbohydrate
Granola bar	1	1 Carbohydrate, 1 Fat
Granola bar, fat-free	1	2 Carbohydrates
Hummus	⅓ cup	1 Carbohydrate, 1 Fat

Food	Serving Size	Exchange(s) per Serving
Ice cream	½ cup	1 Carbohydrate, 2 Fats
Ice cream, light	½ cup	1 Carbohydrate, 1 Fat
Ice cream, fat-free, no sugar added	½ cup	1 Carbohydrate
Jam or jelly, regular	1 tablespoon	1 Carbohydrate
Milk, chocolate, whole	1 cup	2 Carbohydrates, 1 Fat
Pie, fruit, 2 crusts	⅙ pie	3 Carbohydrates, 2 Fats
Pie, pumpkin or custard	⅛ pie	1 Carbohydrate, 2 Fats
Potato chips	12–18 (1 ounce)	1 Carbohydrate, 2 Fats
Pudding, regular, made with low-fat milk	½ cup	2 Carbohydrates
Pudding, sugar-free, made with low-fat milk	½ cup	1 Carbohydrate
Salad dressing, fat-free or low-fat French, ranch, Thousand Island	¼ cup	1 Carbohydrate
Sherbet or sorbet	½ cup	2 Carbohydrates
Spaghetti or pasta sauce, canned or bottled,	½ cup	1 Carbohydrate, 1 Fat
Sweet roll or Danish	1 (2½ ounces)	2½ Carbohydrates, 2 Fats
Syrup, light	2 tablespoons	1 Carbohydrate
Syrup, regular	1 tablespoon	1 Carbohydrate
	¼ cup	4 Carbohydrates
Tortilla chips	6–12 (1 ounce)	1 Carbohydrate, 2 Fats
Vanilla wafers	5	1 Carbohydrate, 1 Fat
Yogurt, frozen, low-fat or fat-free	⅓ cup	1 Carbohydrate, 0–1 Fat
Yogurt, frozen, fat-free, no sugar added	½ cup	1 Carbohydrate
Yogurt, low-fat with fruit	1 cup	3 Carbohydrates, 0–1 Fat

Vegetable Exchanges

Each vegetable serving in this list contains about 5 grams of carbohydrate, 2 grams of protein, 25 calories, and no fat. Most vegetables contain 2 to 3 grams of dietary fiber. Vegetables such as corn, peas, winter squash, and potatoes contain larger amounts of carbohydrate, so they are on the starch list. In general, one Vegetable Exchange equals either of the following amounts:

- ½ cup cooked vegetables or vegetable juice
- 1 cup raw vegetables

If you eat 1 or 2 Vegetable Exchanges at a meal or snack, you do not have to count them. If you eat more than 2 cups cooked or 4 cups raw vegetables at one meal, however, count them as 1 carbohydrate choice. Try to eat at least one or two servings of vegetables with each meal except breakfast.

Vegetables and fruits are the best sources of the antioxidant vitamins C, E, and beta-carotene. Antioxidants have been shown to reduce cell damage and thus lessen the risk of disease and slow the cellular aging process. The National Cancer Institute recommends that everyone eat five servings of vegetables and fruit every day.

This advice is particularly relevant for people with diabetes, who are already at high risk for heart disease. You probably know someone who is taking an antioxidant supplement or eating antioxidant-fortified foods. These products have received a lot of publicity based on the cancer-fighting potential of anti-oxidant vitamins. Most registered dietitians advise getting your vitamins and minerals from foods where they occur naturally. "There is no evidence that antioxidant supplements or fortification affect blood glucose in any way," says Carolyn Leontos, M.S., R.D., C.D.E. "So our recommendation for people with diabetes is the same as for the rest of the population—eat a well-balanced diet."

The same advice holds true for phytochemicals, chemicals that are found in foods and may have disease-preventing potential. Research continues on both antioxidants and phytochemicals. In the meantime, eat plenty of protective vegetables and fruits every day.

Broccoli, brussels sprouts, cauliflower, greens, peppers, and spinach are good sources of vitamin C. Vitamin E can be found in green, leafy vegetables. Dark green and deep yellow vegetables such as spinach, carrots, and winter squash are particularly rich in beta-carotene, which the body converts to vitamin A. Vitamin A promotes growth, is needed for good vision, promotes resistance to infection, and maintains skin tone.

The National Cancer Institute recommends that everyone eat more cruciferous vegetables, the botanical family of vegetables that includes brussels sprouts, cabbage, broccoli, cauliflower, rutabagas, and turnips. Eating plenty of these vegetables has been related to reduced risk of many forms of cancer.

We don't often hear about magnesium, the fourth most abundant trace mineral in the human body. This mineral is needed for metabolism within cells, so lack of adequate magnesium impairs control of blood glucose. Not enough magnesium also can cause sodium retention and potassium depletion. Inadequate magnesium intake is found in up to 25 percent of individuals with diabetes. Eating plenty of vegetables will provide the magnesium you need. Almost all unprocessed foods contain some magnesium, but green leafy vegetables and root vegetables are among the best sources. Other food groups that provide magnesium include legumes, whole grains, nuts, and chocolate.

Fresh and most plain frozen vegetables are naturally low in sodium. Frozen vegetables with sauces or seasoning packets usually have a considerable amount of added salt. The amount is listed on the nutrition label. If you want to reduce salt content, drain and rinse canned vegetables or buy unsalted canned vegetables.

VEGETABLE LIST

One Vegetable Exchange equals 5 grams carbohydrate, 2 grams protein, 0 grams fat, and 25 calories. Vegetables that contain at least 400 milligrams sodium per serving are identified with the symbol 🧂.

Artichoke
Artichoke hearts
Asparagus
Beans (green, wax, Italian)
Bean sprouts
Beets
Broccoli
Brussels sprouts
Cabbage
Carrots
Cauliflower
Celery
Cucumber
Eggplant
Green onions or scallions

Greens (collard, kale, mustard, turnip)
Kohlrabi
Leeks
Mixed vegetables (without corn, peas, or pasta)
Mushrooms
Okra
Onions
Pea pods (snow peas, sugar snaps)
Peppers (all varieties)
Radishes
Salad greens (endive, escarole, lettuce, romaine, spinach)

Sauerkraut 🧂
Spinach
Summer squash
Tomato
Tomatoes, canned
Tomato sauce 🧂
Tomato/vegetable juice 🧂
Turnips
Water chestnuts
Watercress
Zucchini

If vegetables are prepared with fat, count each serving as 1 Vegetable and 1 Fat Exchange. To avoid the fat, use a nonstick pan with nonstick cooking spray or only 1 teaspoon oil to stir-fry vegetables (a great way to add more vegetables to your diet). Also enjoy raw or blanched vegetables as appetizers, snacks, and salads.

Protein Choices

Meat and Meat Substitute Exchanges

The exchanges for meat and meat substitutes each contain about 7 grams of protein. The amount of fat and calories varies depending on how lean the item is. In general, 1 Meat Exchange equals either of the following amounts:

- 1 ounce meat, fish, poultry, or cheese
- ½ cup dried beans, peas, or lentils

Based on fat content, meats are divided into very lean, lean, medium-fat, and high-fat. One ounce (one exchange) of each category of meat contains the following nutrients:

	Carbohydrate (grams)	Protein (grams)	Fat (grams)	Calories
Very Lean	0	7	0–1	35
Lean	0	7	3	55
Medium-Fat	0	7	5	75
High-Fat	0	7	8	100

Your registered dietitian will encourage you to make most of your choices from the lists of very lean and lean meat and meat substitutes. Items from the high-fat list are high in saturated fat, cholesterol, and calories. Limit your choices from this group to three times a week or less. Meat does not contribute any fiber to your meal plan, but dried beans, peas, and lentils are good sources of fiber.

Most grocery stores stock Select and Choice grades of meat. Select grades are usually the leanest meats available. Choice grades contain a moderate amount of fat. Prime cuts of meat, which are usually served in restaurants, have the highest amount of fat. Processed meats, including cold cuts and packaged sausages, carry nutrition labels that will tell you the number of grams of fat. More reduced-fat varieties are available in grocery stores, so the number of very lean and lean options is growing.

When cooking foods from the meat list at home, remember these tips:

- Trim off visible fat before and after cooking.
- Bake, roast, broil, grill, poach, or boil rather than fry.
- Place meat on a rack so the fat will drain away during cooking.
- Use a nonstick cooking spray and nonstick pan to brown or fry foods.
- If you cook poultry with the skin on to retain moisture, remove the skin before eating the poultry.

All foods from the meat list supply protein, which helps to form and maintain all cells of the body. Your diet will probably include 10 to 20 percent of daily calories from protein—the same as recommended for the general population. If your diabetes is complicated by kidney disease, your registered dietitian may lower your protein to 10% of daily calories, the low end of the "normal" range. Diets very low in protein are rarely used anymore.

Lean red meat, liver, egg yolk, and dried peas and beans are also very important sources of iron, a mineral that carries oxygen to the cells and is necessary for blood formation. People, particularly women and teenagers, who do not consume enough iron have low levels of iron in their blood, making them tired, irritable, and less resistant to common illnesses.

Vitamin B_{12}, which is found only in foods of animal origin, also is necessary for blood formation and prevention of another type of anemia. Most foods in the meat group help meet dietary needs for B_{12}.

Zinc, a mineral needed in small amounts to assist in insulin storage, is found in meat, poultry, liver, seafood, eggs, and dried peas. Zinc also influences the ability to taste food, is necessary for metabolism, and promotes resistance to infections.

Meats, dried peas and beans, and peanut butter supply potassium, as do many fruits and vegetables. Potassium helps maintain the body's fluid balance and is necessary for nerve and muscle activity, glycogen formation, and protein usage.

Specific foods in the meat group are excellent sources of other nutrients. Lean pork supplies considerable amounts of thiamin, and seafood supplies iodine, which is also available in iodized salt. The soft, edible bones of canned tuna, salmon, and sardines provide calcium, although most people get most of their calcium from the milk group.

Liver, which is rich in vitamin A and at least 12 other nutrients, is also rich in cholesterol. If you have been advised to limit your sources of dietary cholesterol, limit liver and other organ meats to no more than twice a month.

Some processed meats, seafood, and breaded poultry or meats contain carbohydrate when consumed in a 3-ounce portion. Be sure to read the nutrition label to see if carbohydrate content is close to 15 grams. If so, you will have to count a Carbohydrate Exchange as well.

For each food on the meat list, a 1-ounce portion is based on cooked food with all separable fats removed. Generally, meal plans include several Meat Exchanges at the lunch and dinner meal so you can have a reasonable meat portion. Weigh meat after removing bones and fat and after cooking. Do this occasionally at home so that when you are eating out you can eyeball the right meat portions without having to trim a serving and weigh it. Four ounces raw meat is equal to 3 ounces cooked meat, which is about the size of a deck of cards. Here are some useful examples of meat portions:

2 Meat Exchanges (2 ounces meat): 1 small chicken leg or thigh
½ cup cottage cheese or tuna

3 Meat Exchanges (3 ounces meat): 1 medium pork chop
1 small hamburger
½ chicken breast (1 sidebreast without wing)
1 unbreaded fish fillet

Meat List

VERY LEAN MEAT AND SUBSTITUTES

One exchange equals 0 grams carbohydrate, 7 grams protein, less than 1 gram fat, and 35 calories. Items that have 400 milligrams or more of sodium per exchange are marked with the symbol 🧂.

Poultry

Chicken or turkey (white meat, no skin)
or Cornish hen (without skin)......................1 ounce

Fish

> Cod, flounder, haddock, halibut, or trout
> (fresh or frozen) or tuna (fresh or canned
> in water)..1 ounce

Shellfish

> Clams, crab, lobster, scallops, shrimp,
> or imitation shellfish ....1 ounce

Wild game

> Duck (no skin), pheasant (no skin),
> venison, buffalo, or ostrich ....1 ounce

Cheese with less than 1 gram fat per ounce

> Nonfat cottage cheese or low-fat
> cottage cheese ....¼ cup
> Fat-free cheese ....1 ounce

Other

> Processed sandwich meats with less than
> 1 gram fat per ounce, such as deli thin,
> shaved meats, chipped beef 🧂, turkey ham ...1 ounce
> Egg whites 2
> Egg substitutes, plain.......................................¼ cup
> Hot dogs with less than 1 gram fat
> per ounce 🧂 ....1 ounce
> Kidney (high in cholesterol)............................1 ounce
> Sausage with less than 1 gram fat per ounce ....1 ounce
> *Count as 1 Very Lean Meat plus 1 Starch Exchange:*
> Dried beans, peas, lentils (cooked)...................½ cup

LEAN MEAT AND SUBSTITUTES

One exchange equals 0 grams carbohydrate, 7 grams protein, 3 grams fat, and 55 calories.

Beef

> USDA Select or Choice grades of lean
> beef trimmed of fat, such as round,
> sirloin, and flank steak; tenderloin; rib,
> chuck, and rump roast; T-bone, porter-
> house, and cubed steak; ground round...........1 ounce

Pork

    Lean pork, such as fresh ham; canned,
        cured, or boiled ham; Canadian bacon ;
        tenderloin; center loin chop............................1 ounce

Lamb

    Roast, chop, leg..1 ounce

Veal

    Lean chops and roasts.....................................1 ounce

Poultry

    Chicken or turkey dark meat (without
        skin), chicken white meat (with skin),
        or domestic duck or goose (well drained
        of fat, without skin) ....1 ounce

Fish

    Herring, uncreamed or smoked........................1 ounce
    Oysters..6 medium
    Salmon, fresh or canned, or catfish ....1 ounce
    Sardines, canned ....2 medium
    Tuna, canned in oil, drained ....1 ounce

Wild game

    Goose (without skin) or rabbit.........................1 ounce

Cheese

    4.5% cottage cheese ....¼ cup
    Grated Parmesan..2 tablespoons
    Cheeses with about 2–3 grams fat
        per ounce...1 ounce

Other

    Hot dogs with 3 grams or less fat
        per ounce ....1½ ounces
    Processed sandwich meat with about
        3 grams fat per ounce, such as turkey
        pastrami or kielbasa ....1 ounce
    Liver or heart (high in cholesterol)...................1 ounce

MEDIUM-FAT MEAT AND SUBSTITUTES

One exchange equals 0 grams carbohydrate, 7 grams protein, 5 grams fat, and 75 calories.

Beef

Most beef products, including ground beef,
     meat loaf, corned beef, short ribs, Prime
     grades of meat, trimmed of fat, such as
     prime rib ....1 ounce

Pork

Top loin, chop, Boston butt, cutlets ....1 ounce

Lamb

Rib roast, ground ....1 ounce

Veal

Cutlet (ground or cubed, unbreaded) ....1 ounce

Poultry

Chicken dark meat (with skin), ground
     turkey or chicken, fried chicken
     (with skin) ....1 ounce

Fish

Any fried fish products ....1 ounce

Cheese

Skim- or part-skim-milk cheese, with
     about 4–5 grams fat per ounce ....1 ounce
Feta...1 ounce
Mozzarella ....1 ounce
Ricotta ....¼ cup (2 ounces)

Other

Egg (high in cholesterol; limit to
     3 per week) 1
Sausage with about 5 grams or less fat
     per ounce...1 ounce
Soy milk..1 cup
Tempeh..¼ cup
Tofu ....½ cup (4 ounces)

HIGH-FAT MEAT AND SUBSTITUTES

One exchange equals 0 grams carbohydrate, 7 grams protein, 8 grams fat, and 100 calories. Remember, these items are high in saturated fat, cholesterol, and calories and may raise blood cholesterol levels if eaten on a regular basis.

Pork

　　Spareribs, ground pork, or pork sausage............1 ounce

Cheese

　　All regular cheeses, such as American ▮,
　　　　cheddar, Monterey Jack, Swiss ....1 ounce

Other

　　Processed sandwich meats with about 6–8
　　　　grams fat per ounce, such as bologna,
　　　　pimiento loaf, or salami................................1 ounce
　　Sausage, such as bratwurst, Italian,
　　　　knockwurst, Polish, smoked ....1 ounce
　　Hot dog (turkey or chicken) ▮ 1 (10/pound)
　　Bacon..3 slices (20 slices/pound)
　　Count as 1 High-Fat Meat plus 1 Fat Exchange:
　　Hot dog (beef, pork, or combination) ▮ 1 (10/pound)
　　Peanut butter (contains unsaturated fat) ....2 tablespoons

---

Fat Choices

Fat Exchanges

Fats are divided into three groups based on the main type of fat they contain: monounsaturated, polyunsaturated, or saturated. Each serving in the fat list contains about 5 grams of fat and 45 calories. The sodium content of food on the fat list varies widely. Be sure to check the nutrition label if you are on a restricted-sodium meal plan. In general, 1 Fat Exchange equals:

- 1 teaspoon butter, margarine, or vegetable oil
- 1 tablespoon salad dressing
- 2 to 3 tablespoons light or reduced-calorie salad dressing

All fats—animal or vegetable, hard or liquid—have 9 calories per gram, more than twice the calories of a gram of carbohydrate or protein. Small amounts of monounsaturated and polyunsaturated fats in the diet are linked with health benefits, but high intake of saturated fat is linked with chronic diseases such as heart disease and cancer. Generally, it is wise to limit your fat choices from the saturated fat list. Read Chapter 5, "A New Look at Fats," for an explanation of types of fat and their specific effects on the body.

While we emphasize the negative aspects of eating too much fat, foods with fat do provide some essential nutrients. Margarine, butter, and cream provide vitamin A in a form that is easily used by the body. Vegetable oil is an excellent source of vitamin E. Nuts and seeds provide small amounts of protein, magnesium, and fiber.

The amount and type of salad dressing to use is often very confusing. Generally, regular bottled salad dressings provide 1 Fat Exchange per tablespoon. One teaspoon olive oil or corn oil provides 1 Fat Exchange. One teaspoon regular mayonnaise or 1 tablespoon light or reduced-fat mayonnaise equals 1 Fat Exchange. Reduced-calorie dressings provide about 25 calories per tablespoonful, so 2 tablespoons count as 1 Fat Exchange. If you want to use more dressing, look for fat-free varieties. Most contain less than 10 calories and can be a Free Food. Some fat-free dressings, however, contain carbohydrate to improve texture. These dressings will be found on the Other Carbohydrate list. All bottled dressings carry nutrition labeling. Read the labels and find a dressing that you enjoy.

Unless you have lots of fat calories and Fat Exchanges to use, prepare your own tasty, low-calorie dressings or buy prepared ones and keep them in your refrigerator. Save your Fat Exchanges for cooking, sauces, and spreads. When eating out, ask for low-calorie dressings on the side so you can control the amount you eat.

When selecting regular margarine, choose those with liquid vegetable oil as the first ingredient. Soft margarines are not as saturated as stick margarines and are generally healthier choices. Most hard stick margarines contain hydrogenated or partially hydrogenated fat as the first ingredient. These fats (in a form called trans-fatty acids) may act like saturated fat when eaten and could raise levels of fats in your bloodstream. The law does not require manufacturers to state the amount of trans-fatty acids on the food labels. Look at the ingredient list to see how the fat has been processed. When selecting reduced-fat margarine, look for liquid vegetable oil as the second ingredient; water is usually the first ingredient.

Don't use the lowest-fat margarines for cooking or recipes requiring baking; they contain too much water for dependable results. Use cooking sprays when you can. They are on the Free Foods list and don't add calories. Along with nonstick pots and pans, they reduce the amount of fats needed in many recipes.

Nondairy creamers, whipped toppings, and fat-free products such as margarines, sour cream, and cream cheese can be found on the Free Foods list.

Fat List

One Fat Exchange equals 5 grams fat and 45 calories. Items that have 400 milligrams or more of sodium per exchange are marked with the symbol 🧂.

Monounsaturated Fats

Avocado, medium ....⅛ (1 ounce)
Oil (canola, olive, or peanut)............................1 teaspoon
Olives, ripe (black)..8 large
Olives, green, Spanish stuffed 🧂......................10 large
Nuts:
    Almonds or cashews.....................................6 nuts
    Mixed nuts (50 percent peanuts)...................6 nuts
    Peanuts...10 nuts
    Pecans ....4 halves
Peanut butter, smooth or crunchy ....2 teaspoons
Sesame seeds...1 tablespoon
Tahini (sesame paste)......................................2 teaspoons

Polyunsaturated Fats

Margarine (stick, tub, or squeeze) ....1 teaspoon
Margarine, lower-fat (30–50 percent
    vegetable oil)...1 tablespoon
Mayonnaise, regular...1 teaspoon
Mayonnaise, light or reduced-fat ....1 tablespoon
Miracle Whip salad dressing, regular................2 teaspoons
Miracle Whip salad dressing, light ....1 tablespoon
Oil (corn, safflower, or soybean).......................1 teaspoon
Salad dressings, regular 🧂...............................1 tablespoon

Salad dressings, reduced-fat ....2 tablespoons
Seeds, pumpkin or sunflower ....1 tablespoon
Walnuts, English...4 halves

Saturated Fats

Bacon, cooked..1 slice (20 slices/pound)
Bacon grease ....1 teaspoon
Butter, stick ....1 teaspoon
Butter, whipped ....2 teaspoons
Butter, reduced-fat...1 tablespoon
Chitterlings, boiled ....2 tablespoons (½ ounce)
Coconut, sweetened, shredded ....2 tablespoons
Cream, half-and-half ....2 tablespoons
Cream cheese, regular.......................................1 tablespoon (½ ounce)
Cream cheese, light or reduced-fat ....2 tablespoons (1 ounce)
Fatback or salt pork ....See below*
Shortening or lard..1 teaspoon
Sour cream, regular..2 tablespoons
Sour cream, light or reduced-fat ....3 tablespoons
Sour cream, fat-free ....See Free Food List

*A piece 1 inch × 1 inch × ¼ inch is 1 Fat Exchange if you plan to eat the fatback cooked with vegetables.

A piece 2 inches × 1 inch × ½ inch is 1 Fat Exchange if you eat only the vegetables with the fatback removed.

Free Foods

A Free Food is any food or drink that contains less than 20 calories or less than 5 grams of carbohydrate per serving. Some Free Foods on the list have no specified serving size. You can eat as much as you want of these. For foods listed with a serving size, they are Free Foods only if you eat three or fewer servings spread out over a day. Eating all three servings at one time could affect your blood glucose level. If you eat three or more servings of these at one meal, you will have to reduce carbohydrates elsewhere in the same meal.

Many processed foods now come in sugar-free or fat-free forms or in reduced-fat varieties that can be used as Free Foods. Sugar substitutes and most sugar-free beverages are Free Foods. Most seasonings are Free Foods, but be careful when using seasonings and condiments that contain sodium. They are marked on the list with the salt symbol 🧂.

Sugar Substitutes

Sugar substitutes, alternatives, or replacements that are approved by the Food and Drug Administration (FDA) are safe to use. Common brand names include:

Equal (aspartame)

Sprinkle Sweet (saccharin)

Sweet One (acesulfame K)

Sweet-10 (saccharin)

Sugar Twin (saccharin)

Sweet 'n Low (saccharin)

Although nondairy creamers appear on the Free Foods list, a better and less expensive way of lightening your coffee is to use 1 teaspoon instant nonfat dry milk. This type of milk costs less, needs no refrigeration, provides calcium, and has only 10 calories per teaspoon. You may use 1 teaspoon per meal in your beverage without counting it as an exchange. When using dry milk powder in hot beverages, allow the tea or coffee to cool for a few moments before adding the powder, or "sift" it in by sprinkling it from a shaker so that it will dissolve without a curdled appearance.

Whipped toppings are popular and fairly low in calories and fat. But most are processed in a way that changes monounsaturated fats to trans-fatty acids, so use them in moderation.

FREE FOOD LIST

A Free Food is any food or drink that contains less than 20 calories or less than 5 grams carbohydrate per serving. Foods with a serving size listed should be limited to three servings per day and spread out throughout the day. Foods listed without a serving size can be eaten as often as you like. Items that have 400 milligrams or more of sodium per choice are marked with the symbol 🧂.

Low-Fat or Fat-Free Foods

Cream cheese, fat-free ....1 tablespoon

Creamers, nondairy, liquid ....1 tablespoon

Creamers, nondairy, powdered ....2 teaspoons

Mayonnaise, fat-free ....1 tablespoon

Mayonnaise, reduced-fat ....1 teaspoon

Margarine, fat-free or nonfat ....4 tablespoons

Margarine, reduced-fat..1 teaspoon
Miracle Whip salad dressing, nonfat................1 tablespoon
Miracle Whip salad dressing, reduced-fat.........1 teaspoon
Nonstick cooking spray
Salad dressing, fat-free, ranch or French...........1 tablespoon
Salad dressing, Italian fat-free..........................2 tablespoons
Salsa...¼ cup
Sour cream, fat-free, or reduced-fat ....1 tablespoon
Whipped topping, regular or light....................2 tablespoons

Low-Sugar or Sugar-Free Foods

Candy, hard, sugar-free ....1 candy
Gelatin dessert, sugar-free
Gelatin, unflavored
Gum, sugar-free
Jam/jelly, low-sugar or light ....2 teaspoons
Sugar substitutes
Syrup, sugar-free...2 tablespoons

Drinks

Bouillon, broth, or consommé 🧂
Bouillon or broth, low-sodium
Carbonated or mineral water
Cocoa powder, unsweetened ....1 tablespoon
Coffee
Club soda
Diet soft drinks, sugar-free
Drink mixes, sugar-free
Tea
Tonic water, sugar-free

Condiments

Catsup..1 tablespoon
Horseradish
Lemon juice
Lime juice
Mustard
Pickles, dill 🧂 ....1½ large
Soy sauce 🧂

Soy sauce, light 🧂
Taco sauce..1 tablespoon
Vinegar, flavored vinegars

Seasonings

Flavoring extracts
Garlic
Herbs, fresh or dried
Pimiento
Spices
Tabasco or other hot sauce
Wine, used in cooking.....................................¼ cup
Worcestershire sauce

Most seasonings are also Free Foods. Be aware of seasonings that contain sodium, such as bouillon cubes, or are salts, such as garlic salt or celery salt.

Combination Foods

Much of the food we eat is mixed together in various combinations. These foods do not fall into just one exchange list. Often, it is difficult to tell what is in a casserole or baked dish. This list includes average values for some typical combination foods. It will help you fit these foods into your meal plan. Read the nutrition label of canned and frozen packaged foods to determine exchange values. Ask your registered dietitian for information about combination foods that you eat often.

COMBINATION FOOD LIST

Casseroles

Tuna noodle, lasagna,
   spaghetti with meatballs,
   chili with beans,
   macaroni and cheese 🧂 ......1 cup (8 ounces).........2 Carbohydrates,
                                           2 Medium-Fat Meats

Chow mein
   (without noodles or rice)....2 cups (16 ounces) .....1 Carbohydrate, 2 Lean
                                           Meats

Pizzas and Pot Pies

Pizza, cheese, thin crust.........¼ of 10-inch
pizza (5 ounces) ....2 Carbohydrates, 2
Medium-Fat Meats, 1 Fat

Pizza, meat, topping,
thin crust ....¼ of 10-inch
pizza (5 ounces) ....2 Carbohydrates, 2
Medium-Fat Meats, 2 Fats

Pot pie 🧂 ....1 (7 ounces) ....2 Carbohydrates, 1
Medium-Fat Meat, 4 Fats

Frozen Entrees

Salisbury steak with gravy,
mashed potato 🧂 ....1 (11 ounces) ....2 Carbohydrates, 3
Medium-Fat Meats,
3–4 Fats

Turkey with gravy, mashed
potato, dressing 🧂 ....1 (11 ounces) ....2 Carbohydrates, 2
Medium-Fat Meats, 2 Fats

Entree with less than 300
calories 🧂 ....1 (8 ounces) ....2 Carbohydrates,
3 Lean Meats

Soups

Bean 🧂 ....1 cup..........................1 Carbohydrate, 1 Very
Lean Meat

Cream (made with water)......1 cup (8 ounces).........1 Carbohydrate, 1 Fat

Split pea (made with
water) 🧂 ....½ cup (4 ounces)........1 Carbohydrate

Tomato (made with
water) 🧂 ....1 cup (8 ounces).........1 Carbohydrate

Vegetable beef, chicken
noodle, or other broth
type 🧂 ....1 cup (8 ounces).........1 Carbohydrate

Fast Foods

Burritos with beef 🧂 ....2................................4 Carbohydrates, 2
Medium-Fat Meats, 2 Fats

Chicken nuggets 🧂 ....6................................1 Carbohydrate, 2
Medium-Fat Meats, 1 Fat

Chicken, breaded and fried,
side breast and wing 🧂 ......1 each........................1 Carbohydrate, 4
Medium-Fat Meats, 2 Fats

Fish sandwich with
tartar sauce 🧂 ....1.....................3 Carbohydrates, 1
Medium-Fat Meat, 3 Fats

French fries, thin...................20–25.....................2 Carbohydrates, 2 Fats

Hamburger, regular...............1.....................2 Carbohydrates, 2
Medium-Fat Meats

Hamburger, large 🧂 ....1.....................2 Carbohydrates, 3
Medium-Fat Meats, 1 Fat

Hot dog with bun 🧂 ....1.....................2 Carbohydrates,
1 High-Fat Meat, 1 Fat

Individual pan pizza ....1.....................5 Carbohydrates, 3
Medium-Fat Meats, 3 Fats

Soft-serve cone......................1 medium...................2 Carbohydrates, 1 Fat

Submarine sandwich 🧂 ....1 sub (6 inches)..........3 Carbohydrates,
1 Vegetable, 2 Medium-Fat
Meats, 1 Fat

Taco, hard shell 🧂 ....1 (6 ounces) ....2 Carbohydrates, 2
Medium-Fat Meats, 2 Fats

Taco, soft shell 🧂 ....1 (3 ounces) ....1 Carbohydrate, 1
Medium-Fat Meat, 1 Fat

Other Meal-Planning Considerations

Vegetarian Foods

Vegetarian foods are available on each exchange list. If you are a vegetarian, your registered dietitian can help you design a meal plan to meet your nutrient needs. Whole grains and legumes are excellent sources of vitamins, minerals, fiber, and protein. Vitamin B_{12}, which is essential in preventing one type of anemia, is present only in animal foods. Strict vegetarians (vegans), those who eat no animal protein at all, must get their vitamin B_{12} from a supplement. Vegetarians who eat eggs, cheese, and milk or yogurt (lacto-ovo vegetarians) should be able to get enough B_{12} from their diet. Vegetarians will have more Starch, Fruit, and Vegetable Exchanges and probably fewer exchanges from the meat group than meat eaters will. Some Meat Exchanges will be included, however, because dried beans, peas, and legumes are important nutrient sources for all vegetarians.

Alcohol

Many adults with diabetes ask if they can occasionally drink alcohol. The American Diabetes Association guidelines now state that people whose diabetes is well controlled can have a drink or two with meals. The same precautions regarding the moderate use of alcohol that apply to the general public apply to people with diabetes. Keep in mind that drinking alcohol may delay a meal. Also, after a drink or two, you may be less careful about the amount and type of food you eat.

If you drink alcohol daily, ask your registered dietitian to work it into your regular meal plan. Because the body handles alcohol similarly to fat, one portion may be substituted for 1 or 2 Fat Exchanges. Standard portion sizes are a bottle of beer (12 ounces), a glass of wine (4 ounces), or a shot of distilled spirits (1.5 ounces). Use 1 Fat Exchange for every 45 calories in the alcoholic beverage. If, however, you are at ideal body weight or have Type I diabetes, you may be advised to use occasional alcohol as extra calories without subtracting Fat Exchanges.

You may use some alcohol-containing beverages in cooking and to flavor foods. Dry white or red wine, up to ¼ cup per serving, may be used in cooking as a Free Food. When you use wine or beer in cooking, especially long, slow cooking, some of the alcohol evaporates. When you add wine, liquor, or liqueur at the end of the recipe, it provides some carbohydrate, alcohol, and calories.

Some people may need or want to avoid alcohol altogether, even in cooking. People differ greatly in their reaction to even small amounts of alcohol. Because alcohol lowers blood sugar levels sometimes even small amounts of alcohol can lead to hypoglycemia, which has symptoms that others may mistake for drunkenness. This perception may interfere with appropriate treatment for low blood glucose. In addition, because alcohol contributes seven calories per gram, it can promote weight gain. People with non-insulin-dependent diabetes who take certain oral hypoglycemic agents may feel ill when they drink alcohol. If you have high triglycerides, you may be told to avoid alcohol because it tends to elevate blood triglyceride levels. Pregnant women, people with a history of alcohol abuse, and those with neuropathy (nerve damage) also should avoid drinking alcohol-containing beverages.

If you do drink alcoholic beverages, count any mixers you use as part of your meal plan. Thus, ½ cup orange juice equals 1 Fruit Exchange even when it has vodka in it! Some flavored mineral waters are made with sugars, fruits, and sugar syrups. One peach-flavored water contains 120 calories and about 30 grams of carbohydrate from added syrups and peach nectar. Other fruit-flavored waters and seltzers have few or no calories. Be sure to read the nutrition label. Whenever possible, use calorie-free mixers instead of those with sugar. If you want two drinks instead of one, add lots of club soda to dry wine to make spritzers.

Exchanges for Alcoholic Beverages

Beverage	Serving	Alcohol (grams)	Carbohydrate (grams)	Calories	Exchanges
Beer					
Regular	12 ounces	13	13	150	1 Starch, 2 Fats
Light	12 ounces	11	5	100	2 Fats
Near	12 ounces	1.5	12	60	1 Starch
Distilled Spirits					
80 proof (gin, rum, vodka, whiskey, or scotch)	1½ ounces	14	trace	100	2 Fats
Dry brandy or cognac	1 ounce	11	trace	75	1½ Fats
Table Wines					
Dry white	4 ounces	11	trace	80	2 Fats
Red or Rosé	4 ounces	12	trace	85	2 Fats
Sweet	4 ounces	12	5	105	⅓ Starch, 2 Fats
Light	4 ounces	6	1	50	1 Fat
Wine cooler	4 ounces	13	30	215	2 Fruits, 2 Fats
Sparkling Wines					
Champagne	4 ounces	12	4	100	2 Fats
Sweet kosher	4 ounces	12	12	132	1 Starch, 1 Fat

Appetizer/Dessert Wines

Sherry, dry or sweet	2 ounces	9	2	74	1½ Fats
Port or muscatel	2 ounces	9	7	90	½ Starch, 1½ Fats
Cordials or liqueurs	1½ ounces	13	18	160	1 Starch, 2 Fats

Cocktails

Bloody Mary	5 ounces	14	5	116	1 Vegetable, 1 Fat
Daiquiri	2 ounces	14	2	111	2 Fats
Manhattan	2 ounces	17	2	178	2½ Fats
Martini	2½ ounces	22	trace	156	3½ Fats
Old-Fashioned	4 ounces	26	trace	180	4 Fats
Tom Collins	7½ ounces	16	3	120	2½ Fats

Mixers

Mineral water	Any	—	0	0	Free
Sugar-free tonic	Any	—	0	0	Free
Club soda	Any	—	0	0	Free
Diet soda	Any	—	0	0	Free
Tomato juice	½ cup	—	5	25	1 Vegetable
Bloody Mary mix	½ cup	—	5	25	1 Vegetable
Orange juice	½ cup	—	15	60	1 Fruit
Grapefruit juice	½ cup	—	15	60	1 Fruit
Pineapple juice	½ cup	—	15	60	1 Fruit

Source: M. J. Franz et al., Learning to Live Well with Diabetes (Minneapolis: Chronimed Publishing, 1991).

4

What You Need to Know About Carbohydrates

Your individual meal plan will be based on the percentages of carbohydrate, protein, and fat that should produce the best blood glucose levels for you. Most of your diet will be made up of foods that provide carbohydrates. Your registered dietitian will work with you to develop a meal plan that provides an appropriate amount of calories and the correct amount of carbohydrate depending on your weight and blood levels of glucose and triglycerides.

New Thinking About Sugar

One of the biggest changes in the American Diabetes Association's 1994 guidelines is that they place less emphasis on whether carbohydrates are starches or sugars. The emphasis now is on *total* carbohydrates. Sugar is no longer restricted in meal planning. Gram for gram, simple sugar is processed by the body in much the same way as the starch in rice or a potato. Research has shown that sugar does not affect blood glucose (blood sugar) more dramatically than do other forms of carbohydrate. The rise in blood glucose that occurs after a meal depends on *total* carbohydrates eaten, not on types of carbohydrate eaten.

This new approach, however, does not mean that anything goes when it comes to sugar. In fact, sugary foods can be high in fat and calories and low in essential vitamins and minerals. They can use up your daily carbohydrate quota in no time, and they often contribute to weight gain. Although a ½ cup serving of regular gelatin dessert or ice cream, both of which are Other Carbohydrate Exchanges, have the same amount of carbohydrate as an orange, the orange and the gelatin have only about 60 calories versus the ice cream's 150 or more. Each of the three choices has 15 grams of carbohydrate, but only the orange provides some valuable fiber and many important vitamins and minerals. In contrast, the gelatin provides only sugar, and the ice cream provides small amounts of some vitamins and minerals but requires 2 Fat Exchanges in addition to the Other Carbohydrate Exchange. The bottom line is that most foods with considerable amounts of added sugar don't provide much nutrition bang for the buck. Some sugar is fine as an ingredient, but think twice about using Other Carbohydrate Exchanges.

"The new carbohydrate guideline does tell us we don't need to use more expensive sweeteners, when plain sugar will do," explains Carolyn Leontos, M.S., R.D., C.D.E. "Sugar has certain properties that are important in baking, too, so it's good that we can use some of the real thing." A reasonable approach is to use small amounts of regular or brown sugar in baking and in cooked foods. Sugar substitutes are useful for sweetening fruit, cereal, coffee, tea, and soft drinks when we want sweet flavors but not the calories or extra grams of carbohydrate from sugar.

And as Joan Hill, R.D., C.D.E., points out, being able to have some real sugar helps children and teenagers with diabetes combat the "I'm different" syndrome and cope with peer pressure. Barbara Barry, M.S., R.D., C.D.E., agrees: "Being able to have some sugar makes snacks more fun. And it gives parents a chance to be more flexible."

If you are already comfortably following the former set of guidelines that restrict sugar, you may want to continue on that path. Many individuals with diabetes who are in good control see no reason to add temptations to their usual options. For some people, there is no such thing as a treat now and then. But you should be aware of the changes in thinking about sugar use and discuss them with your registered dietitian.

Types of Carbohydrates

Carbohydrates, which provide four calories per gram, represent an enormous family of nutrients that provide most of the energy in our diet. Carbohydrates come in four forms:

1. *Sugars*—The smallest molecules and sweetest members of the carbohydrate family. Sugars are found naturally in fruits, milk, honey, and table sugar, and they are added to candy, cookies, and many other processed foods.

2. *Starches*—Chemically, long chains of sugar molecules that are usually not sweet. Starches are found in grains, cereals, potatoes, pasta products, breads, and baked goods.

3. *Indigestible carbohydrates*—Cellulose and other fibers that give structure to food. Our body does not have the enzymes to break down these carbohydrates, so no sugar is released when we eat these dietary fibers.

4. *Sugar alcohols*—Synthetic products made from sugars or cellulose. Although the digestive system metabolizes sugar alcohols more slowly than it does sugar, these products do end up in the body as glucose. The most widely used sugar alcohols are sorbitol, mannitol, xylitol, isomalt, and starch hydrolysate.

Sugars

All sugars are *nutritive sweeteners*. You may find the term nutritive sweetener on a food label. This means a sweetener that contains calories. Conversely, *nonnutritive sweetener* refers to a sweetener having few or no calories—for example, aspartame or saccharin. These sugar substitutes are described later in this chapter.

There are hundreds of different sweet substances. The nutrition label on foods lists total grams of carbohydrate followed by the grams of sugar from all sources (both naturally occurring and added sugars). To learn the specific type(s) of sugar check the ingredient list. Note that the names of many forms of sugars end in the suffix *-ose*:

Sucrose: *White sugar* (cane or beet sugar)—whether in the form of granulated, cubed, or powdered sugar—offers nothing but calories. *Brown sugar*, much less refined, is derived from molasses (sorghum cane) and contains very small amounts of a few minerals. *Raw sugar*, very similar to brown sugar, is sometimes crystalline. *Turbinado sugar* is partially refined sugar crystals washed in steam.

Fructose: Sometimes called *levulose*, fructose is found in fruits and honey. It is highly soluble and sweeter than any other sugar in equal amounts. You may see "high-fructose syrup" or "high-fructose corn syrup" on a label; these are concentrated forms of fructose.

Lactose: Because milk is its chief food source, lactose is sometimes called *milk sugar*. It is a combination of glucose and galactose.

Galactose: This simple sugar is found in lactose (milk sugar).

Dextrose: Commercially obtained from starch, dextrose is sometimes called *corn sugar* or *grape sugar.*

Glucose: This sugar is found chiefly in fruits, some vegetables, honey, and corn syrup. Starches break down to glucose, and all other sugars convert to glucose during digestion or metabolism. The phrase *blood sugar* refers to the level of glucose in the blood.

Maltose: This sugar comes from the breakdown of starch in the malting of barley. When starches are digested, they pass through a stage of being maltose before they end up as glucose.

Mannose: Derived from manna and the ivory nut, mannose is used mostly by sugar chemists. The sugar alcohol mannitol (discussed later) is derived from mannose.

In addition to the "-ose sugars," there are other sugars you should be familiar with as well:

Corn syrup: This liquid form of corn sugar is used in baking, candy-making, and some infant feeding formulas. When crystallized, corn syrup may be called *corn syrup solids* or *corn sweetener.* It is relatively inexpensive and is used to sweeten canned fruits and soft drinks. Corn syrup is a blend of fructose and dextrose. *High-fructose corn syrup* has more fructose than dextrose. Studies show that its effect on blood glucose is similar to that of sucrose.

Dextrin: This sugar results from the partial breakdown of starch.

Honey: Derived from flowers from which bees collect nectar, honey may be liquid, creamed, or in combs. It is a more concentrated form of carbohydrate than table sugar. Contrary to some reports, honey does require insulin to be metabolized. It is a carbohydrate and is converted to glucose like all other sugars.

Invert sugar: This sugar is formed when the sugar molecule is split by acids or enzymes. Invert sugar is used in liquid form and is sweeter than sucrose. It helps baked goods stay fresh longer.

Maple syrup and **maple sugar:** Both are made from the sap of maple trees.

Molasses: This strong-flavored sweetener is made from sorghum canes.

More About Fructose

Fructose is naturally found in fruits and honey and can be extracted as a sweetener. It can be used for baking, canning, and freezing and is sold in crystalline form and in individual packets.

In Europe, especially in West Germany and Switzerland, pure fructose, called *nonglucose carbohydrate*, is accepted as a sweetener for use by people with diabetes. Many foods containing fructose are being introduced in the United States as well. Therefore, you should be aware of its advantages and limitations.

Dietary fructose produces a smaller rise in blood glucose than sucrose or starches. Unlike glucose, most fructose is metabolized in the liver, meaning it does not require an initial insulin response to move from the blood directly into the cells for metabolism. During metabolism, part of the fructose molecule may be changed into glucose. The rate of conversion of fructose to glucose varies among individuals. At this point, some insulin is required. But the entire process of fructose absorption and metabolism requires less insulin than does an equal amount of glucose.

So far, research has provided only limited data regarding the long-term effect of high levels of fructose in the diet. However, we do know that large amounts of fructose can adversely affect your total cholesterol, triglycerides, and LDL cholesterol levels. Some medical research also suggests that fructose consumption may increase uric acid production, a potential problem for people with gout. Therefore, if you use fructose as a sweetener, be careful not to use too much. You need not avoid fruits and vegetables where fructose occurs naturally, but aim for a moderate consumption of fructose-sweetened foods, including regular sweetened soft drinks, which are made with high-fructose corn syrup.

Foods with added fructose are never Free Foods. You must substitute them for fruits or other carbohydrates in your meal plan. Thus, you are likely to be giving up Fruit Exchanges and will reduce your vitamin, mineral, and fiber intake. Read the label on a box or individual packet of fructose to find out the carbohydrate and calorie level in the amount you may wish to use. Fructose varies in sweetness according to use. It is somewhat sweeter than other sugars when used in cold, acidic foods. When used in baking, it is less sweet than regular sugar (sucrose).

Fructose is not used in any of the recipes found in this book because it is metabolized at different rates by different people and because it is usually more expensive than other sweeteners and is not in most home kitchens.

Sugar Alcohols

Sugar alcohols—which are chemically alcohols although they are made from sugar—are digested and absorbed much more slowly than other sugars. Nevertheless, they end up in the body as glucose and must be counted in your meal plan. Here are some common sugar alcohols you'll find in commercial products:

- *Hydrogenated starch hydrolysate (HSH)*—HSHs are mixtures of sugar alcohol that have no more than three calories per gram and are used in candy and baked goods.
- *Isomalt*—Both a bulking agent and a sweetener, isomalt is used in hard and soft candies, chewing gum, ice cream, baked goods, and beverages.
- *Mannitol*—Used as a bulking agent in powdered foods, mannitol can also be a dusting agent for chewing gum.
- *Sorbitol*—Commercially made from glucose, sorbitol is used widely in the commercial manufacture of dietetic foods and sugar-free gum.
- *Xylitol*—Derived from fruits and vegetables, plants, and fibrous vegetation, xylitol has the same sweetness, bulk, and calorie value as sucrose. It is used in chewing gum, gumdrops, and hard candy.

Unlike sugar, sugar alcohols do not promote tooth decay. They can, however, cause gastrointestinal distress and diarrhea, even at fairly low intakes. These side effects may cause problems for people with diabetes.

Sugar Substitutes

Three types of nonnutritive (noncaloric), man-made sweeteners are currently sold in the United States: saccharin, aspartame, and acesulfame K. *Cyclamate* was withdrawn from the market in 1970 but is being reviewed again by the Food and Drug Administration. Other sweeteners including *sucralose*, the first sugar substitute made from sugar, have not yet received approval for use in this country. Nonnutritive sweeteners approved by the FDA are considered safe for people with diabetes and for the general public.

It is best to use more than one type of nonnutritive sugar substitute. That way you can take advantage of their varied flavors and cooking properties. Also, you can use different sweeteners in combination to take advantage of the sweetening and cooking properties they have.

Powdered nonnutritive sweeteners are mixed with small amounts of nutritive sweeteners such as dextrose to give them bulk. Nonnutritive sweeteners are so concentrated that it would be impossible to sprinkle them if they were packaged alone.

Saccharin

The granddaddy of nonnutritive sweeteners, saccharin has been used for more than 100 years. It is a white, crystalline powder 375 times sweeter than table sugar. Very little saccharin is broken down by the body; most is excreted in the urine. Saccharin is used in beverages, baked goods, jams, processed fruits, salad dressings, and sauces.

Saccharin is available in tablets, granular, and liquid form. Brands include Sprinkle Sweet®, Sweet-10®, Sweet 'n Low®, Sugar Twin®, and Weight Watchers® Sweet'ner.

The safety of saccharin has been hotly debated. In 1972 it was removed from the Food and Drug Administration's (FDA's) Generally Recognized as Safe (GRAS) list because of its potential link to bladder cancer when used in huge amounts (in male rats). When a ban was proposed, consumers, the American Diabetes Association, and the Juvenile Diabetes Foundation opposed the ban, and saccharin remained available. All products with saccharin carry a warning label that states, "Use of this product may be hazardous to your health. This product contains saccharin, which has been determined to cause cancer in laboratory animals."

Aspartame

Aspartame is a combination of two amino acids, which are the building blocks of protein. It is 180 to 200 times sweeter than table sugar. The FDA approved its use in 1974. The NutraSweet Company sells aspartame under the brand name of NutraSweet® to food manufacturers which use it in many sugar-free soft drinks, puddings, gelatin, cocoa, frozen desserts, drink mixes, and other products. A familiar brand name of aspartame for table use is Equal®.

Most people prefer the flavor of aspartame to the flavor of saccharin. Many people who do not have diabetes use aspartame-containing foods to reduce their calorie intake. Aspartame is available to consumers in packets, tablets, and a granular form.

The label on products containing aspartame must state that the product should not be used in cooking or baking and that it contains phenylalanine (an amino acid): "Phenylketonuric: contains phenylalanine." The notice about phenylalanine is designed to protect people with phenylketonuria (PKU), a rare genetic disease characterized by a sensitivity to phenylalanine, one of the amino acids in aspartame.

Aspartame is stable in dry foods but loses its sweetness when heated or held a long time in liquid form. Heating a soft drink sweetened with aspartame or storing it for several months will not make the drink unsafe, but it can change the drink's taste.

Like saccharin, aspartame's long-term safety has been questioned, especially with regard to use by pregnant women. The courts have ruled and governmental agencies have agreed that aspartame is generally safe in amounts normally eaten. As with any other food, you should avoid aspartame if you have a sensitivity or negative reaction to it.

Acesulfame K

Discovered in Germany in 1967 and approved for use in the United States in 1987, acesulfame K is marketed as Sunette™ to the food industry by Hoechst Food Ingredients. Two hundred times sweeter than sucrose, it is not metabolized by the body and is excreted in the urine. Acesulfame K is used in a number of foods including instant beverages, beverages including alcohol, baked goods, dessert mixes, candies, chewing gums, and tabletop sweeteners. It contains no phenylalanine and is heat-stable. Acesulfame K is available to the general public in packets as Sweet One™.

The safety of acesulfame K has been demonstrated in nearly 90 scientific studies, and the ingredient has been acknowledged as safe by the FDA as well as numerous other regulatory agencies worldwide.

Using Sweeteners in Recipes

One of the advantages of the American Diabetes Association's latest guidelines is that you can use real sugar in baked goods. Sugar is needed in cakes and cookies not only for sweetness but also for the chemical reaction with other ingredients that gives baked products tenderness and lightness. As sugar cooks, it caramelizes, creating that tantalizing browned appearance. Yeast breads and rolls need sugar (or honey) to rise. Sugar substitutes just don't provide the sugar that fuels the action of the yeast. They contribute a sweet taste, but they don't do all the other work of sugar.

Nevertheless, nonnutritive sweeteners are valuable and useful in many recipes, and they will help make your menus more interesting without adding carbohydrates or calories. Most of our recipes that include sugar substitute add it at the end of the directions to maximize its sweetening effect.

You can reduce the sugar in many traditional baked sweets with good results. In some recipes, you can replace part of the sugar with sugar substitute. Saccharin, acesulfame K, and sucralose are heat-stable. You cannot cook with aspartame—heat alters its protein molecules—but a modified heat-stable version is in the development stage.

Facts About Fiber

Twenty years ago, fiber, the indigestible residue of carbohydrate, was considered "roughage"—a nonessential part of the diet. We knew that fiber aided in elimination and relieved constipation, but most people paid little attention to fiber beyond that. Now fiber has been elevated to one of the most important substances in health promotion and disease prevention. The National Cancer Institute recommends that everyone consume 20 to 35 grams of fiber daily from a variety of food sources.

In the past, it was thought that a high fiber intake had a positive effect on blood glucose control. Scientists have since discovered that this theory is correct but only with fiber intake at extremely high levels. You just can't get enough fiber at one meal to create this positive effect. Thus, the fiber recommendation for people with diabetes is now the same as it is for the general public: 20 to 35 grams daily. Most of us eat only 10 to 15 grams each day.

Dietary fiber is the part of plant cells that is resistant to human digestive enzymes. There are many types of fiber—cellulose, hemicellulose, oligosaccharides, pectin, gums, waxes, and lignin. Some occur in grains, others in fruits and vegetables, and others in dried peas and beans. Unlike some animals that can make digestive enzymes to break the chemical bonds of fiber to release energy, we humans cannot completely digest fiber.

The human body uses each type of fiber differently. Insoluble fibers, such as cellulose, pass through the digestive system relatively intact. Insoluble fiber contributes bulk, absorbs water, and helps you feel full. This bulking action also has a laxative effect. Fiber sources like salads and whole grains require chewing, thus allowing time for your brain to get the signal you've eaten enough. Cellulose and the other insoluble fibers protect against constipation, hemorrhoids, irritable bowel syndrome, and diverticulosis, a condition affecting about

Boost Your Fiber

You can increase your fiber intake in a variety of ways. Here are some ideas to get you started:

- Increase your consumption of vegetables of all types, including plenty of raw vegetable salads and cut vegetables.
- Eat whole fruits and dried fruits instead of juice or canned fruits. When the peel is edible (as with apples or pears), eat unpeeled fruits.
- Select breads with visible grain particles—whole wheat, pumpernickel, millet, multigrain, oatmeal, corn tortillas—instead of white bread most of the time. Bread that says wheat or cracked wheat but not whole wheat is usually not a good source of fiber. The brown color often comes from caramel coloring.
- Choose high-fiber starches—corn, winter squash, lima beans, peas—often.
- Eat high-fiber cereals—bran, shredded wheat, oat bran, wheat germ—as Starch Exchanges, and use high-fiber cereal in recipes.
- Have dried peas, beans, or lentils several times a week in soups, casseroles, or salads.
- Eat the edible skins and seeds of vegetables—the skin of a baked potato, the seeds of a cucumber.
- Think nuts and seeds if you can afford the calories and Fat Exchanges.
- Eat brown rice instead of white rice.
- Look for fiber-rich crackers and crackers with seeds.

---

half of all people over age 60. Years ago, when a person had irritable bowel syndrome or diverticulosis, a low-fiber diet was prescribed. Now doctors and dietitians are more likely to recommend a high-fiber diet, including high-fiber cereals and bran products.

Soluble fibers are partially digestible. Although scientists aren't exactly sure how, soluble fibers such as pectin, guar, locust bean gums, oat bran, and legumes can lower blood cholesterol. When we eat soluble fibers, our digestive system seems to trap and excrete more bile and cholesterol, thus reducing blood levels of cholesterol. This is advantageous for people with diabetes, who are at higher risk for heart disease.

Diets high in fiber also have been statistically correlated with reduced frequency of bowel cancer, and fiber helps control weight, too. Many low-calorie fruits and vegetables are rich in fiber and help you feel fuller than calorie-dense foods do.

Food labels list the grams of dietary fiber on the Nutrition Facts panel. A food must have at least 3 grams of fiber to permit a claim that it is a good source of fiber. A food can claim to be an excellent, high, or rich source if it has 5 grams of fiber or more.

When a label tells you that a food is fiber-rich, check the ingredient list for the source of fiber. If you want only the gastrointestinal benefits, wheat bran is fine. If you want cardiovascular benefits, too, look for soluble fiber from oat bran, fruits, and dried beans, peas, and lentils. On some ingredient lists, you will see "guar gum," a soluble fiber used as a thickener and stabilizer. While every bit helps, the amount of guar gum is usually rather small.

Try to eat good sources of fiber at each meal. Individual tolerances vary, so increase your intake gradually. Nature makes ample fiber available year-round. Fiber tablets or supplements are not necessary unless your physician prescribes them.

5

A New Look at Fats

Fats from foods are vital to life. They provide energy and the fatty acids essential for growth. They transport the fat-soluble vitamins A, D, E, and K. Fats also add texture and flavor to food and create that nice feeling of fullness and satisfaction after a meal.

Fats in the diet come in several forms, each of which has a different chemical structure. We describe fats as saturated or unsaturated, depending upon the type and number of bonds within the chemical structure of the fat molecule. Most foods containing fat are combinations of several fatty acids, the basic units of fat.

The amounts and type of fat you eat influence the levels of fats in your bloodstream—primarily *cholesterol* and *triglycerides*. Triglycerides are three units of fatty acids bound by a glycerol molecule. Fats circulate in the bloodstream as triglycerides, and you need insulin to store them in the cells of your body. *Lipid* is the name scientists use for fats, whether in foods or in the blood. Most people, however, refer to the fats in food as fats and the fats in blood as lipids.

When we say a food is a *saturated fat*, we mean that it contains proportionately more saturated fatty acids than unsaturated ones. Saturated fats tend to raise blood cholesterol levels in some people. *Unsaturated fats*, both polyunsaturated and monounsaturated ones, tend to reduce blood cholesterol and triglyceride levels.

Too much fat in the diet, especially saturated fat, can promote heart disease, atherosclerosis, and certain types of cancer. People with diabetes already have three to four times greater risk of heart disease. Too much of all types of fat can also cause weight gain and obesity, which increase the risk of a host of other medical problems.

If you have normal blood fat levels and maintain a reasonable weight, the American Diabetes Association recommends that you follow the same fat guidelines as the general public: 30 percent or less of calories from total fat, with 10 percent or less coming from saturated fat. But if obesity is a problem for you, a reduction in total dietary fat (often 20 to 25 percent of calories) may be recommended—just as it would be recommended for someone without diabetes who wants to lose weight.

Cholesterol Check

Cholesterol is a fatlike substance found in foods of animal origin. It is also made in our bodies, primarily by the liver. We actually make far more cholesterol than we eat. We need some cholesterol to build and maintain brain and nerve cells and to make bile, which helps digest food. But most of us have a lot more than we need. How much cholesterol we make is determined by genetics and by the foods we eat. Both saturated fats and dietary cholesterol tend to raise blood cholesterol levels. Meats, poultry, and dairy products contain cholesterol in varied amounts. Grains, fruits, and vegetables, however, do not contain cholesterol unless it is added in processing or preparation.

The general public is advised to limit dietary cholesterol intake to 300 milligrams a day. Most women are within that limit; most men eat a bit more. Egg yolks (but not whites) contain a large amount of cholesterol, about 215 milligrams per yolk. If you eat more than three whole eggs or yolks a week, switch to egg substitute or egg whites only for eggs beyond three. Liver and other organ meats, although rich in vitamins and minerals, are high in cholesterol, about 330 milligrams per 3-ounce cooked portion. Lean beef and chicken have similar amounts of cholesterol, about 75 mg per 3-ounce cooked portion. Cheeses have 15 to 30 milligrams per ounce. Whole milk provides 33 milligrams per cup; skim milk only 4 milligrams per cup.

Like fat, cholesterol (a waxy fatlike substance) travels through the body in several forms. It is typically bound to fat-protein molecules called *lipoproteins* that circulate in the bloodstream. *Low-density lipoprotein (LDL) cholesterol* is the "bad" cholesterol that increases risk of coronary disease. If your LDL level is elevated, you may be told to limit your saturated fat to less than 7 percent of total calories and your total calories from fat to 30 percent or less.

You should also limit the cholesterol you eat to less than 200 milligrams a day. If your cholesterol does not respond to dietary changes, your physician may prescribe a cholesterol-lowering medication. These medications have side effects, which is why a diet is always the first step and is used in conjunction with medication. This advice is really no different from the guidance given to people who do not have diabetes.

Your plan may differ from that of someone who does not have diabetes, however, if you have elevated levels of triglycerides or *very low density lipoprotein (VLDL) cholesterol.* In this case, your physician or registered dietitian may suggest that you strive for less than 10 percent of calories from saturated fat, less than 10 percent of calories from polyunsaturated fat, and up to 20 percent of calories from monounsaturated fat (olive, canola, and peanut oils, for example). You might also be told to moderate your carbohydrate intake to 40 to 50 percent of calories. All adults, with diabetes or not, should have their blood cholesterol and triglyceride levels tested annually.

Fat and Your Food Plan

Now that you have read about all these numbers and percentages, don't worry too much about them. Your registered dietitian will translate the percentages into food choice lists composed of exchanges (or will incorporate fat guidance in another meal-planning approach). You'll choose a certain number of foods from different lists at each meal. If you eat the recommended amount of food from the recommended lists, you will consume the amount of each type of fat that is most heart-healthy for you. As your blood fat levels change over time, your meal pattern will be adjusted.

Each of the recipes in this book tells you the grams of total fat, grams of saturated and polyunsaturated fats, and milligrams of cholesterol per portion. This data, plus careful reading of food labels, will give you the information you need to help you reduce your fat and cholesterol intake. Remember to look at more than the cholesterol level in food. Total fat, particularly saturated fat and trans-fatty acids (which may act like saturated fat), causes your body to form blood cholesterol.

Oils and Fats

Type of Oil or Fat	Percentage of Polyunsaturated Fat	Percentage of Saturated Fat
Safflower oil	74	9
Sunflower oil	64	10
Corn oil	58	13
Average vegetable oil (soybean plus cottonseed)	40	13
Canola oil*	32	6
Peanut oil	30	19
Chicken fat (schmaltz)	26	29
Vegetable shortening	20	32
Lard	12	40
Olive oil*	9	14
Beef fat	4	48
Butter	4	61
Palm oil**	2	81
Palm kernel oil**	2	81
Coconut oil**	2	86

*Two oils are predominately monounsaturated fatty acids. Olive oil is 77 percent monounsaturated; canola oil is 62 percent monounsaturated. To determine percentage of monounsaturated fats, add polyunsaturated and saturated fats and subtract that number from 100 percent; the remaining percentage is almost all monounsaturated.

**Palm oil, palm kernel oil, and coconut oil are very high in saturated fat. Both are common ingredients in processed foods because they keep products crisp and crunchy. Look for them on the ingredient list of food labels. Granola-type cereals, powdered creamers, baked products, and cookies often contain coconut or palm oil.

What About Fish?

Well-prepared fish tastes great and is a terrific food for people with diabetes. Fish is lower in fat than many meat choices (as long as it's not fried!), and it is especially low in saturated fat. Different species of fish vary from 20 to 100 milligrams of cholesterol per 3-ounce cooked serving. Although shellfish, squid, shrimp, and crabmeat register high in cholesterol, these foods contain a type of cholesterol that does not seem to raise blood fats. Some studies have shown that people who eat at least 7 ounces of fish each week (about two servings) are less likely to die of heart attacks. Other studies do not support this contention, but fish remains an excellent low-fat source of protein, vitamins, and minerals and may have other protective effects.

Fish is also rich in omega-3 fatty acids, a specific polyunsaturated fat that has been shown to decrease triglycerides and cholesterol in the blood. Omega-3 fatty acids can be found in salmon, tuna, canned sardines, mackerel, herring, trout, and shellfish. If your physician advises you to take a fish-oil supplement, you should follow that advice. In general, however, most experts recommend getting omega-3 fatty acids directly from fish. Supplements can have a number of drawbacks. Large amounts of omega-3 fatty acids thin the blood, thus interfering with normal blood clotting, and may promote strokes. Large doses also may provide toxic amounts of the fat-soluble vitamins A and D. Supplements are expensive, and for some people the capsules cause indigestion and "fish breath." Some studies have shown fish oil supplements to impair blood glucose control in people with diabetes.

6

Cutting Down on Salt

The sodium in salt can cause your body to retain water, which may raise your blood pressure. People differ widely in their sensitivity to sodium, but most people can handle almost any amount. Their kidneys regulate and excrete any excess. Other people are somewhat sensitive. Still others are very sodium-sensitive; their blood pressure levels rise and fall with their intake of salt and other forms of sodium. People with diabetes seem to be especially susceptible to high blood pressure, which greatly increases the risk of certain diabetes complications, such as nephropathy. Although sodium restriction may not be part of a typical diabetes meal plan, you should be aware of how sodium fits into your diet and of the general recommendations.

Salt (sodium chloride) is the most common source of sodium in the American diet. Soy sauce, baking powder, and various food ingredients contain other forms of sodium. Most of the sodium in our diets—about 60 percent—comes not from the salt we cook with but from the salt and other sources of sodium added to processed foods. Sodium levels of processed and prepared foods are listed on the food label. The sodium levels for all recipes in this book have been calculated and are provided.

Health experts suggest limiting sodium to 2,400 to 3,000 milligrams daily, less if you have hypertension. That's about 800 to 1,000 milligrams per meal. Most Americans consume 4,000 to 6,000 milligrams of sodium each day. One teaspoon of salt contains 2,300 milligrams of sodium.

We hear so much about cutting back on salt that it's easy to forget why salt is added to food in the first place. Sometimes, of course, we want a food to taste salty. More often, however, salt is used to enhance other flavors and smooth bitterness. Salt can even make some foods taste sweeter. Draining moisture out of eggplant, zucchini, or cucumbers with a sprinkling of salt followed by a rinse intensifies their natural sweetness. Salt in cooking water can help preserve a vegetable's color, improve the texture of pasta and grains, and enhance food aromas.

You may be most familiar with finely ground table salt, which is a processed salt cleared of impurities. Sometimes small amounts of additives are included so the salt flows freely. Iodine may be added as a fortification ingredient. Some cooks feel that *kosher salt* is less harsh and bitter than common table salt. It is a coarser grind, so there is a bit less sodium per teaspoonful because each teaspoonful weighs a bit less. *Sea salt*, produced from the evaporation of sea water, has a stronger flavor than kosher salt while still avoiding the bitterness of table salt. There are many varieties of sea salt, each with a distinctive flavor.

Because it is difficult to assess sodium sensitivity, your doctor will monitor your blood pressure and advise you to reduce your sodium intake if your blood pressure begins to rise. If you are sodium-sensitive, this reduction should have a positive effect.

For those trying to limit sodium, there are blends of salt and salt substitute that have half of the sodium level of table salt. Seasoned salt is another option. Most brands of seasoned salt have 1,200 to 1,300 milligrams of sodium per teaspoon, about half the sodium of table salt. Light seasoned salt is a mixture of herbs and spices with only modest amounts of salt. It provides good flavor with only about 260 milligrams of sodium per teaspoon. Salt substitutes replace sodium with potassium or other minerals. For some people, salt substitutes add a desired salty flavor, but others find substitutes bitter. Taste and flavor perception is highly variable and depends on your taste buds and brain. You may have to experiment to find ways to boost flavor if sodium must be restricted. Instructions on how to modify the recipes in this book to reduce sodium are included after each recipe.

Tips for Cutting Salt

If you need to reduce your intake of sodium, try these ideas:
- Taste your food before adding salt.
- Use fewer canned, packaged, and convenience foods.
- Limit fast foods and salty snacks.
- Substitute fresh, frozen, or unsalted canned vegetables for regular canned vegetables.
- Use reduced-sodium products such as catsup, soy sauce, tomato juice, and soups.
- Use plenty of lemon, garlic, pepper, herbs, vinegar, and other salt-free seasonings to flavor your food instead of relying primarily on salt.

Part II

Living with Diabetes

How well you live with diabetes is influenced by the type of diabetes you have, as well as by your age, family background, education, occupation, and finances. Many emotional factors, including how well you adapt to change and stress, also come into play. Although it's natural to feel some panic and helplessness when you are first diagnosed, you will soon discover that you can control your diabetes. Build your confidence by learning as much as you can. Talk to other people with diabetes, and subscribe to publications about diabetes or look for them regularly at your local public library.

Rely on your health care team—your physicians, registered dietitian, diabetes nurse educator, and other team members—for information and support. Many teams also include exercise physiologists, psychologists, podiatrists, and social workers. If you are not comfortable with the care you are getting, find another doctor or team. Many people and organizations are willing to help you (see Appendix), but the extent to which *you* take control of your diabetes will have the greatest impact on your quality of life and your future. Seek all the information and help you can, but realize that ultimately only you can make the real decisions about your day-to-day care.

7

The Adult with Diabetes

If you are an adult with diabetes, you will make decisions every day about what and how much to eat and about when and how much to exercise. You also may make decisions about prescribed medications. This book, along with advice and guidance from your doctor and registered dietitian, can form the foundation for successful diabetes management. Although scientists are looking for a cure for diabetes, the best we can do now is to control it. Choosing to be in control takes commitment, time, and skill. It pays off by reducing acute emergencies (hypoglycemia and hyperglycemia) and by preventing or delaying the long-term complications of diabetes.

Special Considerations for Women

Sixty percent of all new cases of diabetes are diagnosed in women. Obesity is a greater problem for women than men, and overweight women are particularly at risk for developing non-insulin-dependent (Type II) diabetes. Diabetes increases the risk of heart disease in women five to seven times, versus increasing the risk in men only two to three times. The cause of this discrepancy is not known, although studies indicate that diabetes increases blood pressure more in women than in men. It also lowers women's "good" (HDL) cholesterol more. As a result of ongoing research on women's unique health needs, undoubtedly we will soon better understand the risk factors facing women with diabetes.

Comments Joan Hill, R.D., C.D.E., "Even though a larger percentage of people with diabetes are women, that doesn't mean women automatically find the time to take better care of themselves." In fact, Joan and other registered dietitians who care for women with diabetes observe that quite the opposite is true. "Women tend to put their needs last," says Sue McLaughlin, R.D., L.D., C.D.E. Maggie Powers, M.S., R.D., C.D.E., encourages her clients to find time to take care of themselves. "Remember your mental breaks, exercise breaks, and food breaks," she advises.

Diabetes is also influenced by and influences a woman's reproductive health. According to Susan Thom, R.D., L.D., C.D.E., 30 to 40 percent of women have more insulin resistance during the luteal phase of their menstrual cycle (a week to 10 days before flow begins). "Progesterone and estrogen are elevated at this time," she explains, "and both are insulin antagonists, so it's important to adjust your diet or medication accordingly." If you are pregnant and have Type I or II diabetes, it is critical to keep your blood glucose level in the normal range—to ensure your own health and your baby's.

Gestational diabetes mellitus (GDM) is diagnosed in approximately 90,000 pregnant U.S. women each year. Women with gestational diabetes usually have normal carbohydrate tolerance before pregnancy and return to normal carbohydrate tolerance after delivery. Although temporary, this form of diabetes must be carefully managed. Both mother and baby are at risk if GDM goes undetected or remains untreated.

The most frequent complication of GDM is for the baby to have a high birth weight, which often results in a cesarean delivery. In addition, women with GDM are more likely to develop Type II diabetes later in life. The American Diabetes Association recommends that all pregnant women be screened for GDM at between 24 and 28 weeks. If test results are positive, there will be a lot to learn.

Nutrition intervention is the cornerstone of treatment for gestational diabetes. If you are diagnosed with GDM, your registered dietitian will work closely with you to normalize your blood glucose levels and will develop a personal meal plan to provide the right nutrients for you and your growing baby. You will be taught and encouraged to monitor your glucose levels and ketone levels throughout your pregnancy. Your physician and registered dietitian will counsel you about appropriate weight gain and insulin late in pregnancy. The dietitian will work with you to develop a meal plan and exercise pattern suited to your health needs, preferences, and lifestyle. If you are planning to nurse your baby, don't worry. GDM should have no effect on your ability to breastfeed. Your baby will not be born with diabetes, and your diabetes will disappear after delivery.

It is common to experience anxiety, fear, and even depression when you are first diagnosed with GDM. You probably had no prior clue and feel just fine. It is important to heed the advice of your health care team and to rely on them for support. You will have lots of questions and concerns; this is absolutely normal and expected. Try to follow your care plan diligently but without obsessing over it. While gestational diabetes (and pregnancy in a woman with Type I or Type II diabetes) is stressful, it is manageable. And the results of good management—a healthy baby and good pregnancy—are well worth the effort.

Special Considerations for Men

Some men are quite used to letting others decide for them what they will eat, and they take little responsibility for food purchasing and preparation. According to *Progressive Grocer's* 1995 annual report, only 13 percent of male heads of household do the grocery shopping.

When diagnosed with diabetes, men are often shocked at the notion that they will really have to pay attention to what they eat, how much they eat, and how food is prepared. And they are surprised they should eat at planned mealtimes, too. Even in equal-opportunity households, women still do most of the meal planning and cooking, so many men have a lot to learn.

Often the primary meal preparer—typically a wife, mother, or female friend—is invited to attend counseling sessions on meal planning and food choices for a man with diabetes. A skilled dietitian will assess your needs and tailor a meal plan to those needs, whether you are a man or woman. Your habits, preferences, lifestyle, and even the equipment in your kitchen will be reflected in your personal plan.

You must remember that the diabetes is yours and so is the primary responsibility for control of it. Delegation won't work. Someone else may assist you with the day-to-day and meal-to-meal decision making, but only you can control what you eat and drink. Unless you are in a residential facility that provides all meals, food choices are your responsibility. And, as you know, food choices have a big impact on your health and well-being.

With a Little Help from Your Friends

Managing your diabetes, whether you are 18 or 75, male or female, is by no means easy. Virtually every person who is diagnosed with diabetes will have a lot to learn—about shopping, measuring portions, new cooking skills, and eating out. But diabetes is controllable, and that's more than can be said for some other serious diseases.

Family and friends can be very helpful, but they may not understand diabetes and how to control it. So don't let anyone coax you into making anything less than the best choice—what's right for *you*.

Don't hide the fact that you have diabetes. If you talk about it, you'll be surprised at the consideration and help you will receive. Your friends and coworkers will understand that you must eat at specific times and have certain dietary needs and restrictions. They are far more likely to be supportive if they know that there is a medical reason for your new eating habits and patterns. Also, knowing that you have taken charge of your diet will make it difficult for others to pressure you to eat or drink to excess. As you become increasingly adept at managing your diabetes, you will maintain better blood glucose levels, gain confidence, and feel more in control.

8

The Child with Diabetes

On *Sesame Street*, Kermit the Frog sings the song "It's Not Easy Being Green." The lyrics tell how difficult it is to be different. "Wanting to be more like his or her peers is a big concern for a child with diabetes," says Maggie Powers, M.S., R.D., C.D.E. At some point, almost every child does feel different, maybe because he or she is overweight or skinny, has acne, or wears glasses. But diabetes is harder to grasp—both for the children with this medical problem and for their peers. Furthermore, the treatment—insulin and diet—may restrict schedules, activities, and independence.

"We have to start early with children," says Joan Hill, R.D., C.D.E. "Structure is important, but so is flexibility." Eating patterns for preschool-aged children can be unpredictable. For example, your child may go on food jags and eat only cereal or bananas and peanut butter for days at a time. Although this erratic or finicky eating behavior is quite normal, it does make managing diabetes more difficult. You can give your child some control and yourself some peace of mind by providing reasonable but limited choices.

As children reach school age, they make many food decisions at school and with friends. They need to know what they should eat and need the freedom to choose foods on their own. Once a child learns that blood glucose monitoring reflects what he or she has eaten, the cause-and-effect relationship becomes clearer and can reinforce good food choices.

Children with diabetes also should be encouraged to participate in active sports. "We are seeing a real shift downward in physical activity among children," warns Brenda Broussard, R.D., M.P.H., M.B.A., "and an explosion of obesity. It seems that many kids today would rather watch their favorite sports stars perform on TV than perform themselves."

When a student has diabetes, the student's gym teacher, coach, classroom teacher, school nurse, lunchroom personnel, and school bus drivers should be informed. Give all of them a list of symptoms of hypoglycemia. School personnel

Back-to-School Checklist

School districts are obligated by federal law to accommodate a child's health care needs. Be sure the school is informed that your child has diabetes and has daytime phone numbers for you and your child's doctor. Schedule a conference for you, your child, and school personnel at the start of each school year.

Topics to discuss include:

- Usual causes and signs of hypoglycemia and hyperglycemia in your child
- An explanation of your child's daily management plan
- How changes in daily routine, such as field trips, will be handled
- A review of your child's meal plan and a strategy for handling parties and snacks
- How glucagon will be administered if it is needed

Source: Adapted from A Core Curriculum for Diabetes Education, *2nd ed. (Chicago: American Association of Diabetes Educators, 1993.)*

often have had some experience with children and diabetes, and they want to know how to avoid potential emergencies. You can conduct this briefing discreetly so that the child is not embarrassed or singled out. Send some juice boxes or glucose tablets to the child's teachers, and ask them to be especially watchful just before lunchtime. Before strenuous activity, such as football practice or tennis, the teacher should know that the child may need a source of sugar or may require an insulin adjustment.

Full participation in sports and school activities promotes independence and is very important for all children, whether they have diabetes or not. With some planning, care, and encouragement, the child with diabetes can excel just like any other student in virtually every sport or school activity.

Adolescent Challenges

Adolescence is a particularly hard time for children with diabetes, as well as for their parents and other caregivers. "The hormonal roller coaster of puberty is a challenge," says Susan Thom, R.D., L.D., C.D.E. "Growth hormone is an insulin antagonist, but parents sometimes blame the teen for losing control. Then he or she rebels. Plus all the usual teen issues are at work, too—separation from parents, identity crises, peer pressures, experimentation with smoking, alcohol, and drugs."

Adolescence is also a period in one's life when body image becomes extremely important. "There was a time," recalls Lindsay Leventhal, M.S., R.D., C.D.E., "when the diet for children with diabetes was so restrictive that it could lead to compulsive eating and bulimia in the teen years. Fortunately, meal plans are more flexible now." Even so, teenage girls tend to gain weight after beginning menstruation. "Failure to prepare, to educate, and to monitor the patient during this time may result in unhealthy eating patterns and inappropriate manipulation of insulin doses," notes Deborah V. Edidin, M.D., a pediatric endocrinologist.

Even something as simple as having a soft drink after school with friends can cause a problem for the teen with diabetes. Luckily, diet soft drinks are totally acceptable and available everywhere these days. If the adolescent with diabetes focuses on building a healthy body, rather than on the limitations of diabetes, he or she is more likely to feel like one of the crowd.

The Parent's Role

Basic goals for the child with diabetes are normal growth and development, avoidance of sudden high or low blood glucose levels, minimal complications, and a positive psychological adjustment to having diabetes. "These goals have expanded to include maintenance of blood glucose as close to normal as possible," says Dr. Edidin. "Since the completion of a 10-year study called the Diabetes Control and Complications Trial, we now know conclusively that the better the glucose control, the less likely complications will occur. If complications *do* occur, they may occur later and be milder in the person with well-controlled diabetes."

In the very young child, the responsibility for control of diabetes lies mostly with the parents. Many parents, feeling guilty about the hereditary aspect of diabetes, become overly protective. Children, whether they have diabetes or not, quickly learn that they can manipulate parents by eating or not eating, by eating the right foods or the wrong ones, or by behaving or misbehaving to get attention.

Overly protective parents can be a real problem, explains Susan Thom, R.D., L.D., C.D.E. "Kids are kids first. Don't let diabetes get in the way, she

Tips for Helping Your Child Manage Diabetes

Meal plans for children with diabetes differ from those for adults, because children usually don't need to worry about weight reduction. On the contrary, children need enough calories for growth and development.

- Most children over age 6 need three meals a day plus snacks in the mid-afternoon and at bedtime. Children under age 6 usually require a mid-morning snack, too.
- Unless a child is over his or her healthy body weight, usual caloric guidelines for healthy children are acceptable. For example, very active adolescent boys with diabetes may need 3,500 to 4,500 calories daily.
- Meals and snacks should be timed to correspond with peak action of injected insulin. Children should be encouraged to stick to their eating schedule as much as possible.
- Meal planning and timing, children's variable appetites and food preferences, usual childhood illnesses, and dealing with food allergies can cause parents a lot of stress. When all else fails, offer the child a carbohydrate-containing beverage like milk or juice and pay close attention to blood glucose levels.

---

advises. Even young children can be taught the basic exchanges. It is much like a board game or card game. Children can help prepare meals, weigh and cut food portions, and pack lunches. A registered dietitian can work with you and your child. This ongoing relationship with a dietitian is important. Try to teach your child that he or she can eat the same foods as everyone else, but in different ways. Don't limit choice of foods as much as how much and when your child eats. Concentrate on getting your child's blood glucose under control before you tackle other nutrition issues like eating more fruits and vegetables.

Teach your child that his or her diabetes is a fact, not a secret. Share the fact with others who will be supportive. Let the parents of your child's playmates know that your son or daughter has diabetes. Send appropriate food and snacks to friends' homes and to day care or to school, if necessary. Be sure that others don't misinterpret "I'm not allowed to have candy at home" to mean that your child can have more treats when he comes over to play.

As the child gets older, more self-directed, and more accepting of his or her diabetes, there will be continued peaks and valleys. The adolescent, with or without diabetes, will seek limits, defy authority, and test new behaviors. Hormonal and metabolic changes will alter insulin and food requirements. As a result, the teen's diabetes may be more difficult to control.

Some parents are able to create an emotional environment that makes their child who happens to have diabetes feel special rather than sick or odd. Always remember that the emotional and physical needs of just being a child are far more important than those of being a child with diabetes. But also don't forget Kermit, who said, "It's not easy . . ."

Summer Camps

Summer camps for children with diabetes have helped many kids overcome their feelings of being different. There are more than 50 such camps in the United States. Most include all the usual camping activities, such as swimming, horseback riding, games, and physical exercises, under instruction and supervision. The camps are staffed with complete health teams—doctors, registered dietitians, and nurses—who supervise, teach, and help each child. The camps often have junior counselors who may have diabetes themselves. One of the greatest experiences for children at camp is meeting other children with diabetes—talking together, learning together, and finding out that they are not alone.

In addition to providing your child with social and physical benefits, summer camp is often a good way to let your child get away for a few weeks. During this separation from you, your child can experience a great deal of personal growth and can develop independent behavior and self-confidence in a safe environment. And you can enjoy a much-needed rest or vacation with other family members. It's understandable to want and need a break.

Although there is a charge for attending camp, few refuse a child's application because parents cannot pay. The camp committee's main consideration is which applicants need camp the most. For a list of summer camps for children with diabetes in or near your state, write to the American Diabetes Association (see Appendix).

9

Exercise and Sports

"I know a wonderful exercise," says diabetes educator Carolyn Leontos, M.S., R.D., C.D.E., "and I recommend it for everyone, not just people with diabetes. It's called 'push yourself away from the table.'" All of us, whether we have diabetes or not, maintain a healthy weight by balancing the calories we eat with the energy we use. We can eat more food without gaining weight if we are physically active. Conversely, we must eat less if we don't get enough exercise. Maintaining a healthy weight is especially important to people with diabetes because lean bodies use insulin more effectively. And if insulin injections are necessary, you need less insulin when you are at a healthy weight.

Of course, regular exercise has many benefits beyond weight control. It increases flexibility, builds stamina, boosts energy, and helps beat stress. Exercise also produces hormones that heighten your sense of well-being. In addition, it helps lower blood pressure and decreases risk for cardiovascular disease—both important benefits, especially for the person with diabetes.

The Centers for Disease Control and Prevention and the American College of Sports Medicine recommend that every adult accumulate 30 minutes or more of *moderate-intensity* physical activity every day. For most healthy adults, moderate intensity is equivalent to brisk walking at 3 to 4 miles per hour. This recommendation reflects a new attitude toward fitness that focuses on daily moderate physical activity, not regimented, vigorous, repetitive (boring!) exercise. Experts also say that *accumulation* of physical activity in short bouts—for example, three 10-minute periods—is just as effective as one 30-minute session.

Adding Exercise to Your Life

Lindsay Levanthal, M.S., R.D., C.D.E., has been counseling people with diabetes for nine years. She herself has had Type I diabetes for 31 years. "I have always stressed physical activity over exercise," Lindsay says. "Walk around the mall. Take the stairs instead of the elevator." It's important to be realistic about your limitations, too. "If your neighborhood isn't safe or conditions are icy, you don't want to walk around just for the exercise," cautions Maggie Powers, M.S., R.D., C.D.E. "You have to acknowledge barriers like these and look for solutions. And you should expect your health care counselors to be sensitive to the ramifications of their recommendations. Maybe you can't just walk around the block!"

"If you've got 20 minutes to watch TV, you've got 20 minutes to exercise," says Barbara Barry, M.S., R.D., C.D.E. If you can't tear yourself away from the screen, try doing muscle strengtheners like push-ups, abdominal curls, lunges, and squats while you enjoy your favorite show. Even better, use a treadmill or exercise bike while watching TV. Remember, stronger muscles burn more energy. "And get rid of that remote control," suggests Brenda Broussard, R.D., M.P.H., M.B.A. "Get up to change the channel. Every bit of physical activity counts!"

For her patients who find physical activity difficult for one reason or another, Joan Hill, R.D., C.D.E., recommends two videos. *Armchair Fitness* is available from CCM Productions, P.O. Box 15707D, Chevy Chase, MD 20825. *Chair Dancing* is available from Chair Dancing International, Inc., 2670 Del Mar Heights Rd., Suite 183, Del Mar, CA 92014.

Exercise Tips

Here are some ideas to make exercising easier—even fun!

- Choose activities that you enjoy but are safe for you. If you have foot or joint problems, avoid running.
- Invest in a pair of comfortable, well-fitting shoes appropriate for the sport or activity. Wear cotton socks with shoes to avoid blisters and irritation of sensitive areas on the foot.
- Assemble your workout gear: a diabetes I.D., fruit or crackers, and coins for a phone call or vending machine. Use a fanny pack to keep your gear handy.
- Be sure to drink enough fluids before, during, and after physical activity.
- Warm up and cool down in every exercise session. These steps are key to injury prevention. Stretching muscles properly prevents injuries, too.
- Avoid weight lifting, which can strain the blood vessels in your eyes and increase blood pressure.

Special Considerations

Although the general guidelines for getting enough exercise apply to people with diabetes, some special considerations are also important. These considerations vary according to the type of diabetes.

For People with Type I Diabetes

Although there is no research showing that exercise improves blood glucose control for people with insulin-dependent (Type I) diabetes, exercise is very important in terms of reducing risk for cardiovascular problems. It lowers total serum cholesterol and triglyceride levels while increasing production of HDL cholesterol—the so-called "good" cholesterol that helps protect against coronary heart disease. And research does show that people with Type I diabetes who follow a regular exercise program may require less insulin and tend to take better care of their diabetes.

If you have insulin-dependent diabetes, remember that exercise causes you to burn glucose faster and decreases the need for insulin. Consequently, exercise increases the need for carbohydrates both during and after physical activity. Extra carbohydrates replace muscle and liver glycogen stores depleted by exercise and can prevent delayed hypoglycemic reactions. These extra calories may be needed for up to 24 hours after strenuous or prolonged exercise.

If your blood glucose level is not well controlled, exercise may actually create additional problems. If your blood glucose is already high due to insufficient insulin, exercise may cause it to rise even higher (hyperglycemia) as your muscles signal your liver to release stored carbohydrates. If it is too low, exercise may induce hypoglycemia. Blood glucose monitoring is especially important whenever there are wide swings in blood glucose levels.

If your diabetes is under control, you can either reduce your insulin dosage or consume some carbohydrate—such as a sweetened soft drink or fruit juice—before engaging in vigorous exercise. Always have an additional source of glucose readily available in case you need more as exercise progresses. Your registered dietitian can help you adjust your meal plan and the timing of your insulin injections if necessary. Your physician may want to change the site of your injections based on the type of exercise you do. Exercise can accelerate the rate of insulin absorption from the injection site.

If you exercise at approximately the same time each day, you will maximize the positive effects of physical activity and minimize the negatives. Frequent blood glucose monitoring before, during, and after exercise will help you learn what to expect. It is generally good to exercise after mealtimes or snacks because blood glucose levels are ample. Mild exercise, like walking for 15 minutes, may not require any extra food, but an hour of bicycle riding may require an extra 15 to 50 grams of carbohydrate, depending upon the intensity of the activity and how your body reacts. If you decide to exercise on the spur of the moment—after you've already taken your insulin, so it's too late to adjust your dosage—eat an extra fruit or starch for each 30 to 45 minutes of moderate physical activity.

For People with Type II Diabetes

Research clearly shows that for people with non-insulin-dependent (Type II) diabetes, blood glucose can be lowered with physical activity. If you have Type II diabetes, try monitoring your blood glucose before and after exercise. You will see that exercise acts just like medication. It actually increases the ability of insulin to bind to its receptor sites on the cell membrane, thus helping the body use available insulin. The muscle cells use 10 to 20 times more glucose during exercise than when inactive. If you are overweight, physical activity (coupled with a healthy diet) has the added benefit of helping you reach a healthy weight. But even if you don't lose weight, you'll still see a change in your blood glucose levels after exercise. And, just as it does for people with insulin-dependent diabetes, exercise will help cut your risk of cardiovascular disease.

For Everyone

If you haven't exercised much lately, start slowly and gradually build up your stamina. Emphasize aerobic exercise—moderate-intensity walking, lap swimming, or cycling, for example—because these activities burn calories very effectively. Most important, choose an activity you enjoy, and add some variation so you don't get bored. Exercising with a partner may increase motivation and create a regular time and place to exercise. If you are exercising for weight control, consider spending a bit more time at it and doing it more frequently than you might if cardiovascular fitness were your only goal.

Remember that state of mind is an important part of exercise. You may decide to do some kind of formal exercise on a regular basis. That's great. But also think about making some basic lifestyle changes—using stairs instead of elevators, parking farther away and walking, or getting off the bus a few stops early and walking. Depending on the season and climate, you may enjoy gardening, raking leaves, riding a bike, ice or in-line skating, cross-country skiing, walking the dog, or other ways of actively enjoying the outdoors. You'll find that your attitude toward physical activity will start to change and that a regular program of physical activity may not be difficult to maintain.

Moderate Physical Activity

There are many ways to get moderate-intensity exercise. Here are a few:

- Walking briskly
- Cycling at about 10 miles per hour
- Swimming with moderate effort
- Conditioning exercise, general calisthenics
- Racket sports (tennis, paddleball)
- Golf (pulling cart or carrying clubs)
- Fishing (standing/casting)
- Home care, general cleaning
- Mowing lawn with a power or push mower
- Home repair, painting

Source: Russell R. Pate et al., "Physical Activity and Public Health," Journal of the American Medical Association, *February 1, 1995, pp. 402–408.*

10

Eating Out

An aversion to restaurants is not a symptom of diabetes! Like most Americans, people with diabetes enjoy eating out. And today, more than ever before, the choices are boundless—from classic French and Italian to Middle Eastern, Mexican, Thai, and good old American.

Each year, we spend an increasing percentage of our available food dollars on away-from-home eating (44 percent in 1994). On *average*, we eat out almost four times a week. Some people, particularly young singles and empty nesters, eat out even more often. And many men and women who work outside the home eat at least one meal out every workday.

Not all our "restaurant meals" are consumed in restaurants. In fact, almost half of restaurant orders are for take-out food. We can also bring fully prepared foods home from company cafeterias, supermarkets, and the growing segment of the food service industry that provides "home-style" take-out food. It's no wonder the National Restaurant Association has identified the take-out food service segment as the growth area of the future.

Informed Choices

With so many cuisines and food preparation styles to choose from, it's wise to do some homework. Be familiar with the menu of a restaurant you plan to visit. Call and ask some questions ahead of time so you can plan your choices without pressure. In many communities, the local affiliate of the American Heart Association can tell you which restaurants in your area have heart-healthy menus. These approved menu offerings are low in fats, cholesterol, saturated fats, and sodium. If you choose items identified as heart-healthy, you have a head start in eating foods that are good for you.

If you know the foods and portion sizes of your meal plan and know the major ingredients of the food choices offered, making healthful selections from any menu is not that difficult. And the good news is that thanks to today's emphasis on freshness and flavor, healthful food *tastes* great.

Always remember that you're in control. Here are some basic ground rules to get you moving in the right direction:

- Keep handy a pocket- or purse-sized card showing the number of exchanges or grams of carbohydrate that you're allowed at each meal.

- Just because the restaurant serves large portions doesn't mean you must eat everything at one sitting. Expect the food you order to be more than one meal for you. Share an entree with someone else at the table, or take home the rest to eat another time. "Ask for a take-home bag *before* you begin eating," advises Carolyn Leontos, M.S., R.D., C.D.E. "If you can't keep or don't want leftovers, select the portion of food you plan to eat, then sprinkle the rest with sugar, salt, or pepper so you won't be tempted by it!" Look carefully at your food before you start eating to "guesstimate" the amount that equals your meal plan, or ask the server how big the portion is. Divide the food into eat-now and take-home servings before you start eating.

- Be assertive. Because customers have become more health conscious, restaurants are eager to accommodate special requests. Tell your server you have diabetes. Ask about key ingredients and how foods are prepared. Count at least 1 Fat Exchange if food is fried, sautéed, or sauced.

- Many appetizer portions are equal to exchange amounts. Choose a food listed as an appetizer for your entree. It helps with portion control and saves money, too.

- Ask for all sauces, gravies, condiments, and butter on the side so you can use appropriate amounts. Use diet and low- or reduced-calorie products—for example, salad dressings, jams and syrups, and sugar substitutes—when possible. If they are not listed on the menu, ask if they are available. Carry a small plastic bag with individual packets of salad dressing and sugar substitute along with your emergency hypoglycemia treatment.

- Talk to your registered dietitian to learn which food groups can be interchanged if a meal doesn't exactly fit your plan. Each Carbohydrate Exchange, with 15 grams of carbohydrate, can be used as 1 Fruit, Starch, or Milk Exchange. Look for and order Free Foods as "fillers."

- Always try to eat within an hour of your regular mealtime, especially if you take insulin. Make your reservation earlier than your usual mealtime to allow for preparation. If you know you will be eating dinner much later than usual, consider switching your evening meal with your evening snack, or adjust your medication accordingly.

- If dessert is very important to you, decide on your dessert first, then figure out the rest of your meal based on remaining exchanges. Or plan ahead and share one dessert with others. You'll enjoy some of the dessert and have more exchanges for the rest of your meal.
- Restaurant meals usually contain more fat than at-home meals do. Consider storing up your daily Fat Exchanges if you know you'll be eating out later the same day.
- Try to enjoy some special foods when eating out—foods you would not usually have at home. Why not find new foods you like and let someone else cook them!
- Test your blood glucose at the restaurant before and after your meal. Collecting this data helps you make informed choices in the future.

Restaurant Courses

Now let's take a look at ways you can make smart choices about specific courses.

Appetizers

If you want to use your Fat Exchanges later in the meal, skip cream soups, chips or crackers, creamed herring, and cream cheese spreads. If you choose seafood, count it as part of your total meal's Meat Exchanges. Raw vegetables are free, but go easy on the dip. Clear beef or chicken soups and vegetable soups, including Manhattan clam chowder, are fine. Count tomato juice, vegetable juice, or vegetable soup as a Vegetable Exchange or as a Free Food depending on the amount eaten. Use a Fruit Exchange for a small fresh-fruit cup or melon wedge.

Bread and Other Starches

Count one small, plain roll, a slice of bread, half a large roll, four slices of melba toast, or two bread sticks as 1 Starch Exchange. Choose whole-grain products whenever possible to add fiber. If you use butter or margarine, add Fat Exchanges. Generally avoid fried doughnuts, croissants, sweetrolls, and rich fruit muffins that count as multiple Bread and Fat Exchanges. Be careful with specialty breads that may contain nuts and fruits. Remember to count potatoes, pasta, and other grains and starchy vegetables as Starch Exchanges. Skip the bread or rolls if you are having a pasta or grain entree, because the entree will probably use all of your Starch Exchanges.

Salads and Dressings

Choose a mixed green salad or raw vegetables, and count them as a Vegetable Exchange or a Free Food depending on how your registered dietitian wants you to count vegetables. Ask if a low-fat or reduced-calorie dressing is available. Order dressing on the side so that you can control the amount you eat. Susan Thom, R.D., L.D., C.D.E., has had Type I diabetes for over 25 years. She orders regular salad dressing on the side. She dips her fork in dressing, lets the tines drain, then takes a bite of salad. "I use less than 1 to 1½ tablespoons of dressing," she says, "and have the full flavor spectrum to choose from."

Main Course for Lunch

Depending upon the number of Starch Exchanges you have, consider an open-faced sandwich (one slice), a regular sandwich (two slices), a small bun, or a pita pocket. Sandwiches on large rolls may have 3 or 4 Starch Exchanges. Choose sandwich fillings from foods on the lists of very lean or lean meats, and meat substitutes. Thus, you might choose lean roast beef or steak, ham, fish, sliced chicken, or turkey. Roasted vegetables, with or without some cheese, make a tasty sandwich, too. Look for sandwiches and lunch entrees with medium-fat cheeses like Mozzarella. Look for the words *broiled* and *roasted* for the protein portion of your meal. Limit foods that are fried unless you want to use your fats in this way. Also, look at spreads used on sandwiches. Try mustard or salsa instead of high-fat spreads. Ask for just a little, and remove any extra sauce or mayonnaise.

Other main lunch choices might include cottage cheese and fresh-fruit plate; tuna or salmon salad; a hearty soup, stew, or chili; julienne salad; fajitas; thin-crust pizza; steamed or grilled vegetable plate; chicken, turkey, or fish; or pasta with tomato, vegetable, or meat sauce. Gravies, sauces, cream cheese fillings, and salad fillings with lots of mayonnaise as a binder all require extra Fat Exchanges. Review the meat categories, and choose a meat or meat alternative at the appropriate fat level. Hearty pea or lentil soups can be used if you count each bowl as 2 Starch Exchanges plus 2 Very Lean Meat Exchanges.

Main Course for Dinner

You can enjoy almost any food from the menu for your dinner entree, as long as you eat it in an amount that fits into your meal plan. Most of the time, it's best to choose lean meat, fish, or poultry—roasted, barbecued, baked, grilled, broiled, or poached. Remember that many restaurants use prime meats, which have more fat than similar cuts used at home. Trim off extra fat from chops, steaks, and sliced meats. Avoid thickened gravies and cream sauces. Share an entree, or eat only the portion you are allowed and take home the rest. Consider the whole menu, and mix and match. Maybe you want your main course to be an appetizer, a bowl of soup, a salad featuring meat or cheese, or a pasta with seafood. Don't overlook vegetarian and vegetable- and grain-based entrees.

Vegetables

Ask if the restaurant has a fresh vegetable of the day. Raw, grilled, roasted, or steamed vegetables are often the best choice. Enjoy a variety of seasonal vegetables. Avoid cream or cheese sauces and fried vegetables unless you use Fat Exchanges for them.

Potatoes

Boiled, roasted, baked, and mashed potatoes are great choices, but be mindful of portion size. Consider rice, corn, peas, or pasta alternatives as Starch Exchanges. Limit french fries and potato chips, and count Fat Exchanges if you choose them. Limit butter or sour cream on potatoes unless you plan to use Fat Exchanges for these toppings.

Desserts

Fresh fruit is often the best choice for dessert. If you want frozen yogurt or ice cream, eat only one small (½ cup) scoop. Enjoy angel food cake, puddings, and other desserts, but limit your portion and keep in mind what you have already eaten at that meal. If you reserve 1 Starch, 1 Fruit, and 1 Fat Exchange, you can have a small portion of almost any dessert. Talk to your registered dietitian about your favorite desserts to determine how they can fit into your dining experience.

Beverages

If you have a Milk Exchange to use, low-fat or skim milk is the best choice. If not, drink water, mineral water, club soda with lime, a diet soft drink, coffee, or tea. Choose caffeine-free types if you want to avoid caffeine. If you have a Fruit Exchange, enjoy a small glass of unsweetened fruit juice. Talk to your registered dietitian about how to count a glass of wine or another alcohol-containing beverage in your meal.

Food Exchanges for Fast Food

Although the hamburger remains the king of fast food, chicken, pizza, and submarine sandwiches have a loyal following, too. Fast food is a popular take-out choice, enjoyed by Americans at breakfast, lunch, and dinner.

A step up from traditional fast-food establishments are the so-called quick-comfort restaurants. These self-service places are especially appealing to working people who want a quick home-style family meal that is a cut above burgers and fries. Examples are restaurants that specialize in made-to-order Mexican food, Chinese food, or rotisserie chicken with all the fixins.

Fortunately for people with diabetes—and for others trying to control their weight—it is possible to choose healthful food at a fast-food restaurant. The problem is usually the amount of fat (particularly saturated fat) and sugar and the resulting calories.

Unless you have lots of exchanges to use at a meal, which is sometimes true for teenage boys and athletes, look for lower-calorie options—single burgers, diet soft drinks, grilled chicken or fish sandwiches, a small hot dog, unsweetened juices, low-fat milk, a small order of fries, the salad bar with low-calorie dressing, chili, a roast beef or ham sandwich. Don't be fooled into thinking that chicken and fish sandwiches are automatically low in calories. Anything breaded and fried runs up the fat and calorie count. Chicken nuggets contain ground chicken skin, which adds fat and cholesterol, and they are usually fried. Chicken, tuna, and seafood salad, popular fillings for sub sandwiches, are loaded with mayonnaise. Grilled chicken sandwiches on buns or in pita pockets, without special sauces or mayonnaise, are usually a good choice.

International Flavor

Today's restaurant scene is a crazy quilt of ethnic choices and dining styles. Hope Warshaw, M.M.Sc., R.D., C.D.E., coaches people interested in healthful food—not just people with diabetes—on how to make smart choices when eating out. Here are some restaurant tips from Hope:

- *Chinese*—Stir-fried vegetables are a good choice. White rice is your best bet, but plain fried rice is fine if you're not counting calories. If you're watching sodium, stay away from monosodium glutamate (MSG) and soy sauce.
- *Indian*—Lentils and chickpeas are Indian staples. These legumes are high in soluble fiber, which can help lower blood sugar. Try a chicken tandoori, chicken tikka, or vegetable curry. Fragrant basmati rice is an Indian specialty. One drawback: Indian food can be high in fat. Beware especially of foods sautéed in coconut oil.
- *Italian*—Minestrone or escarole soup is a good starter. Then try a pasta with marinara sauce or primavera (vegetables). Don't overdo it with the garlic bread! Italian food is perfect for sharing. Order a pasta dish and a seafood dish to share for a good balance of protein and carbohydrate.
- *Mexican*—Black bean soup is a healthful choice. Salsa is fine but go easy on the chips. Chicken or beef enchiladas, burritos, fajitas, or soft tacos are good entree choices. You're going to have to watch the fat in a Mexican restaurant, although more and more Mexican establishments are offering low-fat choices. Order a salad instead of a fried appetizer. Use a salsa as salad dressing.
- *Middle Eastern*—Hot or cold dolmas (stuffed grape leaves) and hummus make good appetizers. If you order a Greek salad, ask for the dressing on the side. If your meal plan requires, you can ask for the feta cheese and olives to be left out. Chicken or shrimp kabobs are great; order pita bread and steamed vegetables on the side. Baklava for dessert? Probably not your best choice. But don't miss the Turkish coffee.

Source: Adapted from Hope Warshaw, Eating Out: Your Guide to More Enjoyable Dining *(New York: Diabetes Self-Management Books, 1990). See the Appendix for more information on resources by Hope and others.*

Ask for tomato and lettuce on sandwiches, and skip high-fat spreads or sugary sauces. Be careful with shakes, freezes, turnovers, pancakes with syrup, and pies. Shakes, even the small (16-ounce) ones at McDonald's, have 310 to 350 calories, 5 to 6 grams of fat, and 54 to 63 grams of carbohydrate. A better choice would be a diet soft drink and a vanilla low-fat frozen yogurt cone—120 calories, 24 grams of carbohydrate, and less than 1 gram of fat. "Biggie," "giant," or "super" anything means more calories, fat, and salt. If it says "double" or "triple," believe it!

If you are trying to limit sodium, skip fried chicken and onion rings, because there is a lot of salt in the batter or breading. A large burger with cheese and special sauce often contains more than 1,000 milligrams of sodium—and that's before you eat anything else! Breakfast items and pizza that contain ham or sausage are usually high in sodium, too. Order sandwiches with lettuce and tomato but no sauces, and ask for unsalted french fries. Have it *your* way!

Ethnic fast-food restaurants are starting to offer more healthful options. Taco Bell, for example, currently offers 10 entrees, including chicken and steak tacos, tostadas, MexiMelts, and Pintos 'N Cheese that have under 300 calories and only 5 or 6 grams of fat. New light burritos have only 8 grams of fat and 350 calories. Taco Bell offers fat-free salsas and condiments as well. But watch the taco salad. Even the "light" version has 25 grams of fat and 680 calories—better than the 55 grams of fat and 870 calories found in the original, but still not the best choice.

Although small independent fast-food restaurants may not have nutrient information available, virtually all fast-food chains do. Many also have this information converted into exchanges. Ask the manager if he or she has nutritional information at the restaurant, or write the company's headquarters for it. If you eat at fast-food restaurants on a regular basis, you will want to contact the International Diabetes Center in Minneapolis (see Appendix) for more information on fast-food exchanges. Also see the section on fast foods in Chapter 3, "The Food Exchange System."

Social Gatherings

Your diabetes should never stand in the way of enjoying social gatherings with friends, family, and business associates. Tell yourself ahead of time that you're going to make the best choices you can, then relax and enjoy yourself. Know your meal plan, and proceed with confidence. Remember, not only people with diabetes watch what they eat. Lots of people watch calories, fat, and sodium because they want to follow a healthful diet. Many other people have severe intolerances to wheat or other common foods and must follow diets far more restrictive than yours. Conditions like these require monitoring the ingredients of almost everything they eat.

If you are dining at someone else's home, call the host or hostess ahead of time and explain that because you have diabetes, you have certain dietary preferences and restrictions. Say that you don't require special food but want to let your host know that you may not eat some foods that are served and do not want him or her to be surprised or upset. If the host offers to make a substitution, such as a fruit for dessert for you, be gracious and accept. But don't expect a separate meal.

If you know the menu and the time the meal will be served beforehand, you'll be able to plan your food choices in advance and may adjust the timing or amount of your medication as well. If the party is a potluck affair, bring something you know you can eat. If the event is a cocktail party or light buffet, remember you don't have to eat everything. You can almost always eat something that fits into your plan, but you may need to eat the remaining foods in your meal plan shortly after the party.

Holiday gatherings can be especially stressful. Food is so tied up with our celebration of special times like Thanksgiving, Hanukkah, Kwanza, Easter, Christmas, and New Year's. The tempting aromas and abundance of rich traditional foods can be hard to handle, especially if you are helping with the cooking. At times like these, try not to be too hard on yourself. Just make the best choices you can. Remember portion control. You can enjoy virtually everything—just less of it. Monitor your blood glucose levels and make adjustments as necessary to avoid emergencies.

Holiday festivities can also wreak havoc with the timing of your meals. Talk with your registered dietitian about what adjustments you should make if the main meal of the day comes at an unusual time. For example, many families have Thanksgiving dinner in midafternoon. You need to plan for this, but it need not limit your participation or enjoyment of the celebration.

Brown-Bag Foods

Frequently, it's easier for a child or an adult with diabetes to carry lunch than to choose food in a cafeteria or restaurant. Having what you need readily available means less pressure to make good decisions. When you prepare lunches at home, you can use sugar- or fat-reduced products, and you can take the time to make sure you are including the correct food exchanges. But brown baggers get tired of the sandwich and canned-soup routine! And who blames them?

As you would for any meal, make the brown-bag meal with a combination of foods from your plan. If you are packing a stew with 3 Meat Exchanges and

1 Starch Exchange, and you are allowed 3 Meat Exchanges and 2 Starch Exchanges, fill in with a piece of bread. Double-check to make sure that you use all the food planned for your meal.

Pack pieces of chicken, sliced meat, a pork chop, or cheese in foil or plastic bags. If you bring meat, add some cut vegetables. If you bring a soup or salad, you may need to add a remaining exchange, perhaps as a half sandwich or cheese and a roll. Most breads and sandwich fillings are perfect for brown-bag or picnic lunches. Include fresh fruit, either whole or cut, in plastic bags or small containers.

Children can buy milk at most schools, and low-fat milk is available in cafeterias and vending machines at many work sites. Tomato, vegetable, or fruit juice, coffee, tea, mineral water, and diet sodas are alternative beverages that may be available at work. If you have a Milk Exchange available, carry a thermos of sugar-free hot chocolate in cold weather.

One of the big problems with brown bagging is storage. When a refrigerator is not available, avoid foods that spoil quickly. But if you are willing to carry a wide-mouthed thermos, the problem is more than half solved. Many recipes in this book can be packed into a thermos and kept hot for lunch. All of the soups and most of the pastas and casseroles are perfect. Save leftovers from other home-cooked meals or restaurant meals in the refrigerator or freezer. Leftovers are a boon to brown baggers. The extra servings add great variety beyond sandwiches. As you pack your lunch bag, reheat items to be eaten hot, or if a microwave oven is available for reheating at work or school, include well-chilled or frozen leftovers.

Some people like to put cold packs in their lunch bags or use insulated carriers. You can also freeze individual juice boxes or milk cartons. They keep bag contents cool, and the liquid defrosts but is still chilled by lunchtime. Strategies for keeping food safe and at the right temperature differ according to what equipment is available for cooling and reheating. Many schools and work sites have vending machines and microwaves. You can buy your beverage right there and use the microwave to heat the food you've brought from home.

Some people keep an emergency bag in their desk or locker with an extra meal in case they forget a meal or need extra food because their blood sugar gets too low. This bag might include a single-serving can of water-packed tuna, crackers or simple cookies, vegetable soup, pudding, juice, dried fruit, pretzels, and other foods that don't require refrigeration.

11
Traveling Safely

Planning an overnight trip? How about a family vacation, or maybe that cruise you've always dreamed about? Don't let your diabetes curb your adventurous spirit. Many people with diabetes travel regularly for business and pleasure all over the world. As you plan your trip, remember these pointers:

In your purse or pocket, carry a letter from your physician stating that you have diabetes, your medication, and your doctor's name, address, and telephone number (including country code and area code). For international travel, if you take insulin, the letter should explain to the border customs agent why you are carrying syringes and needles. Do not give yourself insulin injections where strangers may observe you. Someone who does not know you are taking insulin may report you to the police. Your situation may be difficult to explain, especially if you are in another country and don't speak the language. In this age of drug abuse, law enforcement officials are necessarily suspicious.

Wear an identification bracelet or insignia on a neck chain to indicate that you have diabetes. These items are recognized worldwide by medical authorities and institutions. If you have an emergency and cannot communicate that you have diabetes, you may not get the help you need. Proper care can be provided much faster if you are wearing medical alert identification.

Get several diabetes identification wallet cards from your state or local affiliate of the American Diabetes Association. Fill them out, then put one in your purse or pocket and another in a suitcase. Give another to a friend who is traveling with you. Also, ask the American Diabetes Association for its pamphlets about traveling safely.

Carry your insulin, other medications, and a source of sugar with you in carry-on baggage. Luggage can be separated from you or even lost. Remember that insulin should be protected from extreme heat and cold over long periods of time.

For emergencies, carry *on your person* a roll of mints, other hard candy, or glucose tablets. If you suddenly develop hypoglycemia, you may not be able to dig through your luggage. Don't forget that sweetened soft drinks are sold all over the world and are ideal for certain acute diabetes (hypoglycemia) emergencies. Coca-Cola and Pepsi translate to any language!

When making air travel reservations, tell your travel agent or reservations clerk that you have diabetes and will require an appropriate menu on the flight. When you board the plane, tell the flight attendant that you have ordered a special meal. Other passengers may be envious of your healthful food.

Always carry a brown-bag meal in case of emergency. Some travel delays cannot be predicted. Computer glitches or last-minute plane changes may put your specially ordered meal in Salt Lake City when you are on your way to Indianapolis. (If you're traveling for most of the day, carry a full day's supply of food with you.) Avoid stress and emergencies by planning ahead.

If the timing of your meals is strictly regulated and you expect to travel across two or more time zones, ask your doctor or registered dietitian for help in making your mealtime and medication adjustments.

Take copies of your meal plans and food exchange lists with you, and use the suggestions in Chapter 10, "Eating Out." Beware of breakfast! It's easy to overdo this meal when you are on vacation. Fortunately, most hotels offer healthful menus for each meal. For example, Hyatt Hotels offer "Cuisine Naturelle," Hilton Hotels offer "Inspired Cuisine," and the Ritz-Carlton offers "Cuisine Vitale"—just to name a few. Cooked and dry cereals, toast, rolls, fruit, and juice are available everywhere.

If you're going to be staying in one city for an extended time, ask your doctor to recommend a physician in that area, or check with the local or regional Diabetes Association for some names. You can also check with a local pharmacist or the county medical society. If your library has a copy of *The Directory of Medical Specialists*, you can look up endocrinologists or diabetes specialists anywhere in the United States.

If you are staying in a resort, campground, or rental unit, ask at the registration desk if there is a house doctor and how to reach him or her during an emergency.

If you are traveling to a foreign country, read about dining customs and food ahead of time. In some countries, it is customary to eat dinner very late. You will have to adjust your meal plan accordingly. You also may want to have some of the common local food translated into exchanges in advance of your trip. Be careful of food sanitation and quality in underdeveloped countries. If there is any doubt about water quality, choose bottled water. Because gastrointestinal problems are common, especially in international travel, bring medication for diarrhea—just in case.

Have any required immunizations several weeks before your departure, so any side effects will be over before you travel. When you stay in a foreign country, register with the American embassy or consular office; its staff can help you get medical attention if you need it. Also, your doctor can provide you with a list of physicians in each country who assist foreign travelers, speak English and charge standard fees.

Pharmacists in a foreign country may not honor prescriptions written in the United States. You may have to get any prescriptions you need from a local doctor. Your medication may be dispensed under a different name in different countries. Bring a list of the drugs you take, using their *generic* names and the exact quantity you are supposed to take. Ask your doctor's office to prepare this list for you at your next regularly scheduled appointment.

When you are on vacation, your exercise level may increase with activities like sightseeing, backpacking, hiking, tennis, golf, swimming, or skiing. Remember that a change in physical activity will affect your meal plan. You may need to add some snacks and/or decrease medication.

If you are following an exercise plan, don't let travel interfere. Most hotels have some kind of exercise facility. Ask your travel agent to check whether a pool or workout room is available. Pack a jump rope or hand weights you can fill with water. Channel surf to find a morning workout show on television and follow along. The Residence Inn "Shape Program" provides guests with an exercise book that outlines how to do an in-room workout using towels, chairs, a phone book, and other common items.

If you belong to one of the on-line computer services, check to see if there is a diabetes discussion group you can join. CompuServe's Diabetes Forum offers lots of helpful information. You will be able to post a message asking other people with diabetes about their travel experiences. And you'll be able to share what you learn about managing your diabetes on the road.

Although you may not need the doctor, the packed meal, or the medical identification, it is best to plan ahead for every possible contingency. Think of it as free travel insurance. Unfortunately, you can't take a vacation from diabetes, but you can travel with peace of mind, knowing your safety net is in place.

Part III

Recipes

A well-designed meal plan for the person with diabetes can be the basis for economical, nutritious meals for the whole family. Foods prepared for someone with diabetes can also be enjoyed by everyone else sharing the same meal. The recipes in this book will tantalize your family and your friends. In fact, every recipe has passed the taste test by several people who do not have diabetes.

During recipe development for this revised edition of *The Art of Cooking for the Diabetic*, every ingredient was weighed and measured. Yields and serving sizes were noted carefully. Weights and portions are expressed in household measures to make your cooking faster and easier. Cooking for the person with diabetes can't be a haphazard effort. Ingredients and portions must be measured. Although using more or less of any ingredient changes the nutrient profile, do feel free to substitute ingredients that are nutritionally similar, like different herbs or salad greens. If you are cooking for one, you may want to reduce the recipes by half or plan on freezing individual portions to save cooking time later.

Measuring portions at serving time is the only way to become proficient at judging how much food equals an exchange or portion. If you conscientiously weigh and measure your foods for a few weeks, you will develop this expertise. Even after you can easily eyeball a 3-ounce portion of meat, test yourself once a month or so to be sure your "guesstimate" of 3 ounces hasn't grown to 4 or 5 ounces. Even if you are not the person doing the cooking in your household, you must be savvy about what constitutes a portion. This knowledge will be vital when you serve yourself food from platters or bowls at the table or when you eat away from home.

It's a big help to have the right equipment as you prepare healthful recipes. Here is a list of kitchen tools specified in our recipes that will help you to measure and prepare healthy foods:

- Nonstick skillets, large and small—These are great for low-fat sautéeing and stir-frying because you can use less oil.
- Basic set of small, medium, and large pots with lids—Choose nonstick surfaces. These cut down on the need for fat in recipes and are easier to clean.
- Measuring tools—You'll need a kitchen scale that shows grams and ounces, standard measuring spoons, metal measuring cups for dry ingredients, and cup- and quart-sized glass measuring cups for liquids.
- Food processor—This handy machine speeds chopping, slicing, dicing, and mixing.
- Regular or hand-held mixer—This is useful for preparing baked goods, whipping potatoes, and beating egg whites.
- Grill rack—Use this to keep fat drippings away from broiled foods.
- Sharp knives, knife sharpener, and nonporous cutting board: Sharp tools speed slicing and dicing. A nonporous cutting board can be sanitized more easily.
- Steamer basket—Steaming is a quick way to cook fish and vegetables, and it minimizes the loss of nutrients.
- Multipurpose grater—Get the full taste of cheese with just a little bit by grating or shredding instead of slicing it. A grater is also useful for grating lemon or orange zest and fresh gingerroot.
- Fat separator—This is a handy watering-can-like pitcher that you use to skim the fat off liquids and pan juices.
- Pastry brush—A brush reduces the amount of oil in cooking by allowing you to gently brush it on rather than pour it.
- Baking and roasting pans, cookie tins, and cupcake tins—Select nonstick surfaces, which make cleanup easier and cut down on the need for fat.
- Colander or large strainer—Use this to drain pasta and vegetables and to separate solids from soup stock.
- Wire cooling rack—The rack not only cools cookies and baked goods, it is perfect for putting in a roasting pan to "dry" toast, tomatoes, etc., on all sides without burning.

- Outdoor barbecue or indoor stovetop grill—Many foods benefit from the smoke and sizzle of grilling. This cooking method adds flavor and reduces fat.

In this edition of *The Art of Cooking for the Diabetic*, you'll find hundreds of recipes, most of which reflect the growing interest in bolder-flavored ethnic foods and American regional cuisines. Fresh ingredients are used whenever possible. Comments topping most recipes share ideas for alternative ingredients and menu and serving ideas. If you have enjoyed past editions of this book, you'll also find some old favorites from them—many with a new twist.

Under each recipe you will see a nutrient analysis for one serving. These values are for the portion size stated. (Generally carbohydrate—abbreviated as CHO—fat, and protein have been rounded to the nearest gram, calories have been rounded to the nearest 5 calories, sodium and cholesterol to the nearest 5 milligrams, and fiber and saturated fat reported at the nearest .5 gram.) You may want more or less than one serving; just remember that nutrient levels and exchanges go up and down based on the portion you eat.

The nutrients in each recipe have been converted to the newly revised food exchanges. Generally, exchanges have been assigned based on the levels of carbohydrate, protein, and fat and the major ingredients in the recipe. For example, if fruit is the major ingredient, the recipe will count as 1 or more Fruit Exchanges. Because carbohydrates may be substituted for each other, if you have Starch or Milk Exchanges available at that meal, you can count the Fruit Exchange recipe as a starch or Milk Exchange instead. You will want to discuss how to do this—and how often to do it—with your registered dietitian.

Depending on your unique needs and meal plan, you may look specifically at levels of particular nutrients within each recipe's nutrient profile. For example, if you are on a low-sodium diet or low-cholesterol diet, you will want to take a closer look at the sodium or cholesterol levels of the recipes. A note under each recipe describes how to modify it for a low-sodium diet.

Vegetarians and individuals who keep kosher can substitute Vegetable Stock (see Index) for recipes calling for Chicken Stock or broth as an ingredient. This variation is not listed every time Chicken Stock is included as an ingredient.

Sometimes recipes list a choice of ingredients. The first ingredient listed is the one included in the calculated nutrient value. The calculated values do not include ingredients listed as optional. When a recipe calls for cooking a vegetable, pasta, or seafood in boiling water, the salt is not included as a recipe ingredient. An estimate of the sodium absorbed by that food is included in the calculated value.

You can make your life a lot easier by having reduced-fat and reduced-sodium items in your refrigerator or pantry. If you are on a low-cholesterol diet, have egg substitutes handy. Try reduced-fat and reduced-sodium cheeses to find ones that you like. Salt-free herb blends, fresh herbs, fresh lemon, and fresh garlic all provide a boost of flavor that is especially welcome when you must limit fat and salt.

Today, nutritionists and chefs are meeting on common ground. The recipes in this book reflect that partnership. They were developed with both *good taste* and *good health* in mind. As an individual with diabetes, you do have special dietary needs—and surely one of those needs is to enjoy fresh, flavorful food. Start right here, right now, with *The Art of Cooking for the Diabetic.*

12

Appetizers

Dilled Salmon on Endive

For an elegant presentation, arrange the stuffed endive in circles, like petals of a flower, on a platter.

2 medium heads (5–6 ounces total) Belgian endive

1 recipe Lox Spread (see Index) 2–4 sprigs fresh dill

Cut base from each head of endive, wash and separate leaves. Fill bottom half of each leaf with Lox Spread.

Break dill into very small sprigs. Garnish each endive boat with a small sprig of dill.

8 servings
1 serving = 3 stuffed endive leaves

CAL.	CHO*(g)*	PRO.*(g)*	TOTAL FAT*(g)*	SAT. FAT*(g)*	CHOL.*(mg)*	FIBER*(g)*	SODIUM*(mg)*
35	2	4	1	0.5	5	0.5	140

Food exchange per serving: 1 Very Lean Meat
Low-sodium diets: This recipe is acceptable.

Artichoke Flowers

These artichokes are festive and delicious with Buttermilk Ranch Dressing, or you can substitute bottled dressing if you prefer. (Check the label on bottled dressings to determine exchange values.) They can be served tepid or chilled. The artichoke has virtually no calories. The oil added to the cooking water is not absorbed but improves the appearance of the leaves.

*2 large (1½ pounds total)
  artichokes
1 tablespoon lemon juice
1 tablespoon vegetable oil*

*6 tablespoons light ranch dressing
  or Buttermilk Ranch Dressing
  (see Index)*

Trim tough bottom of stem and bottom tough outer leaves from each artichoke. Trim tops of artichoke leaves with scissors or sharp knife to remove burrs on artichoke leaves.

Add lemon juice and vegetable oil to a large pot of boiling salted water. Add artichokes. Cover and simmer about 20 minutes, until the artichokes are cooked. (The stems should be tender when pierced with a sharp knife.) Drain the artichokes.

Strip off artichoke leaves, arranging them in slightly overlapping circle in a flower pattern. Leaves of both artichokes should fill 6 small plates. Stop stripping leaves when you get to cone of leaves covering the choke. Cut off these tough leaves and cut out and discard the hairy choke.

Slice artichoke heart and bottom. Arrange slices in center of artichoke leaves.

Drizzle 1 tablespoon of dressing over bases of leaves and hearts on center of each plate.

6 servings
1 serving = leaves and heart of ⅓ artichoke plus 1 tablespoon dressing

CAL.	CHO(g)	PRO.(g)	TOTAL FAT(g)	SAT. FAT(g)	CHOL.(mg)	FIBER(g)	SODIUM(mg)
40	7	1	1	0	0	2.5	250

Food exchange per serving: 1 Vegetable
Low-sodium diets: Omit salt in boiling water.

Caviar-Topped New Potatoes

Elegant and easy, this recipe can be easily doubled for company.

½ pound (about 8) small red new potatoes
3 tablespoons sour half-and-half or Yogurt Cheese (see Index)

1 scallion, finely minced, or 1½ teaspoons snipped fresh dill
1½ tablespoons red lumpfish caviar

Place potatoes in a medium-sized pot of boiling salted water. Boil 15 minutes or until tender when pierced with a fork. Drain potatoes and cool 5–10 minutes.

Cut each potato in half. With a small melon baller, scoop about ½ teaspoon of potato from center of each potato half and discard. Cool potatoes to room temperature or chill them.

In a small bowl mix sour half-and-half and minced scallion. Spoon 1 rounded teaspoon of the half-and-half mixture onto each potato half. Top each with ¼ teaspoon caviar.

4 servings
1 serving = 4 stuffed potato halves

CAL.	CHO*(g)*	PRO.*(g)*	TOTAL FAT*(g)*	SAT. FAT*(g)*	CHOL.*(mg)*	FIBER*(g)*	SODIUM*(mg)*
70	11	2	2	1	25	1	150

Food exchange per serving: 1 Starch
Low-sodium diets: This recipe is suitable.

Eggplant Provençale

Serve this as an appetizer or light entree. You can use our Chunky Tomato Sauce, or bottled pasta sauce—the varieties with extra spices, garlic, herb, onion, etc.—works very well, too.

1 cup spicy pasta sauce or Chunky Tomato Sauce (see Index)	4 lettuce leaves
2 small (about 1 pound total) eggplants	1 tablespoon snipped fresh parsley
2 tablespoons reduced-calorie Italian dressing	1 teaspoon drained capers

Preheat oven to 350°F. Chill pasta sauce. Slice hard top off each eggplant, but leave skin on. Slice eggplants in half lengthwise. Pierce eggplant halves over all sides and through skin with a fork. Brush all surfaces of eggplant with Italian dressing; place in a baking pan.

Bake 25–30 minutes, turning and basting after 15 minutes.

Chill eggplant. When ready to serve, line plates with lettuce, add a piece of eggplant, and top with ¼ cup chilled pasta sauce. Sprinkle each with parsley and a few capers.

4 servings
1 serving = 1 eggplant half plus ¼ cup sauce

CAL.	CHO(g)	PRO.(g)	TOTAL FAT(g)	SAT. FAT(g)	CHOL.(mg)	FIBER(g)	SODIUM(mg)
100	18	2	3	0.5	0	2	435

Food exchanges per serving: 3 Vegetables plus ½ Fat *or* 1 Other Carbohydrate plus ½ Fat
Low-sodium diets: Substitute unsalted pasta sauce; omit capers.

Roasted Onion Confiture

As an appetizer, this recipe is delicious served atop Garlic Sourdough Toasts (see Index) or in Herbed Phyllo Cups (see Index) garnished with chopped parsley. You can also serve it with fish, beef, or chicken breasts.

2 (about 1 pound total) sweet onions such as Vidalia, WallaWalla, or sweet Spanish, chopped

2 teaspoons olive oil

¼ teaspoon salt

¼ teaspoon freshly ground pepper

3 tablespoons raisins

1 tablespoon + 1 teaspoon balsamic vinegar

2 teaspoons drained capers

Preheat oven to 350°F. In a mixing bowl, toss onions with oil, salt, and pepper. Prepare flat baking pan with cooking spray. Spread onions on the pan.

Cover with foil and bake 30 minutes. Turn onions; bake uncovered another 15 minutes until onions are tender and begin to brown.

Stir in raisins, vinegar, and capers. Put into small container and refrigerate several hours before using, to allow flavors to blend.

8 servings (makes 2 cups)
1 serving = ¼ cup

CAL.	CHO*(g)*	PRO.*(g)*	TOTAL FAT*(g)*	SAT. FAT*(g)*	CHOL.*(mg)*	FIBER*(g)*	SODIUM*(mg)*
50	8	1	2	0	0	1	90

Food exchange per serving: 1 Vegetable *or* ½ Starch
Low-sodium diets: Omit salt.

Grilled Vegetable Terrine

Although the recipe takes a while to prepare and must be assembled in advance, it's beautiful to serve as an appetizer or vegetable. And it is rich in Vitamin A and potassium.

Marinade

2 tablespoons balsamic vinegar
2 tablespoons water
1 tablespoon chopped fresh basil or other fresh herbs
1 tablespoon virgin olive oil
½ teaspoon minced fresh garlic
½ teaspoon salt
¼ teaspoon freshly ground pepper

Terrine

1 medium (1 pound total) eggplant, peeled
3 medium (1 pound total) zucchini
3 (1 pound total) yellow summer squash
3 medium (1 pound total) leeks
1 large red bell pepper
1 (6-ounce) can tomato paste with Italian seasoning
¼ cup freshly grated Parmesan cheese
10 herb sprigs to garnish (basil, tarragon, rosemary, or parsley)

Mix marinade ingredients in a small bowl.

Cut eggplant, zucchini, and summer squash lengthwise into thin slices (¼–½ inch thick). Wash leeks well, trim off stem end and tough greens, and slice lengthwise. Remove core from pepper, and cut pepper into several flat slices. Brush all vegetables with marinade.

Grill vegetables over coals or using indoor grill until vegetables are tender and marked with grill marks. Peel skin from grilled red pepper.

Preheat oven to 350°F. Prepare an 8″ × 4″ loaf pan with cooking spray. Layer grilled vegetables in pan, alternating vegetables. Spread some tomato paste and sprinkle some Parmesan cheese between layers. There should be three or four layers. Cover top with foil and press down firmly to compress vegetable terrine. Bake terrine 30–40 minutes. Allow to cool 10 minutes.

Run knife around pan edges and turn terrine out of pan. If serving warm, slice carefully with serrated knife in ¾-inch slices. If serving at room temperature, refrigerate terrine, then slice immediately before serving. Garnish each slice with herb sprig.

10 servings
1 serving = 1 ¾-inch slice

CAL.	CHO*(g)*	PRO.*(g)*	TOTAL FAT*(g)*	SAT. FAT*(g)*	CHOL.*(mg)*	FIBER*(g)*	SODIUM*(mg)*
75	12	3	3	0.5	2	2.5	295

Food exchanges per serving: 2 Vegetables *or* 1 Starch
Low-sodium diets: Omit salt; substitute unsalted tomato paste.

Scallops Seviche

Seviche is usually marinated raw seafood. Because we are concerned about the food safety of raw seafood, this recipe calls for cooking the scallops. Substitute shrimp for the scallops if you wish.

12 ounces fresh or frozen sea
   scallops, thawed
½ cup cider vinegar
¼ cup water
1½ teaspoons mixed pickling spices

1 tablespoon finely chopped onion
½ teaspoon salt
Lettuce leaves to line plates
2 lemons, sliced thin

Preheat oven to 350°F. Separate scallops and spread in a small baking dish.

In a small bowl or jar, combine vinegar, water, pickling spices, onion, and salt. Pour over scallops. Cover dish with foil and bake 15 minutes.

Chill scallops in liquid. Drain and serve on lettuce leaves. Garnish with lemon slices.

8 servings
1 serving = about 4 scallops

CAL.	CHO(g)	PRO.(g)	TOTAL FAT(g)	SAT. FAT(g)	CHOL.(mg)	FIBER(g)	SODIUM(mg)
40	1	7	0.5	0	15	0	105

Food exchange per serving: 1 Very Lean Meat
Low-sodium diets: Omit salt.

Prosciutto with Papaya

Papaya, like mango and cantaloupe, is an excellent source of antioxidant vitamins A and C. This recipe supplies a whole day's worth of several vitamins and lots of potassium.

1 large, ripe papaya   *8 ripe black olives (optional)*
4 leaves green leaf lettuce
2 ounces paper-thin slices of
*   prosciutto or lean smoked ham*

*P*are papaya and remove seeds. Slice lengthwise into eight slices.

Line four plates with lettuce leaves, and arrange two strips of papaya on each plate. Gently wrap center of each papaya strip with prosciutto. Garnish with olives.

4 servings
1 serving = 2 papaya strips

CAL.	CHO*(g)*	PRO.*(g)*	TOTAL FAT*(g)*	SAT. FAT*(g)*	CHOL.*(mg)*	FIBER*(g)*	SODIUM*(mg)*
70	10	5	2	0.5	10	1	265

Food exchanges per serving: 1 Fruit plus 1 Lean Meat (prosciutto); 1 Fruit plus 1 Very Lean Meat (lean ham, chicken, or turkey)
Low-sodium diets: Substitute thinly sliced chicken or turkey for prosciutto; omit olives.

Chevre and Sun-Dried Tomato Spread

Goat cheese, also called chevre, has 5 or 6 grams of fat per ounce. Enjoy this tasty spread on crackers or as a dip for raw vegetables.

½ ounce sun-dried tomatoes, not packed in oil
4 ounces herbed chevre (goat cheese)
1 teaspoon snipped fresh basil or tarragon

2 leaves of fresh basil or 1 sprig of tarragon for garnish

Method 1: Soften tomatoes in warm water for 15 minutes; drain well. Put tomatoes, cheese, and snipped herbs in food processor; blend well. Garnish with herb sprig.

    Method 2: Soften tomatoes in warm water for 15 minutes; drain well. Finely chop tomatoes. Whip cheese with tomatoes and snipped herbs. Garnish with herb sprig.

4 servings (makes ½ cup)
1 serving = 2 tablespooons

CAL.	CHO(g)	PRO.(g)	TOTAL FAT(g)	SAT. FAT(g)	CHOL.(mg)	FIBER(g)	SODIUM(mg)
90	3	6	6	4	15	1	110

Food exchange per serving: 1 Medium-Fat Meat
Low-sodium diets: This recipe is acceptable.

Cremini Mushroom Spread

8 ounces cremini or brown
    mushrooms
¼ *cup chopped fresh parsley*
3 *scallions, cut in several pieces*
⅔ *cup Yogurt Cheese (see Index)*

2 ounces fat-free cream cheese,
    Fromage Blanc, or Neufchâtel
    cheese
¼ *teaspoon salt*
⅛ *teaspoon freshly ground pepper*

Spray a large nonstick skillet with butter-flavored cooking spray. Sauté mushrooms until they release some liquid and are lightly browned.

Chop mushrooms, parsley, and scallions together in a food processor. Remove 2 tablespoons vegetable mixture and set aside. To mushrooms in processor, add Yogurt Cheese, cream cheese, salt, and pepper. Pulse to blend. Do not overprocess; tiny mushroom chunks should remain. Place in serving bowl and top with reserved chopped mushrooms.

6 servings (makes 1½ cups)
1 serving = ¼ cup

CAL.	CHO(g)	PRO.(g)	TOTAL FAT(g)	SAT. FAT(g)	CHOL.(mg)	FIBER(g)	SODIUM(mg)
40	5	4	0	0	0	1	155

Food exchange per serving: 1 Vegetable
Low-sodium diets: Omit salt.

Lox Spread

This is a classic spread for bagels. Supermarket deli counters often have "ends" and bits of lox at reduced prices. You don't need beautifully cut slices.

¾ cup creamed (4% milk fat) cottage cheese

3 scallions with greens, cut in pieces

2 ounces smoked salmon (lox)

¼ teaspoon freshly ground pepper

*P*lace all ingredients in a blender or food processor. Whip about 30 seconds, until mixture is well blended but flecks of salmon and scallion are visible. Place in bowl, cover, and refrigerate at least 2 hours for flavors to blend.

8 servings
1 serving = 2 tablespoons

CAL.	CHO*(g)*	PRO.*(g)*	TOTAL FAT*(g)*	SAT. FAT*(g)*	CHOL.*(mg)*	FIBER*(g)*	SODIUM*(mg)*
30	1	4	1	0.5	5	0	135

Food exchange per serving: 1 Very Lean Meat
Low-sodium diets: This recipe is acceptable.

Parmesan-Scallion Dip

I like this as a dip for veggies. Try it with broccoli, carrots, green beans, and zucchini or with 94 percent fat-free potato crisps. The dip can be used to stuff cherry tomatoes, Belgian endive leaves, or celery, too.

1 cup Whipped Cottage Cheese and Chives (see Index)

5 tablespoons grated Parmesan cheese

4 scallions, including greens, chopped fine

1 tablespoon prepared horseradish

Dash cayenne pepper

Combine all ingredients in a small bowl; mix well. Taste and add more cayenne if desired. Cover and chill at least 2 hours before serving.

12 servings (makes 1½ cups)
1 serving = 2 tablespoons

CAL.	CHO(g)	PRO.(g)	TOTAL FAT(g)	SAT. FAT(g)	CHOL.(mg)	FIBER(g)	SODIUM(mg)
30	1	3	1.5	1	5	0	135

Food exchange per serving: ½ Lean Meat
Low-sodium diets: Omit salt from Whipped Cottage Cheese and Chives.

Yogurt Dill Dip

This dip is also a great sauce for Dilled Lamb in Pita Pockets (see Index) or for grilled or poached fish.

1 cup (8 ounces) plain low-fat
    yogurt
1 tablespoon chopped fresh dill

½ teaspoon salt
¼ teaspoon freshly ground pepper

Combine all ingredients in a small bowl. Cover and chill at least 2 hours before serving.

8 servings (makes 1 cup)
1 serving = 2 tablespoons

CAL.	CHO(g)	PRO.(g)	TOTAL FAT(g)	SAT. FAT(g)	CHOL.(mg)	FIBER(g)	SODIUM(mg)
20	2	1	0.5	0	0	0	155

Food exchange per serving: a Free Food
Low-sodium diets: Omit salt.

Vegetable Dip for Crudités

Serve this dip with an assortment of fresh vegetables: jicama sticks, celery sticks, carrot sticks, scallions, cauliflower pieces, kohlrabi coins, mushrooms, broccoli florets, red pepper strips, summer squash strips.

1 cup low-fat (2% milk fat) cottage
　　cheese
1 cup shredded carrot
½ cup seeded, chopped green pepper
¼ cup minced onion
¼ cup plain low-fat yogurt

2 tablespoons catsup
1 teaspoon fresh lemon juice
½ teaspoon salt
½ teaspoon freshly ground pepper
½ teaspoon celery seed

Combine all ingredients in a food processor fitted with a steel blade or in a blender; process until smooth. Place in a bowl, cover, and refrigerate at least 2 hours before serving.

10 servings (makes 2½ cups)
1 serving = ¼ cup

CAL.	CHO(g)	PRO.(g)	TOTAL FAT(g)	SAT. FAT(g)	CHOL.(mg)	FIBER(g)	SODIUM(mg)
35	4	4	0.5	0	0	0.5	245

Food exchange per serving: 1 Vegetable
Low-sodium diets: Omit salt.

West Indies Dip

Delightful as a dressing for a fresh-fruit plate or with sliced apples, oranges, or bananas.

1 cup plus 2 tablespoons Whipped
Cottage Cheese and Chives
(see Index)
2 tablespoons chopped onion

3 tablespoons prepared chutney
2 teaspoons curry powder
⅛ teaspoon ground nutmeg

Combine all ingredients in a blender and cover tightly. Blend at low speed about 30 seconds or until smooth. Chill at least 2 hours before serving.

10 servings (makes 1¼ cups)
1 serving = 2 tablespoons

CAL.	CHO(g)	PRO.(g)	TOTAL FAT(g)	SAT. FAT(g)	CHOL.(mg)	FIBER(g)	SODIUM(mg)
40	4	3	1	0.5	0	0	135

Food exchange per serving: ½ Skim Milk
Low-sodium diets: This recipe is fine.

Crostini

The recipe is for basic crostini. Feel free to add finely chopped tomatoes, roasted pepper, sliced olives, or a dab of Chunky Salsa (see Index) or Roasted Onion Confiture (see Index) as additional toppings. Fresh mozzarella provides a wonderful delicate taste and soft texture, but you can use packaged part-skim mozzarella.

*2 (about 4 ounces) brown-and-
    serve soft bread sticks*
2 teaspoons virgin olive oil
1 small clove garlic, crushed

Dash cayenne pepper
2 ounces fresh mozzarella cheese
*2 tablespoons slivered fresh basil
    leaves*

Preheat oven to 350°F. Cut each bread stick, on the diagonal, into eight ½-inch slices. In a small bowl, mix oil, garlic, and cayenne. Arrange bread slices on cookie sheet, and brush tops with oil mixture.

Cut mozzarella into small, thin slices. Top each bread slice with a piece of cheese. Bake about 5 minutes or until cheese melts and bread browns around edges.

Top each of the crostini with a small mound of slivered basil.

4 servings (makes 16 crostini)
1 serving = 4 crostini

CAL.	CHO(g)	PRO.(g)	TOTAL FAT(g)	SAT. FAT(g)	CHOL.(mg)	FIBER(g)	SODIUM(mg)
140	15	5	6	0.5	10	1	175

Food exchanges per serving: 1 Starch plus 1 Fat *or* 1 Whole Milk plus ½ Starch
Low-sodium diets: This recipe is fine.

Garlic Sourdough Toasts

These crunchy toasts are wonderful with salads and soups or as a base for hors d'oeuvre spreads. Try them topped with Roasted Onion Confiture (see Index) or Chevre and Sun-Dried Tomato Spread (see Index). Use 2 teaspoons of either to top each toast.

1 tablespoon + 1 teaspoon olive oil   1-pound loaf sourdough bread, long
1 teaspoon crushed fresh garlic   style

Preheat oven to 300°F. Mix oil and garlic in a small bowl. Cut crusts off each end of bread, and trim sides to form a rectangular block. (Bread will trim to a block about 2½″ × 1¾″ × 9″ long and weigh about 9 ounces.) Cut bread into ¼-inch slices.

Place a cooling rack on top of a cookie sheet. Arrange slices on rack; brush tops lightly with garlic oil. Bake until crisp and slightly toasted, about 15 minutes. Cool and store in tightly covered container.

12 servings (makes about 36 toasts)
1 serving = 3 toasts

CAL.	CHO(g)	PRO.(g)	TOTAL FAT(g)	SAT. FAT(g)	CHOL.(mg)	FIBER(g)	SODIUM(mg)
70	11	2	2	0.5	0	0.5	130

Food exchange per serving: 1 Starch
Low-sodium diets: This recipe is fine.

Refried Bean Dip

Serve this tasty high-fiber dip with whole-grain crackers, tortillas, or reduced-fat tortilla chips.

1 16-ounce can red kidney beans, including liquid
¼ cup finely chopped scallions with tops
½ cup low-fat (2% milk fat) cottage cheese

1 4-ounce can chopped mild green chilies, drained
½ teaspoon ground cumin
Dash chili powder (optional)

*P*uree beans and bean liquid in a blender or food processor fitted with steel blade. Lightly spray cooking spray in a nonstick pan. Sauté pureed beans and scallions over medium heat until hot, stirring often. Stir in cottage cheese, chilies, cumin, and chili powder if desired.

Cover and refrigerate for flavors to blend.

10 servings (makes 2½ cups)
1 serving = ¼ cup

CAL.	CHO(g)	PRO.(g)	TOTAL FAT(g)	SAT. FAT(g)	CHOL.(mg)	FIBER(g)	SODIUM(mg)
50	8	4	0	0	0	3	225

Food exchange per serving: ½ Starch plus ½ Very Lean Meat
Low-sodium diets: Substitute unsalted canned beans, or drain and rinse kidney beans and add 1–2 tablespoons water to replace liquid from can.

Herbed Phyllo Cups

Enjoy these pretty herbed cups filled with Hot Crab Dip (see next recipe), Roasted Onion Confiture (see Index), or the filling of your choice. Each holds about ¼ cup filling. Although you must count the filling, the lovely cups are a Free Food, at only 15 calories each.

3 leaves (14″ × 18″) phyllo dough   2 tablespoons minced mixed fresh
Butter-flavored cooking spray   herbs

*P*reheat oven to 350°F.

Put 1 leaf of phyllo dough on a cutting board. Lightly spray with cooking spray. Sprinkle with half the herbs. Gently lay second leaf of dough over herbs. Spray again and spread with remaining herbs. Top with third leaf. Lightly spray top layer. With scissors or a sharp knife, cut layered phyllo into 4½-inch squares.

Coat inside of 12 muffin cups with butter-flavored cooking spray. Gently place phyllo squares into muffin cups with pointed edges up, forming small fluted-edge cups. You may want to do this in two batches, leaving alternating cups empty so edges of Phyllo cups don't touch.

Bake 6–8 minutes until cups are crisp and lightly browned. If not used immediately, store in a tightly covered container.

12 servings
1 serving = 1 phyllo cup

CAL.	CHO(g)	PRO.(g)	TOTAL FAT(g)	SAT. FAT(g)	CHOL.(mg)	FIBER(g)	SODIUM(mg)
15	3	0	0.5	0	0	0	25

Food exchange per serving: a Free Food
Low-sodium diets: This recipe is excellent.

Hot Crab Dip

Serve this dip in many ways—in Herbed Phyllo Cups (see preceding recipe), as a dip with fat-free black-pepper crackers, or as a filling for cherry tomatoes. Or, for stuffed mushrooms, fill mushrooms with the unheated mixture, then bake until hot.

8 ounces crabmeat, fresh or frozen, drained
4 ounces Neufchâtel cheese, fat-free cream cheese, or Fromage Blanc
⅓ cup light ricotta cheese
1 tablespoon snipped fresh chives

1 tablespoon fresh lemon juice
2 teaspoons snipped fresh dill or
½ teaspoon dried dill
1 teaspoon seasoned salt
1 teaspoon finely minced garlic
¼ teaspoon hot-pepper sauce

*I*n a medium-sized bowl, combine all ingredients and mix well. Transfer mixture to a small nonstick saucepan. Heat over low heat about 2 minutes, stirring constantly, just until mixture is hot.

6 servings
1 serving = ¼ cup

CAL.	CHO(g)	PRO.(g)	TOTAL FAT(g)	SAT. FAT(g)	CHOL.(mg)	FIBER(g)	SODIUM(mg)
105	2	11	6	3	55	0	410

Food exchanges per serving: 1 Medium-Fat Meat (made with Neufchâtel cheese) *or* 1 Lean Meat (made with fat-free cream cheese)
Low-sodium diets: Substitute light seasoned salt.

Broiled Portobello Mushrooms

Serve a whole mushroom as an appetizer or under polenta. These hearty mushrooms are also great grilled. If you like garlic, add a crushed clove to the oil.

4 (about 1 pound total) Portobello mushrooms, each about 5 inches in diameter

1 tablespoon virgin olive oil
¼ teaspoon salt
⅛ teaspoon freshly ground pepper

Wash mushrooms well; trim off stems for another use.

Put mushrooms on a broiler pan or disposable pan, cap side up. Brush tops with half of oil, and season with half of salt and pepper. Broil 2 minutes.

Turn mushrooms over so the stem side is up. Brush with remaining oil; season with remaining salt and pepper. Broil 3 minutes more until mushrooms soften.

4 servings
1 serving = 1 mushroom

CAL.	CHO(g)	PRO.(g)	TOTAL FAT(g)	SAT. FAT(g)	CHOL.(mg)	FIBER(g)	SODIUM(mg)
50	4	2	3	0.5	0	1	140

Food exchanges per serving: 1 Vegetable plus ½ Fat
Low-sodium diets: Omit salt.

Easy Quesadillas

If you like spicy foods, use peppered Monterey Jack cheese or spiced Chihuahua, a Mexican-style white cheese that melts easily. Use Chunky Salsa (see Index), Cilantro Salsa (see Index), or a commercial prepared salsa.

1 teaspoon corn oil or melted margarine
2 8-inch-diameter flour tortillas
⅔ cup shredded Chihuahua or peppered Monterey Jack cheese

⅓ cup chunky salsa—mild, medium, or spicy as you prefer

Preheat oven to 350°F.

Brush corn oil or margarine on a cookie sheet to oil an 8-inch circle. Put 1 tortilla on oiled cookie sheet. Spread cheese evenly over tortilla, then press remaining tortilla on top.

Bake 6–8 minutes or until cheese melts. Press tortillas together. Flip tortillas so oiled side is up.

Cut into eight wedges with a knife or pizza cutter. Return to oven 2 more minutes. Serve wedges with salsa as dip or topping.

2 servings
1 serving = 4 wedges, each with salsa

CAL.	CHO(g)	PRO.(g)	TOTAL FAT(g)	SAT. FAT(g)	CHOL.(mg)	FIBER(g)	SODIUM(mg)
295	23	12	17	7	40	1	845

Food exchanges per serving: 1 Starch plus 1 Vegetable plus 1 Medium-Fat Meat plus 2 Fats
Low-sodium diets: Substitute reduced-sodium cheese; prepare salsa without salt.

Gorgonzola Triangles

My neighbor Linda Garcin was a taste-tester for this recipe. She loved it, as will other fans of Gorgonzola.

½ cup (2 ounces) crumbled
    Gorgonzola cheese
¼ cup light ricotta cheese
2 teaspoons minced fresh basil or
    oregano or ½ teaspoon dried
    basil or oregano

4 leaves (each 14″ × 18″) phyllo
    dough
1 tablespoon sesame seeds
Butter- or olive oil–flavored
    cooking spray

In a small bowl, mix Gorgonzola, ricotta, and herbs with a fork.

Preheat oven to 375°F. On a cutting board, lay out 1 leaf phyllo, and spray top with cooking spray. Sprinkle with 1 teaspoon sesame seeds. Gently lay a second leaf of phyllo on top of the first; spray with cooking spray. Cut phyllo layers into 10 long strips, each 1½ inches wide.

Place small scoop of cheese filling (about 2 teaspoons) 1 inch from end of each strip. Fold corner of one strip diagonally across to opposite edge to form triangle. Spray top of triangle with cooking spray; sprinkle with a few sesame seeds. Fold triangle end over end until entire phyllo strip is folded. Continue to fold triangles end over end, spraying each triangle and sprinkling with sesame seeds. Repeat entire process with remaining phyllo leaves, filling, and seeds.

Bake triangles until phyllo is crisp and lightly browned, about 8–10 minutes.

10 servings
1 serving = 2 triangles

CAL.	CHO(g)	PRO.(g)	TOTAL FAT(g)	SAT. FAT(g)	CHOL.(mg)	FIBER(g)	SODIUM(mg)
60	5	2	4	1.5	5	0	120

Food exchanges per serving: ½ Starch plus 1 Fat
Low-sodium diets: This recipe is fine.

13
Soups

Chicken Stock

This rich stock adds great flavor to many recipes in this book. It's much tastier than canned chicken broth. Don't salt the stock during cooking. It may get too salty as the liquid cooks and becomes more concentrated. You may want to add salt to taste when you eat the stock as soup.

Freeze the stock in small containers so you can defrost it as needed for a recipe ingredient or for a bowl of soup. I like to prepare the stock while I make dinner so that it is finished late in the evening. It can be chilled overnight, defatted in the morning, and put in the freezer before I go to work.

1 3½-pound chicken, cut up
2 medium carrots, cut lengthwise
1 medium onion, skin on, cut in
    half
1 rib celery

1 leek, well washed, cut lengthwise
    (optional)
1 bay leaf
1 teaspoon peppercorns

Combine all ingredients in a large stockpot. Add 3 quarts water. Bring to a boil. Lower heat and let soup simmer for 3½ hours, skimming off any foam that rises.

Strain soup through a fine sieve. Discard vegetables; skin chicken, and save cooked chicken for chicken salad or other recipes.

Refrigerate soup overnight.

Remove all fat from the top of the stock. Use, refrigerate, or freeze defatted stock. Stock keeps four to five days in the refrigerator and two months in the freezer.

8 servings (makes 2 quarts)
1 serving = 1 cup

CAL.	CHO(g)	PRO.(g)	TOTAL FAT(g)	SAT. FAT(g)	CHOL.(mg)	FIBER(g)	SODIUM(mg)
30	3	3	2	0.5	0	0	110

Food exchange per serving: ½ Lean Meat; amounts less than 1 cup are Free Foods
Low-sodium diets: This recipe is suitable.

Vegetable Stock

You can substitute this tasty Vegetable Stock in any recipe calling for
Chicken Stock (the preceding recipe)—a substitution that is especially
helpful for vegetarians, those who have a vegetarian in their household, and
those who keep kosher. Freeze stock in 1-cup portions for use in recipes
when you need just a little. Add salt to taste at serving time if desired.

*2 large onions, chopped (about 4
    cups total)*
*2 large leeks, well washed and
    chopped (about 2½ cups total)*
3 ribs celery, chopped
2 large carrots, chopped
*1 ¾- to 1-pound celery root, peeled
    and diced*

½ cup chopped shallots
3½ quarts water
1 cup fresh parsley stems and leaves
2 bay leaves
2 tablespoons black peppercorns

*I*n a large pot, combine vegetables and 3½ quarts water. Bring to a simmer,
skimming foam from surface. Add parsley, bay leaves, and peppercorns.
Simmer gently about 3 hours until stock is reduced to about 6 cups; add more
water as necessary to keep ingredients covered. Strain stock through a fine
sieve.

Stock keeps 3 days in the refrigerator or 1 month if frozen.

6 servings
1 serving = 1 cup

CAL.	CHO(g)	PRO.(g)	TOTAL FAT(g)	SAT. FAT(g)	CHOL.(mg)	FIBER(g)	SODIUM(mg)
15	4	0	0	0	0	0	15

Food exchange per serving: a Free Food
Low-sodium diets: This recipe is excellent.

Tomato Florentine Soup

Hearty enough for a light entree, this soup is nice with crusty rolls and a wedge of cheese. I like the flavor and texture of evaporated milk, which makes the soup quite creamy, but you can substitute 2% milk or evaporated skim milk.

1 28-ounce can crushed tomatoes, Italian-style, no salt added
1 medium onion, chopped fine
2 tablespoons tomato paste
2 cups Chicken Stock (see Index) or chicken or vegetable broth
1 bay leaf

½ teaspoon salt
¼ teaspoon freshly ground pepper
¾ cup (½ of 10-ounce box) frozen chopped spinach, thawed and well drained
1 cup evaporated milk

*P*ut tomatoes with liquid, onion, tomato paste, Chicken Stock, bay leaf, salt, and pepper in a large pot. Bring to a boil; simmer, uncovered, for 5 minutes. Add spinach. Simmer 3 more minutes.

Add milk and heat, stirring constantly, only until hot enough to serve. Remove bay leaf.

6 servings (makes 6 cups)
1 serving = 1 cup

CAL.	CHO(g)	PRO.(g)	TOTAL FAT(g)	SAT. FAT(g)	CHOL.(mg)	FIBER(g)	SODIUM(mg)
115	15	6	4	2	15	2.5	340

Food exchanges per serving: 1 Vegetable plus 1 Low-Fat Milk
Low-sodium diets: Omit salt.

Chilled Cucumber Soup

A delicious cold soup for hot weather.

2 (1 pound total) cucumbers,
   slender and firm
2¾ cups low-fat (1½% milk fat)
   buttermilk
1 teaspoon salt

1 teaspoon fresh lemon juice
1 tablespoon finely minced onion
Paprika or snipped dill weed for
   garnish

*R*emove ends of cucumbers. Pare one, then slice into ¼-inch slices. If skins feel waxy, pare both cucumbers. Select four unpared slices for garnish. Cut these again to yield eight very thin slices. Wrap and store in refrigerator.

   Pour 1 cup buttermilk into blender or food processor; add half the cucumber slices. Blend at high speed for 30–40 seconds, until smooth. Add remaining cucumber slices, salt, lemon juice, and onion; blend for about 1 minute. Stir in remaining buttermilk to mix thoroughly. Pour into a 1-quart jar.

   Cover and refrigerate for at least 2 hours. (Do not keep longer than 48 hours before using.) Serve garnished with thin slices of cucumber and a sprinkling of paprika or dill.

4 servings (makes 4 cups)
1 serving = 1 cup

CAL.	CHO(g)	PRO.(g)	TOTAL FAT(g)	SAT. FAT(g)	CHOL.(mg)	FIBER(g)	SODIUM(mg)
96	15	7	2	1	5	1.5	735

Food exchanges per serving: 1 Vegetable plus 1 Skim Milk
Low-sodium diets: Omit salt. Substitute skim milk for buttermilk, and increase lemon juice to 1 tablespoon. Add 2 teaspoons fresh snipped dill or ½ teaspoon dried dill before blending.

Tex-Mex Corn Soup

Our taste-testers loved this soup, and it is quick and easy to prepare.

1 tablespoon margarine
½ cup chopped onion
1 cup chopped red bell pepper
1 teaspoon crushed red pepper
    flakes
4 cups Chicken Stock (see Index) or
    chicken or vegetable broth

1 17-ounce can creamed corn,
    including liquid
1 16-ounce can whole kernel corn,
    including liquid
¼ teaspoon salt
¼ teaspoon freshly ground pepper

Melt margarine in a large saucepan. Add onion, sweet red bell pepper, and red pepper flakes; sauté until tender, stirring occasionally, about 2 minutes.

Stir in Chicken Stock and both cans of corn. Continue cooking until the soup is very hot. Add salt and pepper. Serve immediately.

8 servings
1 serving = 1 cup

CAL.	CHO(g)	PRO.(g)	TOTAL FAT(g)	SAT. FAT(g)	CHOL.(mg)	FIBER(g)	SODIUM(mg)
110	23	4	3	0.5	0	1.5	455

Food exchanges per serving: 1 Starch plus 1 Vegetable
Low-sodium diets: Omit salt; substitute unsalted broth and canned corn.

Gazpacho

A favorite summer soup loaded with protective vitamins A and C; rich in potassium as well.

1 large clove garlic, peeled
1 pound ripe tomatoes
2 large (1½ pounds total) cucumbers
1 cup finely diced green pepper
¾ cup finely diced celery
½ cup finely diced onion
2 cups tomato juice or tomato vegetable juice

1 tablespoon corn oil
1 cup cold water
3 dashes hot-pepper sauce
1 teaspoon salt
½ teaspoon coarsely ground pepper
½ cup seasoned croutons
Chopped fresh parsley for garnish

Crush garlic into the bottom of a 2½-quart bowl. Core tomatoes, and discard cores and seeds; finely dice tomatoes. Pare cucumbers, cut lengthwise, and discard centers and seeds; finely dice remaining cucumber. Measure all ingredients, except croutons and parsley, into the bowl containing garlic. Mix thoroughly.

Cover bowl tightly and chill for 2 hours or longer. Serve soup in chilled bowls; garnish with croutons and parsley.

7 servings (makes 7 cups)
1 serving = 1 cup

CAL.	CHO(g)	PRO.(g)	TOTAL FAT(g)	SAT. FAT(g)	CHOL.(mg)	FIBER(g)	SODIUM(mg)
75	16	2	2	0.5	0	2	620

Food exchanges per serving: 3 Vegetables *or* 1 Starch
Low-sodium diets: Omit salt. Substitute unsalted tomato juice.

Green Goddess Soup

This soup looks beautiful and creamy, tastes delicious, yet contains not a bit of cream! It's great hot or chilled. The National Cancer Institute recommends cruciferous vegetables (including broccoli and cauliflower) to protect against cancer. Add this bonus to plenty of vitamins A, C, and calcium, and you have a soup that protects your whole body.

1 recipe Herbed Broccoli
    Cauliflower Puree (see Index)
2 cups skim milk
¼ teaspoon grated or ground
    nutmeg

1 tablespoon snipped fresh herbs
    (oregano, basil, chives, thyme,
    or marjoram)

In a medium pot, combine Herbed Broccoli Cauliflower Puree, milk, and nutmeg. Stir to blend. Heat over low heat until mixture begins to simmer.
    Serve garnished with snipped herbs.

4 servings (makes 4 cups)
1 serving = 1 cup

CAL.	CHO(g)	PRO.(g)	TOTAL FAT(g)	SAT. FAT(g)	CHOL.(mg)	FIBER(g)	SODIUM(mg)
110	13	8	4	1	0	2.5	425

Food exchanges per serving: 1 Low-Fat Milk *or* 1 Vegetable plus ½ Low-Fat Milk
Low-sodium diets: Omit salt from the puree.

Sweet Potato and Red Pepper Bisque

This recipe is adapted from one supplied to chefs by Club Corporation of America. If you want a fancy presentation, core large, sweet red peppers, and serve the bisque in the peppers.

1 bunch scallions	2 (1 pound total) sweet potatoes,
1 large (8-ounce) red bell pepper	peeled and sliced thin
2 teaspoons olive oil	1 teaspoon salt
1 large shallot, sliced	¼ teaspoon white pepper
4 cups Chicken Stock (see Index),	
Vegetable Stock (see Index), or	
chicken broth	

*T*rim stem ends from scallions and cut into 1-inch lengths. Discard top half of greens. Core and slice red pepper.

In a large nonstick skillet or Dutch oven, heat olive oil. Add scallions, red pepper, and shallot; sauté until tender, about 5 minutes.

Add Chicken Stock and sweet potatoes. Bring to a boil, cover, and simmer 30 minutes until sweet potatoes are tender.

Put mixture in a food processor or blender in batches. Puree until smooth. Season with salt and white pepper. Reheat if necessary.

6 servings (makes 4½ cups)
1 serving = ¾ cup

CAL.	CHO(g)	PRO.(g)	TOTAL FAT(g)	SAT. FAT(g)	CHOL.(mg)	FIBER(g)	SODIUM(mg)
105	19	4	3	0.5	0	3	450

Food exchanges per serving: 1 Starch plus 1 Vegetable
Low-sodium diets: Omit salt.

Tortilla Soup

4 cups (½ recipe) Chicken Stock
    (see Index) or unsalted chicken
    broth
6 cherry tomatoes
1 small zucchini
1 rib celery
1 carrot, peeled
½ small green bell pepper

½ small jalepeño pepper, seeded
1 clove garlic
1 cup diced, cooked, skinless chicken
1½ teaspoons ground cumin
½ teaspoon salt
¼ teaspoon freshly ground black
    pepper
24 baked tortilla chips

Heat Chicken Stock in a medium pot.

Cut tops off tomatoes; squeeze out seeds and liquid. Put tomatoes, zucchini, celery, carrot, green pepper, jalepeño pepper, and garlic into bowl of a food processor; process until vegetables are finely chopped.

Add chopped vegetables to stock; simmer 20 minutes. Add chicken and cumin; simmer 10 more minutes. Season with salt and black pepper.

To serve, put 4 tortilla chips in the bottom of each bowl. Pour soup over chips.

6 servings
1 serving = 1 cup soup plus 4 chips

CAL.	CHO(g)	PRO.(g)	TOTAL FAT(g)	SAT. FAT(g)	CHOL.(mg)	FIBER(g)	SODIUM(mg)
110	11	11	4	1	20	1.5	290

Food exchanges per serving: 1 Lean Meat plus 1 Starch *or* 1 Lean Meat plus 1 Vegetable plus ½ Starch
Low-sodium diets: Omit salt.

French Onion Soup

1 tablespoon olive oil
1 pound sweet yellow onions,
   sliced thin
4 cups beef broth
½ cup dry red wine

1 teaspoon finely chopped garlic
6 thin slices (2 ounces total) French
   bread (baguette)
2 tablespoons grated Parmesan
   cheese

*H*eat oil in a Dutch oven or deep pot. Add onions; sauté over medium heat, stirring often, about 10 minutes or until well browned. Add broth, wine, and garlic. Reduce heat; simmer 20 minutes.

While soup is cooking, preheat oven to 300°F. Set a wire cooling rack on top of a cookie sheet, and place bread on rack. Bake about 15 minutes to dry toasts. Top each toast with 1 teaspoon Parmesan cheese. Return to oven for 5 minutes until cheese melts and browns slightly.

Divide soup among 6 bowls. Top each with a cheese toast. Serve hot.

6 servings
1 serving = 1 cup soup with 1 cheese toast

CAL.	CHO(g)	PRO.(g)	TOTAL FAT(g)	SAT. FAT(g)	CHOL.(mg)	FIBER(g)	SODIUM(mg)
110	12	3	3	0.5	0	1.5	1,185

Food exchanges per serving: 1 Starch plus ½ Fat
Low-sodium diets: Substitute unsalted beef broth.

Onion Soup Gratinée

This hearty and scrumptious soup is best used as an entree. You can add an additional Medium-Fat Meat exchange by putting an extra ounce of sliced cheese atop each crock. It's even better!

1 recipe French Onion Soup (preceding recipe)
10 ounces sliced part-skim mozzarella cheese or sliced Gruyère

¼ cup shredded or grated Parmesan cheese

Preheat oven to 350°F. Pour soup into six 8-ounce ovenproof serving bowls or soup crocks. Top with cheese toasts from French Onion Soup recipe. Arrange mozzarella or Gruyère cheese over tops of bowls to cover entire opening. Sprinkle Parmesan cheese over mozzarella. (The soup can be refrigerated at this point and baked later if you wish.)

Put soup bowls on a jelly roll pan. Bake 15–20 minutes or until soup is very hot and cheese is lightly browned. Allow additional cooking time if soup has been chilled.

6 servings
1 serving = 1 crock soup

CAL.	CHO(g)	PRO.(g)	TOTAL FAT(g)	SAT. FAT(g)	CHOL.(mg)	FIBER(g)	SODIUM(mg)
250	14	16	12	6	30	1.5	1,480

Food exchanges per serving: 2 Medium-Fat Meats plus 1 Starch
Low-sodium diets: Substitute unsalted beef broth and reduced-sodium cheese.

Mushroom Vegetable Soup

A mushroom lover's delight! Served with cheese and fruit, this hearty, healthful, and delicious soup will make a full meal.

1 pound fresh mushrooms	*¼ cup tomato paste*
2 tablespoons margarine, divided	*¼ cup minced fresh parsley* or *1½*
1 cup finely chopped carrots	*tablespoons parsley flakes*
1 cup finely chopped celery	*1 bay leaf*
1 cup finely chopped onion	*½ teaspoon salt*
1 clove garlic, minced	*¼ teaspoon freshly ground pepper*
1 13¾-ounce can beef broth	*2 tablespoons dry sherry*
2 cups water	

*W*ash mushrooms; slice half of them and set aside. Chop remaining mushrooms. Melt 1 tablespoon of the margarine in a large pot. Add chopped mushrooms and sauté until tender. Add carrots, celery, onion, garlic, beef broth, water, tomato paste, parsley, bay leaf, salt, and pepper. Simmer, covered, 1 hour. Puree soup in a blender or a food processor fitted with a steel blade.

Sauté sliced mushrooms in remaining 1 tablespoon margarine. Return pureed soup to pot; add sautéed mushrooms and sherry. Reheat over moderate heat, stirring often, until soup is hot.

6 servings (makes 6 cups)
1 serving = 1 cup

CAL.	CHO*(g)*	PRO.*(g)*	TOTAL FAT*(g)*	SAT. FAT*(g)*	CHOL.*(mg)*	FIBER*(g)*	SODIUM*(mg)*
100	11	4	4	0.5	0	3	670

Food exchanges per serving: 2 Vegetables plus 1 Fat
Low-sodium diets: Omit salt. Substitute unsalted beef broth and unsalted margarine.

Minestrone Soup

½ cup dry navy beans

4 cups Chicken Stock (see Index) or chicken broth

¾ cup peeled, sliced carrots

½ cup sliced potato (with peel)

1 tablespoon corn oil

½ cup sliced onion

1 16-ounce can Italian tomatoes, including liquid

2 cups thinly sliced cabbage

1 cup sliced zucchini

½ cup sliced celery

½ cup drained, canned chickpeas (garbanzo beans)

½ cup uncooked rotini or other pasta

1 tablespoon finely minced fresh parsley

2 teaspoons crumbled dried basil

¼ teaspoon salt

¼ teaspoon freshly ground pepper

Cover navy beans with water in a large pot. Over medium heat, bring just to the boiling point. Remove pan from heat, cover, and let stand for 1 hour.

Drain navy beans and return to pot. Add Chicken Stock, carrots, and potato. Cover and cook over medium heat until vegetables are almost tender, about 35 minutes.

Heat oil in a small skillet. Add onion; sauté until tender.

Add onion and all remaining ingredients to soup pot. Cook 15 minutes more or until pasta is cooked. Serve hot.

6 servings (makes 6 cups)
1 serving = 1 cup

CAL.	CHO(g)	PRO.(g)	TOTAL FAT(g)	SAT. FAT(g)	CHOL.(mg)	FIBER(g)	SODIUM(mg)
185	31	10	5	1	0	5	335

Food exchanges per serving: 2 Starches plus ½ Lean Meat
Low-sodium diets: Omit salt; substitute unsalted canned vegetables and broth.

Split Pea Soup

Of all the recipes in this book, this soup is among the richest in fiber, vitamins, and minerals. Delicious, too!

1 pound dry split peas, washed
1½ quarts water
½ cup chopped onion
2 cups sliced celery
1 cup sliced carrots
½ teaspoon ground white pepper
½ teaspoon salt

1 teaspoon minced garlic
1 16-ounce can stewed tomatoes,
*   including liquid*
1 10¾-ounce can chicken broth or
*   1¾ cups Chicken Stock (see*
*   Index)*
1 tomato, diced fine

Combine the peas, water, onion, celery, and carrots in a large pot; bring mixture to a boil. Reduce heat to simmer; cover and continue cooking 2 hours, stirring occasionally. Add more water if mixture becomes too thick.

Season soup with pepper, salt, and garlic. Continue cooking 15 minutes or until peas are tender. Add canned tomatoes with liquid and chicken broth; allow to cool.

Puree soup in a blender or a food processor fitted with a steel blade. Return pureed soup to pot; reheat over moderate heat, stirring. Serve garnished with diced tomato.

10 servings (makes 10 cups)
1 serving = 1 cup

CAL.	CHO(g)	PRO.(g)	TOTAL FAT(g)	SAT. FAT(g)	CHOL.(mg)	FIBER(g)	SODIUM(mg)
190	34	13	1	0	0	4.5	450

Food exchanges per serving: 2 Starches plus 1 Very Lean Meat
Low-sodium diets: Omit salt. Substitute unsalted canned tomatoes and broth.

Cuban Black Bean Soup

2 strips bacon
½ cup chopped onion
1 cup chopped celery
2½ cups cooked or canned black
    beans, drained
2½ cups water

½ teaspoon ground cumin
½ teaspoon salt
½ teaspoon freshly ground pepper
6 tablespoons chopped onion for
    garnish

Fry bacon over medium heat in a small, heavy frying pan; crumble and set aside. Heat bacon drippings over medium heat. Add onion and celery; sauté until tender, stirring occasionally.

Puree beans in a blender or a food processor fitted with a steel blade; stir into vegetables. Add crumbled bacon, water, cumin, salt, and pepper. Cook over medium heat, stirring occasionally, until soup is hot. Soup will thicken as it stands and can be thinned with additional water, if desired. Serve soup hot, topped with chopped onion.

6 servings (makes 6 cups)
1 serving = 1 cup

CAL.	CHO(g)	PRO.(g)	TOTAL FAT(g)	SAT. FAT(g)	CHOL.(mg)	FIBER(g)	SODIUM(mg)
150	20	7	5	1.5	5	2	255

Food exchanges per serving: 1 Very Lean Meat plus 1 Starch plus 1 Vegetable
Low-sodium diets: Omit salt.

Rio Grande Kidney Bean Soup

1 strip bacon	3 cups beef broth
1 teaspoon minced garlic	3 bay leaves
½ cup chopped onion	½ teaspoon salt
2½ cups canned kidney beans with liquid	⅛ teaspoon freshly ground pepper
	¼ teaspoon crumbled dried basil

*F*ry bacon in a heavy frying pan over medium heat; drain, crumble, and set aside. Reheat bacon drippings over medium heat. Add garlic and onion; sauté until tender, stirring occasionally.

Puree beans in a blender or a food processor fitted with a steel blade. Stir into onion mixture. Blend in crumbled bacon and remaining ingredients. Cook over medium heat, stirring occasionally, until soup is hot. Remove and discard bay leaves.

Soup will thicken as it stands and can be thinned with water or additional beef broth, if desired.

6 servings (makes 6 cups)
1 serving = 1 cup

CAL.	CHO(g)	PRO.(g)	TOTAL FAT(g)	SAT. FAT(g)	CHOL.(mg)	FIBER(g)	SODIUM(mg)
125	18	7	3	1	5	7	990

Food exchanges per serving: 1 Starch plus 1 Lean Meat
Low-sodium diets: This recipe is not suitable.

Greek Egg-Lemon Soup

4 cups Chicken Stock (see Index) or
    chicken broth
2 tablespoons uncooked white rice
2 medium eggs, beaten
2 tablespoons fresh lemon juice

¼ teaspoon mixed herb seasoning
    (dried green herbs, oregano,
    etc.)
Dash coarsely ground pepper
Parsley sprigs for garnish

Heat Chicken Stock to a rolling boil; add rice slowly so as not to stop the boiling. Cover, reduce heat to low, and let simmer gently 15 minutes or until rice is tender but firm.

Combine eggs and lemon juice in a medium bowl. Slowly pour half of soup into egg mixture, stirring quickly. Return egg and soup mixture to remaining soup, and cook over very low heat 3–4 minutes, stirring constantly, until mixture is smooth and coats the spoon. (Boiling or high heat can cause curdling.) Stir in herb seasoning and pepper.

Spoon into bowls, and garnish with parsley. Serve immediately.

4 servings (makes 3 cups)
1 serving = ¾ cup

CAL.	CHO(g)	PRO.(g)	TOTAL FAT(g)	SAT. FAT(g)	CHOL.(mg)	FIBER(g)	SODIUM(mg)
85	8	6	5	1.5	95	0.5	140

Food exchanges per serving: ½ Starch plus ½ Medium-Fat Meat
Low-sodium diets: Use unsalted chicken broth.

Tuscan White Bean Soup

This hearty soup makes a nice entree and is an excellent source of fiber and potassium.

¼ cup chopped onion
½ teaspoon minced garlic
3 tablespoons olive oil, divided
½ pound dry Great Northern
    beans, washed
2 quarts water

2 large bay leaves
1 teaspoon crumbled dried basil
½ teaspoon salt
½ teaspoon ground white pepper
2 tablespoons chopped fresh parsley
2 scallions, chopped

Sauté onion and garlic in 2 tablespoons of the olive oil until soft, stirring often. Add beans, water, bay leaves, and basil. Bring mixture to a boil. Reduce to a simmer, cover, and continue cooking until beans are tender, about 2 hours. Add more liquid if mixture becomes thick and stir occasionally. Season with salt and pepper.

Cool soup. Puree beans in a blender or a food processor fitted with a steel blade.

Return pureed soup to pot; reheat over moderate heat, stirring often. Blend in remaining 1 tablespoon olive oil. If soup is too thick, add water or chicken broth.

Serve soup hot, garnished with chopped parsley and scallions.

4 servings (makes 4 cups)
1 serving = 1 cup

CAL.	CHO(g)	PRO.(g)	TOTAL FAT(g)	SAT. FAT(g)	CHOL.(mg)	FIBER(g)	SODIUM(mg)
295	38	13	11	1.5	0	23	285

Food exchanges per serving: 2½ Starches plus 1 Lean Meat plus 1 Fat
Low-sodium diets: Omit salt.

Old-Fashioned Chicken Noodle Soup

The calculated values are based on a generous portion—just like Grandma would serve.

4 cups (½ recipe) Chicken Stock (see Index)

1 cup (about 4½ ounces) finely cut, cooked skinless chicken (from Chicken Stock)

1 cup cooked thin noodles or spaghetti

2 teaspoons chopped fresh parsley

½ teaspoon salt

⅛ teaspoon ground white pepper

Put all ingredients into a medium-sized pot. Bring to a boil. Reduce heat and simmer 3–5 minutes. Taste and adjust seasoning if necessary.

4 servings (makes 6 cups)
1 serving = 1½ cups

CAL.	CHO(g)	PRO.(g)	TOTAL FAT(g)	SAT. FAT(g)	CHOL.(mg)	FIBER(g)	SODIUM(mg)
140	13	14	5	1.5	40	1	415

Food exchanges per serving: 1 Starch plus 1½ Lean Meats
Low-sodium diets: Omit salt from recipe and from cooking water of spaghetti.

Chinese Chicken Corn Soup

3 cups Chicken Stock (see Index) or
    unsalted chicken broth
1 8¾-ounce can creamed corn
1 cup diced, cooked, skinless chicken
1 tablespoon cornstarch

2 tablespoons cold water
2 egg whites
2 tablespoons finely minced fresh
    parsley for garnish

Combine Chicken Stock, corn, and chicken in a large saucepan. Bring
mixture to a boil over medium heat, stirring occasionally.

In a small bowl or cup, blend cornstarch with cold water; add to soup.
Continue cooking, uncovered, 3 minutes.

Beat egg whites until foamy; stir into soup. Reduce heat and simmer 3
minutes.

Ladle soup into individual bowls, and garnish with parsley. Serve hot.

4 servings (makes 4 cups)
1 serving = 1 cup

CAL.	CHO(g)	PRO.(g)	TOTAL FAT(g)	SAT. FAT(g)	CHOL.(mg)	FIBER(g)	SODIUM(mg)
145	15	14	4	1	30	1	315

Food exchanges per serving: 1 Starch plus 1½ Lean Meats
Low-sodium diets: Substitute unsalted canned creamed corn.

Shortcut Beef and Bean Soup

It takes only a half hour to make this soup. The canned stock and beans save time; the prepared salsa saves time and labor. You can reduce the fat in this recipe by using extra-lean ground beef and rinsing the cooked meat. If you do this, you can count the recipe as 1 Starch plus 2 Lean Meat Exchanges.

1 pound lean ground beef
1 onion, chopped fine
1 13¾-ounce can beef broth
1 15-ounce can black beans,
   including liquid

1 cup mild chunky salsa
2 tablespoons finely chopped
   scallions for garnish

*I*n a large pot or dutch oven, brown beef and onion over medium heat. Pour off drippings. Add broth and black beans; simmer 10 minutes. Add salsa and 1½ cups water; cook another 5 minutes.

Garnish each bowl of soup with a sprinkling of chopped scallions.

8 servings (makes 8 cups)
1 serving = 1 cup

CAL.	CHO(g)	PRO.(g)	TOTAL FAT(g)	SAT. FAT(g)	CHOL.(mg)	FIBER(g)	SODIUM(mg)
185	13	14	8	3	35	2	800

Food exchanges per serving: 1 Starch plus 2 Medium-Fat Meats
Low-sodium diets: Substitute unsalted beef broth and Chunky Salsa (see Index) prepared without salt.

Fish Chowder

This hearty entree soup is an excellent source of many vitamins and minerals, and leftovers are even better the next day.

1 pound fresh or frozen fish fillets	⅓ cup catsup
4 thin slices bacon	2 teaspoons Worcestershire sauce
¾ cup chopped onions	1 teaspoon salt
1 16-ounce can tomatoes with liquid	¼ teaspoon coarsely ground pepper
2 cups water	⅛ teaspoon dried thyme
1 cup diced potato	⅛ teaspoon dried marjoram
½ cup diced carrots	1 tablespoon minced fresh parsley
½ cup finely chopped celery with leaves	

Thaw fish fillets if frozen. Remove bones and skin from fish; cut into 1-inch pieces. Cut bacon into ½-inch pieces.

In a large saucepan over medium heat, fry bacon until crisp, turning frequently. Add onion; cook, stirring, over medium heat until tender and translucent.

Cut tomatoes into bite-sized pieces. Add tomatoes, tomato liquid, water, potato, carrots, celery, catsup, Worcestershire sauce, salt, pepper, thyme, and marjoram to the onions; bring to a boil. Reduce heat to low; cover and simmer about 45 minutes. Add fish; cover and simmer another 10–12 minutes, until fish flakes and is tender.

Serve garnished with a sprinkling of parsley.

6 servings (makes 6 cups)
1 serving = 1 cup

CAL.	CHO(g)	PRO.(g)	TOTAL FAT(g)	SAT. FAT(g)	CHOL.(mg)	FIBER(g)	SODIUM(mg)
210	15	17	9	3.5	40	2	825

Food exchanges per serving: 2 Medium-Fat Meats plus 1 Starch
Low-sodium diets: Omit salt. Use unsalted canned tomatoes and reduced-sodium catsup.

14

Salads and Dressings

Asparagus Salad with Pecans

If you make this salad with Buttermilk Ranch Dressing, you can count it as only 1 Vegetable Exchange and save 5 grams of fat.

24 medium-sized fresh asparagus
    spears
6 crisp leaves red leaf lettuce
6 tablespoons light ranch dressing
    or Buttermilk Ranch Dressing
    (see Index)

2 tablespoons chopped pecans,
    lightly toasted

Bring a large pot of water to boil. Wash asparagus; snap off tough bottoms of stems. Add asparagus and let water return to a boil. Cook about 3 minutes, until asparagus is crisp but tender. Remove asparagus, run under cold water or immerse in ice water, then refrigerate until chilled.

At serving time, line six salad plates with lettuce, and arrange 4 asparagus spears on each. Top each salad with 1 tablespoon dressing, and sprinkle with 1 teaspoon toasted pecans.

6 servings
1 serving = 4 spears plus 1 tablespoon dressing plus 1 teaspoon pecans

CAL.	CHO(g)	PRO.(g)	TOTAL FAT(g)	SAT. FAT(g)	CHOL.(mg)	FIBER(g)	SODIUM(mg)
85	4	2	7	1	5	1	155

Food exchanges per serving: 1 Vegetable plus 1 Fat
Low-sodium diet: This recipe is acceptable.

Jicama and Pepper Salad with Orange Dressing

This sweet and crunchy salad is perfect with spring foods, especially Mexican flavors.

½ medium (8 ounces) jicama, peeled
½ small or ¼ large red bell pepper
½ small or ¼ large green bell pepper
½ small or ¼ large yellow bell pepper

Orange Dressing

2–3 scallions, cut in 2-inch sections
½ small jalapeño pepper
1 medium orange, peeled and cut in sections
1 tablespoon olive oil
½ teaspoon salt
Sugar substitute equivalent to 2 teaspoons sugar

Cut jicama into julienne strips. Cut peppers into thin strips, cutting long strips in half. Combine jicama and peppers in a bowl.

Put scallions, jalapeño, orange sections, olive oil, and salt in a blender or food processor. Process 1–2 minutes to make dressing. Add sugar substitute to taste.

Pour dressing over vegetables; toss well to mix. Serve on individual salad plates.

6 servings
1 serving = ½ cup

CAL.	CHO(g)	PRO.(g)	TOTAL FAT(g)	SAT. FAT(g)	CHOL.(mg)	FIBER(g)	SODIUM(mg)
50	7	1	2	0.5	0	1.5	185

Food exchanges per serving: 1 Vegetable plus ½ Fat
Low-sodium diets: Omit salt in dressing.

Spinach Salad

The sweet dressing on this salad provides contrast to the greens. If you want to serve this salad as an entree, top it with Sesame Pork Coins or Pan-Grilled Scallops (see Index).

12 ounces fresh spinach, well washed	2 hard-boiled eggs
1 cup fresh or canned and drained bean sprouts	1 cup fat-free French dressing
1 8½-ounce can water chestnuts, drained and sliced	Sugar substitute equivalent to 1 tablespoon sugar or 1 tablespoon sugar

*R*emove and discard stems of spinach; tear leaves into bite-sized pieces. Pat spinach dry with paper towels and put in a large salad bowl. Spread a layer of bean sprouts, then a layer of water chestnuts, over spinach. Slice eggs and distribute over salad.

Cover salad with a damp paper towel; refrigerate until chilled. Meanwhile, mix together sweetener and French dressing.

Toss salad with dressing immediately before serving.

8 servings
1 serving = 1 cup

CAL.	CHO(g)	PRO.(g)	TOTAL FAT(g)	SAT. FAT(g)	CHOL.(mg)	FIBER(g)	SODIUM(mg)
85	14	3	1	0.5	55	2.5	280

Food exchange per serving: 1 Starch *or* 1 Other Carbohydrate
Low-sodium diets: Substitute a reduced-sodium salad dressing.

Mushroom Delight

This recipe is a favorite from earlier editions of this book.

1½ tablespoons canola or corn oil

1 tablespoon fresh lemon juice

1 tablespoon wine vinegar

1–2 tablespoons finely chopped dill pickle

½ teaspoon dry mustard

¼ teaspoon salt

⅛ teaspoon coarsely ground pepper

1 clove garlic, crushed

12 ounces (about 4½ cups) fresh mushrooms, washed and sliced thin

6 lettuce leaves

2 tablespoons snipped fresh parsley

Place all ingredients except mushrooms, lettuce, and parsley in a small jar. Cover the jar; shake well.

Place mushrooms in a mixing bowl. Drizzle dressing over mushrooms, and toss gently so that dressing thoroughly coats them. Serve on lettuce leaves, and garnish with parsley.

4 servings (makes 3 cups)
1 serving = ¾ cup

CAL.	CHO(g)	PRO.(g)	TOTAL FAT(g)	SAT. FAT(g)	CHOL.(mg)	FIBER(g)	SODIUM(mg)
70	5	2	5	0.5	0	1	185

Food exchanges per serving: 1 Vegetable plus 1 Fat
Low-sodium diets: Omit salt.

Indian Carrot Salad

This recipe is a vitamin A bonanza!

1 tablespoon corn oil	*½ teaspoon minced garlic*
1 tablespoon lime juice	*4 cups sliced cooked carrots*
½ teaspoon ground cumin	*¼ cup wheat sprouts or cooked*
½ teaspoon ground cinnamon	*wheat berries for garnish*
¼ teaspoon salt	

*W*hisk oil and lime juice together in a large bowl. Whisk in cumin, cinnamon, salt, and garlic. Stir in carrot.

Cover and refrigerate until cold. Serve chilled, garnished with wheat sprouts.

8 servings (makes 4 cups)
1 serving = ½ cup

CAL.	CHO(g)	PRO.(g)	TOTAL FAT(g)	SAT. FAT(g)	CHOL.(mg)	FIBER(g)	SODIUM(mg)
60	10	1	2	0	0	2	120

Food exchange per serving: 2 Vegetables
Low-sodium diets: This recipe is suitable.

Carrot and Raisin Salad

Carrots, along with pumpkins and sweet potatoes, are an excellent source of protective vitamins.

½ cup fat-free mayonnaise	3 cups shredded carrots
¼ teaspoon salt	⅓ cup (1½-ounce box) seedless
Sugar substitute equivalent to 2	raisins
tablespoons sugar	Lettuce leaves

*I*n a large bowl, mix mayonnaise, salt, and sugar substitute. Add carrots and raisins; toss. Cover and chill at least 2 hours.

Serve on crisp lettuce leaves.

6 servings (makes 3 cups)
1 serving = ½ cup, lightly packed

CAL.	CHO(g)	PRO.(g)	TOTAL FAT(g)	SAT. FAT(g)	CHOL.(mg)	FIBER(g)	SODIUM(mg)
60	15	1	0	0	0	2	250

Food exchanges per serving: 3 Vegetables *or* 1 Fruit
Low-sodium diets: Omit salt.

Middle Eastern Salad

Try this salad served in Whole-Wheat Pita Bread (see Index).

1 medium green bell pepper,
   chopped
2 medium tomatoes, chopped
1 medium cucumber, peeled and
   chopped
3 scallions, with tops, chopped

1 cup plain low-fat yogurt
1 tablespoon fresh dill or 1½
   teaspoons dried dill
½ teaspoon salt
½ teaspoon freshly ground pepper

*T*oss green pepper, tomatoes, cucumber, and scallions in a medium-sized bowl. In a small bowl, combine yogurt, dill, salt, and pepper.

   Spoon yogurt mixture over salad and toss.

6 servings (makes 4½ cups)
1 serving = ¾ cup

CAL.	CHO*(g)*	PRO.*(g)*	TOTAL FAT*(g)*	SAT. FAT*(g)*	CHOL.*(mg)*	FIBER*(g)*	SODIUM*(mg)*
45	7	3	1	0.5	0	1	215

Food exchange per serving: 1 Vegetable
Low-sodium diets: Omit salt.

Pineapple Coleslaw

1 cup fresh ripe pineapple chunks
    or canned juice-packed crushed
    pineapple
4 cups (7 ounces) finely chopped
    shredded cabbage
8 ounces low-fat pineapple yogurt

1 carrot, peeled and grated
¼ cup finely chopped scallions
1 teaspoon caraway seeds
½ teaspoon dry mustard
½ teaspoon salt

If using fresh pineapple, put in a food processor and process until finely chopped but not pureed. Place pineapple, including any liquid, in a large bowl with cabbage, and toss. Add all other ingredients; mix well.

6 servings (makes 3 cups)
1 serving = ½ cup

CAL.	CHO(g)	PRO.(g)	TOTAL FAT(g)	SAT. FAT(g)	CHOL.(mg)	FIBER(g)	SODIUM(mg)
70	14	2	1	0	0	1.5	215

Food exchanges per serving: 1 Fruit *or* 1 Vegetable plus ½ Fruit
Low-sodium diets: Omit salt.

Slaw Rouge

¾ cup cider vinegar
¼ cup cold water
½ teaspoon salt
½ teaspoon crushed dried tarragon
    or *2 teaspoons snipped fresh
    tarragon*

*Sugar substitute equivalent to 4
    teaspoons sugar*
2 cups shredded red cabbage
1 cup finely chopped celery
½ cup chopped onion

Combine vinegar, water, salt, and tarragon in a small saucepan. Heat almost to a boil. Remove from heat, add sweetener, and stir to dissolve.

Mix vegetables in a large bowl; pour vinegar mixture on top. Toss gently several times to mix well. Cover bowl and chill for a few hours for flavors to blend.

Just before serving, toss gently again.

8 servings (makes about 4 cups)
1 serving = ½ cup

CAL.	CHO(g)	PRO.(g)	TOTAL FAT(g)	SAT. FAT(g)	CHOL.(mg)	FIBER(g)	SODIUM(mg)
15	4	1	0	0	0	1	150

Food exchange per serving: a Free Food
Low-sodium diets: Omit salt.

Waldorf Salad

Tart apples include Rome, Jonathan, and Granny Smith varieties. If fat is a major concern, substitute fat-free mayonnaise and count a serving as 1 Fruit plus 1 Fat Exchange.

3 medium (1 pound) tart apples
⅔ cup thinly sliced celery
½ cup walnuts, halves and pieces
⅓ cup light or reduced-fat mayonnaise

⅓ cup unsweetened applesauce
2 teaspoons lemon juice
¼ teaspoon salt
¼ teaspoon freshly ground pepper
Crisp lettuce leaves

Wash and core apples. Cut them into bite-sized slices with peel on. Put apples in a large bowl; add celery and walnuts.

To make the dressing, mix remaining ingredients in a small bowl. Gently toss apple mixture with dressing. Serve on lettuce leaves.

6 servings (makes 4½ cups)
1 serving = ¾ cup

CAL.	CHO(g)	PRO.(g)	TOTAL FAT(g)	SAT. FAT(g)	CHOL.(mg)	FIBER(g)	SODIUM(mg)
150	15	2	10	1.5	5	2.5	175

Food exchanges per serving: 1 Fruit plus 2 Fats
Low-sodium diets: Omit salt.

Jackstraw Salad

1 medium (about 4 ounces) red
    apple
½ cup thin strips green bell pepper
½ cup thin celery sticks, ⅛ inch
    wide × 1 inch long

¾ cup shredded cabbage
¼ cup thinly sliced onion rings
⅓ cup Poppy Seed Dressing
    (see Index)
Crisp lettuce leaves

Remove core and stem of apple; leave skin on. Cut apple into thin sticks about ⅛ inch wide. Combine all ingredients except lettuce in a large bowl, and toss lightly to coat with dressing.

Serve on crisp lettuce.

4 servings (makes 3 cups)
1 serving = ¾ cup

CAL.	CHO(g)	PRO.(g)	TOTAL FAT(g)	SAT. FAT(g)	CHOL.(mg)	FIBER(g)	SODIUM(mg)
35	8	1	0.5	0	0	1.5	105

Food exchanges per serving: 1 Vegetable
Low-sodium diets: Omit salt in dressing recipe.

Tomato Aspic Salad

½ cup cold water
1 tablespoon granulated gelatin
1½ cups tomato juice or vegetable
    juice cocktail
1½ teaspoons fresh lemon juice or
    white vinegar

2 drops hot-pepper sauce
½ teaspoon minced onion
Crisp lettuce
1 green bell pepper, cut in rings

Pour cold water into a small saucepan; sprinkle gelatin on top. Stir over low heat 3–4 minutes or until gelatin is completely dissolved. Remove from heat. Add tomato juice, lemon juice, hot-pepper sauce, and onion. Mix well.

Chill until aspic is the consistency of unbeaten egg whites. Turn carefully into four ½-cup molds. Chill until firm.

Unmold on crisp lettuce and garnish with green pepper rings.

4 servings
1 serving = ½ cup

CAL.	CHO(g)	PRO.(g)	TOTAL FAT(g)	SAT. FAT(g)	CHOL.(mg)	FIBER(g)	SODIUM(mg)
25	5	2	0	0	0	1	335

Food exchanges per serving: 1 Vegetable
Low-sodium diets: Substitute unsalted tomato juice.

Fennel and Red Grapefruit Salad

This crunchy salad is particularly nice served on red leaf or Boston lettuce.

1 large red grapefruit, cut in half　　*1 large fennel bulb, sliced thin*
2 tablespoons fat-free Italian　　　　*1 tablespoon snipped fennel greens*
　　dressing
Sugar substitute equal to
　　2 teaspoons sugar or
　　2 teaspoons sugar

Cut segments from unpeeled grapefruit halves and place in a medium-sized bowl.

Squeeze any remaining juice into a small bowl. Add dressing and sugar substitute to the juice; mix well. Toss fennel and greens with grapefruit segments. Pour dressing over grapefruit and fennel; mix well.

4 servings
1 serving = ⅔ cup

CAL.	CHO*(g)*	PRO.*(g)*	TOTAL FAT*(g)*	SAT. FAT*(g)*	CHOL.*(mg)*	FIBER*(g)*	SODIUM*(mg)*
35	8	1	0	0	0	1	115

Food exchange per serving: ½ Fruit
Low-sodium diets: This recipe is acceptable.

Romaine, Red Onion, and Fennel Salad with Tart Lime Dressing

Tart Lime Dressing	Salad
¼ cup fresh lime juice	6 ounces romaine lettuce
1 tablespoon olive oil	1½ cups (about 1 large bulb)
1 clove garlic, minced	fennel, shredded
¼ teaspoon salt	1 cup cauliflower, cut into bite-
¼ teaspoon freshly ground pepper	sized pieces
¼ teaspoon paprika	½ cup sliced red onion

Combine all dressing ingredients; mix well.

Wash, dry, and tear lettuce into bite-sized pieces. Place lettuce, fennel, cauliflower, and onion in a salad bowl; toss. Pour dressing over salad and toss just before serving.

4 servings
1 serving = 1 cup salad plus 1 tablespoon dressing

CAL.	CHO(g)	PRO.(g)	TOTAL FAT(g)	SAT. FAT(g)	CHOL.(mg)	FIBER(g)	SODIUM(mg)
65	7	2	4	0.5	0	2	185

Food exchanges per serving: 1 Vegetable plus 1 Fat
Low-sodium diets: Omit salt from dressing.

Thai Cucumber Salad

You can substitute ⅓ cup rice wine vinegar plus 2 teaspoons sugar and ¼ teaspoon salt for the sweet cooking rice wine.

2 medium (about 1¼ pounds total) cucumbers	⅓ cup sweet cooking rice wine, sometimes called Mirin
4 scallions, chopped	¼ teaspoon crushed red pepper flakes
1 large shallot, minced	¼ teaspoon salt
2 tablespoons chopped cilantro	

*P*eel cucumbers, and halve them lengthwise; remove seeds, and slice cucumbers thinly. In a large bowl, combine all ingredients; toss to mix. Put salad in a refrigerator container and chill at least 1 hour.

Shake to distribute rice wine through cucumbers. Drain liquid before serving.

4 servings (makes 1¾ cups)
1 serving = scant ½ cup

CAL.	CHO(g)	PRO.(g)	TOTAL FAT(g)	SAT. FAT(g)	CHOL.(mg)	FIBER(g)	SODIUM(mg)
30	6	1	0	0	0	1	175

Food exchange per serving: 1 Vegetable
Low-sodium diets: Omit salt.

Creamy Cucumber Salad

To make a Cucumber Sauce (see Index), whip this creamy salad in a blender or food processor. To make Cucumber Riata as a topping for Tandoori Chicken Breasts (see Index), finely chop the cucumber instead of slicing it. Three recipes in one!

1 large cucumber, peeled
1 cup plain low-fat yogurt
2 teaspoons white or cider vinegar
1 tablespoon snipped fresh dill or 1
    teaspoon dried dill weed

½ teaspoon salt
¼ teaspoon freshly ground pepper

Slice cucumber lengthwise and remove seeds. Thinly slice cucumber and place in a salad bowl. Add remaining ingredients. Mix thoroughly and chill at least ½ hour before serving.

5 servings (makes 2½ cups)
1 serving = ½ cup

CAL.	CHO(g)	PRO.(g)	TOTAL FAT(g)	SAT. FAT(g)	CHOL.(mg)	FIBER(g)	SODIUM(mg)
35	5	3	1	0.5	0	0.5	255

Food exchanges per serving: 1 Vegetable
Low-sodium diets: Omit salt.

Italian White Bean Salad

1 cup fresh or frozen chopped broccoli	*¼ cup low-calorie Italian dressing*
1 16-ounce can Great Northern or cannellini beans	*2 tablespoons minced fresh parsley*
	1 clove garlic, minced fine
	1 teaspoon freshly ground pepper

*B*lanch and chop fresh broccoli, or thaw frozen broccoli. Drain and rinse beans. Combine all other ingredients; mix well. Refrigerate at least 2 hours before serving to blend flavors.

5 servings (makes about 2½ cups)
1 serving = about ½ cup

CAL.	CHO(g)	PRO.(g)	TOTAL FAT(g)	SAT. FAT(g)	CHOL.(mg)	FIBER(g)	SODIUM(mg)
60	11	4	0.5	0	0	3	320

Food exchange per serving: 1 Starch
Low-sodium diets: Substitute Kay's Dressing (see Index) prepared without salt or reduced-sodium, fat-free Italian dressing for the low-calorie dressing.

Green Bean and Romano Salad

1 pound fresh green beans
2 large shallots, minced
1 tablespoon balsamic vinegar
¼ teaspoon freshly ground pepper

2 tablespoons olive oil
⅓ cup chopped fresh basil leaves
⅓ cup grated Romano cheese,
    divided

Snap stem ends from beans and discard any blemished beans.

Cook beans in a large pot of boiling salted water just until crisp tender, about 3–4 minutes. Plunge beans into a bowl of ice water to stop cooking and keep the bright green color. Drain beans and set aside.

Combine shallots, vinegar, and pepper in a small bowl. Gradually mix in oil. Stir in basil and half of the grated cheese. Place beans in a salad bowl and toss with dressing. Refrigerate at least 2 hours.

At serving time, top salad with remaining cheese.

8 servings (makes 5⅓ cups)
1 serving = ⅔ cup

CAL.	CHO(g)	PRO.(g)	TOTAL FAT(g)	SAT. FAT(g)	CHOL.(mg)	FIBER(g)	SODIUM(mg)
60	5	2	4	0.5	5	1	45

Food exchanges per serving: 1 Vegetable plus 1 Fat
Low-sodium diets: This recipe is excellent.

Latin Banana Lentil Salad

Different colored lentils taste the same, and all are very nutrient-rich, but the brightly colored ones make prettier salads. This salad is a great addition to a buffet. If you want to make less, the recipe can easily be divided in half.

1 cup red lentils

1 tablespoon canola or corn oil

1½ cups diced onions

1 cup diced red bell pepper

1½ teaspoons minced garlic

2 medium-sized ripe bananas, peeled and sliced into thin rounds

2 tablespoons chopped cilantro

2 tablespoons chopped fresh parsley

2 tablespoons sherry vinegar

¾ teaspoon salt

¼ teaspoon freshly ground black pepper

Cover lentils with water; soak for at least 8 hours. Drain and rinse well.

Put lentils in a large pot, cover with fresh water, and bring to a boil. Cook 8 minutes; drain and cool.

Heat oil in a nonstick skillet. Add onions and red pepper; sauté until tender. Add garlic; remove from heat.

Toss lentils with bananas, onion mixture, and all remaining ingredients. Stir well to mix. Chill salad for 1 hour for flavors to blend.

12 servings (makes 6 cups)
1 serving = ½ cup

CAL.	CHO(g)	PRO.(g)	TOTAL FAT(g)	SAT. FAT(g)	CHOL.(mg)	FIBER(g)	SODIUM(mg)
90	16	5	1	0	0	2.5	140

Food exchange per serving: 1 Starch
Low-sodium diets: Omit salt.

Black Bean and Corn Salad

This salad provides great color, texture, and nutrient value—and it doesn't need a dressing. It travels well and adds to any picnic, outdoor meal, pot-luck or buffet.

1 15-ounce can black beans
2 cups frozen corn kernels, thawed, or 2 cups fresh corn cut from cob, blanched, and chilled

¼ cup chopped red bell pepper
¼ cup chopped cilantro

*R*inse and drain beans in a colander or strainer. Put in a salad bowl. Add all other ingredients and mix well.

8 servings (makes 4 cups)
1 serving = ½ cup

CAL.	CHO(g)	PRO.(g)	TOTAL FAT(g)	SAT. FAT(g)	CHOL.(mg)	FIBER(g)	SODIUM(mg)
65	14	3	1	0	0	2.5	85

Food exchange per serving: 1 Starch
Low-sodium diets: This recipe is suitable.

Tomato, Basil, and Mozzarella Salad

Make this salad only in the summer or when you can get very large, red, ripe tomatoes. It's one of our favorite warm-weather salads and a great appetizer or part of an antipasto platter.

2–3 (1 pound) large, red, very ripe tomatoes
2 ounces shredded mozzarella cheese
8 leaves fresh basil
2 teaspoons olive oil
Dash cracked pepper

Slice tomatoes crosswise into ½-inch-thick slices, 4 slices per tomato. Arrange 2–3 slices on each salad plate. Sprinkle mozzarella on top of each tomato.

Cut fresh basil leaves into strips, and top each tomato with basil. Drizzle olive oil over the tops, and add a dash of pepper. Enjoy!

4 servings
1 serving = 2–3 slices tomato with topping

CAL.	CHO(g)	PRO.(g)	TOTAL FAT(g)	SAT. FAT(g)	CHOL.(mg)	FIBER(g)	SODIUM(mg)
85	6	4	6	2	10	1.5	65

Food exchanges per serving: 1 Vegetable plus 1 Fat
Low-sodium diets: This recipe is suitable.

Greek Salad

Yes, there is quite a bit of fat in the recipe, but most of it is a heart-healthy olive oil. You just can't make great-tasting Greek Salad without some olives, olive oil, and feta cheese. Serve the salad with crusty bread and maybe simply grilled or broiled fish.

Salad

*½ head iceberg lettuce, washed and
     torn*
½ cucumber, peeled and sliced
1 cup cherry tomatoes, halved
½ cup thinly sliced onions
*½ cup thinly sliced green bell
     pepper rings*
2 ounces feta cheese, crumbled
1 teaspoon dried oregano

Dressing

3 tablespoons olive oil
2 tablespoons water
1 tablespoon white wine vinegar
2 teaspoons dried oregano
2 teaspoons chopped fresh parsley
1 teaspoon lemon juice
½ teaspoon salt
*¼ teaspoon freshly ground black
     pepper*

Topping

6 anchovies, drained
12 Calamata (Greek) olives

Layer salad ingredients in a salad bowl.

Put dressing ingredients in a small jar; cover and shake well to mix. Pour over salad and toss.

Top salad with anchovies and olives.

6 servings (makes 7½ cups)
1 serving = 1¼ cup

CAL.	CHO(g)	PRO.(g)	TOTAL FAT(g)	SAT. FAT(g)	CHOL.(mg)	FIBER(g)	SODIUM(mg)
160	7	4	13	3.5	15	1	675

Food exchanges per serving: 2 Vegetables plus 2 Fats
Low-sodium diets: Omit salt from dressing. Serve ½ anchovy and 1 olive on each salad.

Roasted Pepper and Goat Cheese Salad

Red peppers, whether roasted or not, are a terrific source of many protective vitamins.

1 tablespoon virgin olive oil
1 clove garlic, crushed
1 small head leaf lettuce
1 recipe Roasted Red Peppers
  (see Index)

6 ounces goat cheese or fresh
  mozzarella cheese, sliced thin
1 tablespoon snipped fresh basil

In a small bowl, mix oil and garlic.

Wash and drain lettuce leaves, and arrange on a platter or individual salad plates. Arrange pepper slices on lettuce. Top peppers with thin slices of cheese.

Brush tops of peppers and cheese with garlic oil. Garnish salads with snipped basil.

6 servings
1 serving = 1 salad with lettuce, ½ pepper, 1 ounce cheese

CAL.	CHO(g)	PRO.(g)	TOTAL FAT(g)	SAT. FAT(g)	CHOL.(mg)	FIBER(g)	SODIUM(mg)
130	2	6	10	6	20	0.5	150

Food exchanges per serving: 1 Vegetable plus ½ Medium-Fat Meat plus 1 Fat
Low-sodium diets: This recipe is suitable.

Spicy Orange Noodle Salad

8 ounces fine egg noodles
⅔ cup sliced scallions, cut on
    diagonal
½ cup chopped cilantro
1 large orange
3 tablespoons cider vinegar
¼ cup peanut oil
1 tablespoon reduced-sodium soy
    sauce

2 teaspoons Oriental dark-roasted
    sesame oil
1 teaspoon salt
½ teaspoon crushed red pepper
    flakes
⅓ cup dry roasted peanuts, chopped
    coarse

Cook noodles in 2 quarts boiling water for 3–5 minutes. Drain in strainer and rinse in cool water. Mix with scallions and cilantro.

Grate zest from orange (about 2 tablespoons) and set aside. Squeeze juice from orange into a small bowl. Add vinegar, peanut oil, soy sauce, sesame oil, salt, and pepper flakes. Toss pasta with dressing, ⅔ of the orange zest, and ⅔ of the chopped peanuts. Before serving, top noodles with remaining zest and peanuts.

9 servings (makes 4½ cups)
1 serving = ½ cup

CAL.	CHO(g)	PRO.(g)	TOTAL FAT(g)	SAT. FAT(g)	CHOL.(mg)	FIBER(g)	SODIUM(mg)
200	21	5	11	1.5	25	1.5	315

Food exchanges per serving: 1½ Starches plus 2 Fats
Low-sodium diets: Omit salt.

Panzanella

This Italian bread salad is a good use for leftover bread and a nice change from potato or pasta salad. It's sort of a sandwich and salad in one dish.

Salad

1 1-pound loaf firm Italian bread
2 small red onions, thinly sliced
1 cucumber, peeled and sliced
4 ripe tomatoes, cut into wedges
1 small head romaine lettuce, torn
  into bite-sized pieces
10 fresh basil leaves or ¾ teaspoon
  dried basil

Dressing

¼ cup olive oil
2 tablespoons red wine vinegar
1 teaspoon salt
½ teaspoon freshly ground pepper

Cut off bread crust; cut or tear bread into cubes. Let bread stand uncovered until it dries out, about 3 hours.

Sprinkle bread with about 1 cup cold water. Bread should be wet but not soggy. Refrigerate several hours.

Combine dressing ingredients in a small bowl or jar. Place bread cubes in a large salad bowl; add remaining salad ingredients, and mix. Drizzle with dressing and toss.

9 servings (makes 9 cups)
1 serving = 1 cup

CAL.	CHO*(g)*	PRO.*(g)*	TOTAL FAT*(g)*	SAT. FAT*(g)*	CHOL.*(mg)*	FIBER*(g)*	SODIUM*(mg)*
225	33	6	8	1	0	3.5	550

Food exchanges per serving: 2 Starches plus 1 Fat
Low-sodium diets: Omit salt.

Picnic Macaroni Salad

3 cups hot macaroni, cooked al
 dente and drained
⅓ cup light or reduced-fat
 mayonnaise
⅓ cup thinly sliced celery
2 tablespoons minced fresh parsley
2 tablespoons chopped scallions
 with tops

2 tablespoons chopped red bell
 pepper
2 hard-boiled eggs, sliced
½ teaspoon salt
¼ teaspoon coarsely ground pepper

Mix all ingredients together in a large bowl. Cover and refrigerate several hours for flavors to blend.

8 servings (makes about 4 cups)
1 serving = ½ cup

CAL.	CHO(g)	PRO.(g)	TOTAL FAT(g)	SAT. FAT(g)	CHOL.(mg)	FIBER(g)	SODIUM(mg)
122	16	4	4	1	55	1	210

Food exchanges per serving: 1 Starch plus ½ Fat
Low-sodium diets: Omit salt.

Red Potato Salad

2½ cups quartered red new
    potatoes, cooked
½ cup finely chopped onion
¼ cup chopped fresh parsley
½ cup finely chopped celery
½ cup plain low-fat yogurt

1 tablespoon prepared mustard
¾ teaspoon mixed herb, pizza, or
    Italian seasoning
1 hard-boiled egg, sliced
Paprika for garnish

Combine potatoes, onion, parsley, and celery in a large bowl; mix. In a small bowl, stir together yogurt, mustard, and seasoning; add to vegetables and mix carefully. Cover and chill several hours to allow flavors to blend.

To serve, garnish with egg slices and paprika.

6 servings (makes almost 4 cups)
1 serving = ⅔ cup

CAL.	CHO(g)	PRO.(g)	TOTAL FAT(g)	SAT. FAT(g)	CHOL.(mg)	FIBER(g)	SODIUM(mg)
85	15	4	1	0.5	35	1.5	75

Food exchanges per serving: 1 Starch
Low-sodium diets: This recipe is acceptable.

Norwegian Chef Salad

Sardines are a good source of omega-3 fatty acids, a heart-healthy form of fat found in some seafood. The portion is generous because you will use this as an entree salad.

1 head romaine lettuce
1 small red onion, sliced thin
6 radishes, sliced
1 small cucumber, peeled and sliced
    thin
1 cup halved cherry tomatoes
3 ounces light Jarlsberg cheese, cut
    in strips

1 3¾-ounce can sardines packed in
    water, drained
¼ cup fat-free red French dressing
    or Lemon Shaker Dressing
    (see Index)

Wash lettuce and tear into bite-sized pieces. In a salad bowl, toss together greens, onion, radishes, and cucumber.

Arrange tomatoes, cheese strips, and sardines on top of salad. Drizzle dressing over salad.

4 servings (makes about 6 cups)
1 serving = 1½ cups

CAL.	CHO(g)	PRO.(g)	TOTAL FAT(g)	SAT. FAT(g)	CHOL.(mg)	FIBER(g)	SODIUM(mg)
200	13	13	9	3.5	40	3.5	235

Food exchanges per serving: 2 Medium-Fat Meats plus 2 Vegetables
Low-sodium diets: This recipe is suitable.

Smoked Turkey Salad with Chutney Dressing

This salad is a grand way to use leftover cooked chicken or turkey. It is best when refrigerated at least an hour to allow the flavors to blend. Use Mango Chutney, Apple Pear Chutney (see Index), or a prepared chutney. For a lower-fat version, substitute fat-free mayonnaise and reduce the nuts to 2 tablespoons.

½ cup Mango Chutney (see Index)
⅓ cup light or reduced-fat
*   mayonnaise*
2 teaspoons lemon juice
½ teaspoon freshly ground pepper

¾ pound cooked smoked turkey, cut
*   into cubes*
1 cup halved seedless red grapes
½ cup walnut pieces
½ cup thinly sliced celery

*I*n a large bowl, mix chutney, mayonnaise, lemon juice, and pepper. Add remaining ingredients; toss to coat turkey with dressing. If time permits, refrigerate for 1 hour for flavors to blend.

4 servings (makes 4 cups)
1 serving = 1 cup

CAL.	CHO(g)	PRO.(g)	TOTAL FAT(g)	SAT. FAT(g)	CHOL.(mg)	FIBER(g)	SODIUM(mg)
360	34	19	18	3.5	50	1.5	1,050

Food exchanges per serving: 2 Fruits plus 2 Lean Meats plus 2 Fats
Low-sodium diets: Substitute cooked chicken or turkey for smoked turkey. Omit salt from chutney if using homemade chutney.

Chicken and Barley Salad

As a special treat, serve this salad in a seeded red or green bell pepper.

⅔ cup uncooked quick-cooking   ½ cup chopped tomatoes
    barley   ½ cup chopped red onion
2 cups water   2 tablespoons fresh lemon juice
2 cups diced cooked chicken   1 teaspoon Dijon mustard
½ cup diced celery   5 lettuce leaves

Bring 2 cups water to a vigorous boil in a medium saucepan over high heat.
Stir in barley; return to a boil. Reduce heat, cover, and simmer 8–10 minutes
or until barley is tender, stirring occasionally. Drain if necessary; cool.

   Toss barley with remaining ingredients except lettuce. Serve on lettuce
leaves.

5 servings (makes 5 cups)
1 serving = 1 cup

CAL.	CHO(g)	PRO.(g)	TOTAL FAT(g)	SAT. FAT(g)	CHOL.(mg)	FIBER(g)	SODIUM(mg)
190	18	19	4	1	50	3	85

Food exchanges per serving: 2 Lean Meats plus 1 Starch plus 1 Vegetable
Low-sodium diets: This recipe is excellent.

Classic Tuna Salad

2 6-ounce cans water-packed tuna,
    drained
½ cup chopped onion
½ cup chopped celery
⅓ cup light or reduced-fat
    mayonnaise

1 teaspoon lemon juice
½ teaspoon salt
¼ teaspoon freshly ground pepper

Combine all ingredients in a medium-sized bowl. Mix well.

5 servings (makes 2½ cups)
1 serving = ½ cup

CAL.	CHO(g)	PRO.(g)	TOTAL FAT(g)	SAT. FAT(g)	CHOL.(mg)	FIBER(g)	SODIUM(mg)
130	3	18	5	1	30	0.5	530

Food exchanges per serving: 2½ Lean Meats
Low-sodium diets: Omit salt; add ½ teaspoon unsalted herb blend.

Tuna Salad with Grapes and Almonds

For chicken salad, substitute 1 cup cooked, diced, skinless chicken for the can of tuna.

1 6-ounce can water-packed tuna, drained
⅓ cup chopped scallions
½ cup chopped celery
3 tablespoons light or reduced-fat mayonnaise

1 teaspoon lemon juice
¼ teaspoon salt
⅛ teaspoon freshly ground pepper
1 cup small red seedless grapes
¼ cup slivered almonds, toasted

Combine all ingredients in a medium mixing bowl; mix well. If serving immediately, reserve 1 tablespoon almonds to sprinkle on top.

5 servings (makes 2½ cups)
1 serving = ½ cup

CAL.	CHO(g)	PRO.(g)	TOTAL FAT(g)	SAT. FAT(g)	CHOL.(mg)	FIBER(g)	SODIUM(mg)
120	6	11	6	1	15	1	275

Food exchanges per serving: 2 Lean Meats plus ½ Fruit
Low-sodium diets: Omit salt.

Spicy Sesame Beef Salad

As you will use steak from the Sesame-Ginger Beef Steak recipe, save time by saving some grilled peppers from that recipe, too. This wonderful one-dish meal is not only beautiful, it is also loaded with vitamins A and C, niacin, and the minerals zinc and potassium.

6 ounces cooked Sesame-Ginger
    Beef Steak (see Index)
12 snow peas, blanched
2 grilled pepper halves (from
    Sesame-Ginger Beef Steak
    recipe)
1 tablespoon reduced-sodium soy
    sauce
1 tablespoon red wine vinegar

1 teaspoon Oriental dark-roasted
    sesame oil, divided
½ teaspoon sugar
⅛ teaspoon hot-pepper sauce
1 tablespoon corn or canola oil
1 cup cooked vermicelli or other
    noodles
1 tablespoon unsalted roasted
    peanuts

Carve beef diagonally across the grain into thin slices; cut each slice in half. Cut snow peas in half diagonally, if large. Cut grilled pepper into thin strips 2″ × ¼″. In a medium-sized mixing bowl, combine beef, snow peas, and pepper strips.

In a small bowl, stir together soy sauce, vinegar, ½ teaspoon of the sesame oil, sugar, and pepper sauce. Whisk in vegetable oil. Add dressing to beef mixture, tossing to coat; set aside.

Toss vermicelli with remaining ½ teaspoon sesame oil; arrange on a platter. Top with beef mixture. Garnish with peanuts.

2 servings
1 serving = ½ cup vermicelli plus 1 cup meat-vegetable mixture

CAL.	CHO(g)	PRO.(g)	TOTAL FAT(g)	SAT. FAT(g)	CHOL.(mg)	FIBER(g)	SODIUM(mg)
415	27	29	21	5	55	2.5	400

Food exchanges per serving: 3 Medium-Fat Meats plus 1½ Starches plus 1 Vegetable plus 1 Fat
Low-sodium diets: This recipe is acceptable.

Mustard Dressing

This dressing is excellent with seafood or ham or when you want tangy mustard flavor.

1½ teaspoons dry mustard
1 tablespoon water
2 tablespoons all-purpose flour
1 teaspoon salt
Dash cayenne pepper
2 egg yolks, well beaten

¾ cup water
2 tablespoons cider or white
    vinegar
Sugar substitute equivalent to
    1 tablespoon of sugar

Mix mustard and 1 tablespoon water in a small container until smooth; let stand 5 minutes. Mix together flour, salt, and cayenne pepper in top of a double boiler. Add egg yolks and ¾ cup water to mustard, blend together. Add egg-mustard mixture to dry ingredients and mix well. Cook and stir over simmering water about 10 minutes or until thick and smooth.

Remove from heat. Add vinegar and sweetener; blend well. Pour into a ½-pint jar; cover and chill. Stir before using.

8 servings (makes 1 cup)
1 serving = 2 tablespoons

CAL.	CHO(g)	PRO.(g)	TOTAL FAT(g)	SAT. FAT(g)	CHOL.(mg)	FIBER(g)	SODIUM(mg)
25	2	1	1	0.5	53	0	275

Food exchange per serving: a Free Food
Low-sodium diets: Omit salt.

Lemon Shaker Dressing

This tasty, very low calorie dressing can also be used as a marinade for vegetables and meat.

½ cup fresh lemon juice

¾ cup water

¼ teaspoon salt

1 teaspoon grated lemon zest

½ teaspoon Worcestershire sauce

¼ teaspoon celery seed

⅛ teaspoon freshly ground pepper

¼ teaspoon dry mustard

Sugar substitute equivalent to

    2 tablespoons sugar

Combine all ingredients in a pint jar; cover tightly and shake vigorously. Store in refrigerator. Shake well before using.

14 servings (makes 1¾ cups)
1 serving = 2 tablespoons

CAL.	CHO(g)	PRO.(g)	TOTAL FAT(g)	SAT. FAT(g)	CHOL.(mg)	FIBER(g)	SODIUM(mg)
2	0	0	0	0	0	0	20

Food exchange per serving: a Free Food
Low-sodium diets: Omit salt.

Kay's Dressing

This dressing is a variation of the old standard "Zero Dressing." Kay Middleton, the original coauthor of this book, was especially proud of this one.

½ cup water
½ cup white vinegar
½ teaspoon salt
½ teaspoon dry mustard

⅛ teaspoon freshly ground pepper
1/16 teaspoon paprika
Sugar substitute equivalent to
    4 teaspoons sugar

Combine all ingredients in a pint jar; cover tightly. Shake vigorously and store in refrigerator. Shake before using.

8 servings (makes 1 cup)
1 serving = 2 tablespoons

CAL.	CHO(g)	PRO.(g)	TOTAL FAT(g)	SAT. FAT(g)	CHOL.(mg)	FIBER(g)	SODIUM(mg)
4	1	0	0	0	0	0	135

Food exchange per serving: a Free Food
Low-sodium diets: Omit salt.

Poppy Seed Dressing

This is a variation of Kay's Dressing (see preceding recipe). Delicious over fruit salads.

½ cup water	⅛ teaspoon freshly ground pepper
½ cup cider vinegar	1 tablespoon poppy seeds
½ teaspoon salt	Sugar substitute equivalent to
½ teaspoon dry mustard	4 teaspoons sugar

Combine all ingredients in a pint jar; cover tightly. Shake vigorously and store in refrigerator. Shake before using.

8 servings (makes 1 cup)
1 serving = 2 tablespoons

CAL.	CHO(g)	PRO.(g)	TOTAL FAT(g)	SAT. FAT(g)	CHOL.(mg)	FIBER(g)	SODIUM(mg)
10	1	0	0.5	0	0	0	135

Food exchange per serving: a Free Food
Low-sodium diets: Omit salt.

Curry Dressing

Try this easy and delicious dressing on chicken or fish salads or as a dip for assorted raw vegetables.

1 cup plain low-fat yogurt   ½ teaspoon salt
1½ teaspoons curry powder   ¼ teaspoon cayenne pepper
½ teaspoon ground ginger

*B*lend all ingredients until smooth. Chill in a covered container at least 1 hour before serving.

8 servings (makes 1 cup)
1 serving = 2 tablespoons

CAL.	CHO(g)	PRO.(g)	TOTAL FAT(g)	SAT. FAT(g)	CHOL.(mg)	FIBER(g)	SODIUM(mg)
20	2	1.5	0.5	0.5	0	0	155

Food exchange per serving: a Free Food
Low-sodium diets: Omit salt.

Buttermilk Ranch Dressing

This low-fat dressing tastes better than most bottled varieties. It takes only about 5 minutes to make. The buttermilk gives it a nice, creamy consistency.

½ small onion, cut in chunks
2 tablespoons cider vinegar
1 tablespoon olive oil
1 tablespoon Dijon mustard
1 tablespoon chopped fresh parsley

1 teaspoon minced garlic
½ teaspoon coarsely ground pepper
1 cup cultured low-fat (1½% milk
    fat) buttermilk

Combine all ingredients except buttermilk in bowl of a food processor or blender. Process 2 minutes or until mixture is of even consistency.

Put mixture into a pint jar. Add buttermilk, and shake to mix. Chill at least 1 hour for flavors to blend.

14 servings (makes 1⅔ cups)
1 serving = 2 tablespoons

CAL.	CHO*(g)*	PRO.*(g)*	TOTAL FAT*(g)*	SAT. FAT*(g)*	CHOL.*(mg)*	FIBER*(g)*	SODIUM*(mg)*
21	1	1	1	0	0	0	45

Food exchange per serving: a Free Food
Low-sodium diets: This recipe is suitable.

Roasted Shallot and Pepper Dressing

This dressing is ideal for entertaining. It's also great as a dip for vegetables, baked pita chips, or low-fat potato chips. If you are using it as a dip, plan on ¼ cup per serving (6 servings), and count it as 1 Vegetable Exchange.

1 (⅓ recipe) Roasted Red Pepper
    (see Index or use bottled
    roasted red peppers)
⅓ cup Roasted Shallots (see Index)
1 cup cultured low-fat (1½% milk
    fat) buttermilk

1 teaspoon coarsely ground pepper
2 teaspoons balsamic vinegar
½ teaspoon salt

*F*inely chop roasted shallots and peppers in a food processor or blender. Add other ingredients; process about 1 minute.

Refrigerate at least 1 hour for flavors to blend.

12 servings (makes 1½ cups)
1 serving = 2 tablespoons

CAL.	CHO(g)	PRO.(g)	TOTAL FAT(g)	SAT. FAT(g)	CHOL.(mg)	FIBER(g)	SODIUM(mg)
17	2	1	0	0	0	0	125

Food exchange per serving: a Free Food
Low-sodium diets: Omit salt.

Gazpacho Dressing

A great way to use leftover grilled or roasted vegetables or a portion of Grilled Vegetable Terrine (see Index). Don't use roasted potatoes, winter squash, or other starchy vegetables. Peppers, eggplant, leeks, zucchini, onions, and/or mushrooms work best. This dressing is loaded with vitamins and minerals.

4 ounces mixed grilled or roasted vegetables
1½ cups vegetable juice cocktail or tomato juice

½ teaspoon hot pepper sauce

*C*oarsely puree vegetables (several varieties are best) in a food processor or blender. Add juice and pepper; process about 1 minute until well blended. Taste and add more pepper sauce if desired.

24 servings (makes 3 cups)
1 serving = 2 tablespoons

CAL.	CHO*(g)*	PRO.*(g)*	TOTAL FAT*(g)*	SAT. FAT*(g)*	CHOL.*(mg)*	FIBER*(g)*	SODIUM*(mg)*
6	1	0	0	0	0	0	95

Food exchange per serving: a Free Food
Low-sodium diets: Substitute unsalted vegetable juice cocktail or tomato juice.

Thai-Style Vinaigrette

Use this dressing over cucumbers or Thai rice noodles or as a marinade for grilled vegetables or seafood.

¼ cup white wine or rice vinegar	1 tablespoon Oriental dark-roasted sesame oil
¼ cup Chicken Stock (see Index) or chicken broth	1 shallot, peeled and cut into pieces
¼ cup Thai fish sauce (Nam pla)	1 clove garlic
1 tablespoon lime juice	1-inch cube fresh gingerroot

Combine all ingredients in a food processor or blender. Process 2 minutes or until well blended.

8 servings (makes 1 cup)
1 serving = 2 tablespoons

CAL.	CHO(g)	PRO.(g)	TOTAL FAT(g)	SAT. FAT(g)	CHOL.(mg)	FIBER(g)	SODIUM(mg)
40	2	1	3	0.5	0	0	300

Food exchange per serving: ½ Fat
Low-sodium diets: This recipe is not suitable. Thai fish sauce has a lot of sodium, and that is an important part of the recipe's flavor.

15

Breads, Crepes and Pancakes, Pizzas, and Sandwiches

Breads

Cracked-Wheat Carrot Loaf

½ cup boiling water
¼ cup cracked wheat
1 package active dry yeast
¼ cup warm (110–115°F) water
⅓ cup warm (110–115°F) skim
    milk
¼ cup margarine

¼ cup firmly packed brown sugar
1 teaspoon salt
1 cup shredded carrot
1 egg
2⅓–2⅔ cups all-purpose flour,
    divided
⅔ cup oat bran cereal

*I*n a small bowl, pour boiling water over cracked wheat; let stand 15 minutes. Drain excess water; set aside. In another small bowl, dissolve yeast in warm water.

In a large bowl, combine milk, margarine, brown sugar, salt, carrot, and egg. Add dissolved yeast and cracked wheat. The margarine may not melt completely.

In a small bowl, combine 1 cup of the all-purpose flour and oat bran cereal; add to yeast mixture. Beat 1 minute at medium speed with an electric mixer. Add enough of the remaining all-purpose flour to make a moderately stiff dough.

Turn out onto a lightly floured surface. Knead about 10 minutes or until dough is smooth and elastic. Shape into a ball. Grease a large bowl. Place dough in bowl, turning once to coat surface. Cover; let rise in a warm place about 1½ hours or until nearly double in size.

Prepare an 8½″ × 4½″ × 2½″ loaf pan with nonstick cooking spray. Punch dough down; shape into a loaf. Place in a prepared pan. Cover; let rise in a warm place about 1 hour or until nearly double in size.

Meanwhile, heat oven to 375°F. Bake 25–30 minutes, shielding crust with aluminum foil after 20 minutes of baking. Remove from pan; cool on a wire rack.

16 servings (1 loaf)
1 serving = 1 ½-inch slice

CAL.	CHO*(g)*	PRO.*(g)*	TOTAL FAT*(g)*	SAT. FAT*(g)*	CHOL.*(mg)*	FIBER*(g)*	SODIUM*(mg)*
145	26	4	4	0.5	15	2	190

Food exchanges per serving: 1 Starch plus 1 Other Carbohydrate
Low-sodium diets: Omit salt.

Dilly Bread

1 cup creamed (4% milk fat) cottage cheese, at room temperature

1 teaspoon salt

1½ tablespoons sugar

2 tablespoons margarine, melted

2 tablespoons fresh snipped dill or 1 tablespoon dried dill

1 teaspoon grated lemon zest

2 tablespoons finely minced scallion

½ cup lukewarm (110–115°F) water

1 package instant active dry yeast

2½ cups all-purpose flour, divided

2 teaspoons margarine, divided, at room temperature

*W*hen cottage cheese is warmed to room temperature, add salt, sugar, melted margarine, dill, lemon zest, and scallion. Mix thoroughly, then set aside.

Pour the lukewarm water into a large bowl. Sprinkle yeast on top; stir to dissolve. Stir in cottage cheese mixture; blend thoroughly. Add 1¼ cups of the flour gradually, beating until smooth. Stir (do not beat) in the remaining 1¼ cups flour gradually, mixing well.

Turn onto a lightly floured board; knead until smooth and elastic (about 7–8 minutes). Use 1 teaspoon of the softened margarine to grease a large bowl. Place dough in this bowl and turn it around to grease lightly on all sides. Cover bowl and place in a warm place, free from drafts, until dough doubles in bulk, about 1 hour. (The oven, turned off, works well for this.)

Punch down dough in four or five places; turn out on board, and let rest for 15 minutes. Meanwhile, grease a 9″ × 5″ × 3″ loaf pan with remaining 1 teaspoon softened margarine.

Shape dough into a loaf and place in the prepared pan. Cover; let rise in a warm place until center is slightly higher than edge of pan (about 1 hour).

Preheat oven to 400°F 10 minutes before end of rising time. Bake loaf about 50 minutes.

18 slices (makes a 22-ounce loaf)
1 serving = 1 ½-inch slice

CAL.	CHO(g)	PRO.(g)	TOTAL FAT(g)	SAT. FAT(g)	CHOL.(mg)	FIBER(g)	SODIUM(mg)
95	15	3	2	0.5	0	0.5	190

Food exchange per serving: 1 Starch
Low-sodium diets: Omit salt.

California Sunshine Bread

If the water or orange juice is very hot, the yeast will be destroyed. If the liquid is too cold, the yeast action will be too slow. Sugar is needed for the yeast to work, so don't use a sugar substitute.

¼ cup lukewarm (110–115°F) water

3 tablespoons sugar

1 package instant active dry yeast

⅔ cup fresh orange juice, warmed to room temperature

2½ cups unsifted all-purpose flour, divided

1 teaspoon salt

3 tablespoons margarine, melted

1 tablespoon finely grated fresh orange zest

1 teaspoon finely grated fresh lemon zest

Combine lukewarm water, sugar, and yeast in a large bowl, stirring until completely dissolved. Add warm orange juice and beat until well blended. Add 1 cup of the flour gradually, beating gently until smooth. Cover bowl and set in a warm place until bubbly and light (30–40 minutes). Add salt, margarine, and grated orange and lemon zest; beat gently to mix. Stir in remaining flour gradually, mixing well.

Turn onto a lightly floured board and knead until smooth and elastic (about 10 minutes). Place in a large, oiled bowl, turning dough around to coat all over. Cover bowl; place in a warm place until dough has doubled in size (1–2 hours). Punch dough down in several places. Knead on board for 5 minutes. Prepare an 8½″ × 4½″ × 2½″ loaf pan with nonstick cooking spray. Shape dough into a loaf and place in pan. Cover and let rise in a warm place about 1 hour.

Preheat oven to 375°F. When bread has risen, bake 35–45 minutes. Remove bread from pan and cool on a wire rack.

15 slices (makes 1¼-pound loaf)
1 serving = 1 ½-inch slice

CAL.	CHO(g)	PRO.(g)	TOTAL FAT(g)	SAT. FAT(g)	CHOL.(mg)	FIBER(g)	SODIUM(mg)
115	20	2	3	0.5	0	0.5	175

Food exchange per serving: 1 Starch
Low-sodium diets: Omit salt.

Mustard Whole-Wheat Bread

This bread is wonderful for sandwiches.

2 packages instant active dry yeast
¾ cup lukewarm (110–115°F)
    water
2 teaspoons sugar
1⅓ cups unsifted all-purpose flour

1 teaspoon salt
3 tablespoons margarine, melted
⅓ cup Dijon mustard
1⅓ cups whole-wheat flour

Combine yeast, lukewarm water, and sugar in a large bowl; stir until yeast is completely dissolved. Add all-purpose flour gradually, beating until smooth. Cover bowl, set in a warm place, and let rise until surface is bubbly and batter is light (30–40 minutes). Add salt, margarine, and mustard; mix well. Add whole-wheat flour gradually, mixing thoroughly.

Turn dough onto a lightly floured board, and knead for 10 minutes or until light and elastic. Place in a large oiled bowl, turning dough over several times to form a ball that is well coated. Cover bowl and set in a warm place until the dough is doubled in size, about 1–2 hours.

Punch down dough in several places; turn onto a lightly floured board, and knead 5 minutes. Let rest, covered, 10 minutes. Prepare an 8½″ × 4½″ × 2½″ loaf pan with nonstick cooking spray. Shape dough into a loaf and place in pan. Cover and let rise until doubled in size.

When almost ready, preheat oven to 375°F. Bake 40–45 minutes. Remove bread from pan, and cool on a wire rack.

15 slices (makes 1¼-pound loaf)
1 serving = 1 ½-inch slice

CAL.	CHO(g)	PRO.(g)	TOTAL FAT(g)	SAT. FAT(g)	CHOL.(mg)	FIBER(g)	SODIUM(mg)
110	17	3	3	0.5	0	2	300

Food exchange per serving: 1 Starch
Low-sodium diets: Omit salt; substitute unsalted margarine.

Three-Pepper Cheese Bread

This quick, easy bread requires no kneading or rising time.

2 cups whole-wheat flour
1½ teaspoons baking powder
½ teaspoon baking soda
¼ teaspoon salt
1½ cups shredded sharp cheddar
    cheese
¼ cup finely chopped jalapeño
    pepper

¼ cup finely chopped red bell pepper
¼ cup finely chopped green bell
    pepper
1 cup skim milk
2 eggs, beaten
2 tablespoons corn oil

Preheat oven to 375°F.

In a large bowl, stir together flour, baking powder, baking soda, and salt. Stir in cheese and peppers.

In a separate bowl, combine milk, eggs, and oil. Add to dry ingredients, stirring just until dry ingredients are moistened.

Prepare an 8½″ × 4½″ × 2½″ loaf pan with nonstick cooking spray; add batter. Bake 40 minutes or until toothpick inserted in center comes out clean. Cool 15 minutes before removing from pan. Bring to room temperature before slicing.

16 servings
1 serving = 1 ½-inch slice

CAL.	CHO(g)	PRO.(g)	TOTAL FAT(g)	SAT. FAT(g)	CHOL.(mg)	FIBER(g)	SODIUM(mg)
125	12	6	6	2.5	40	2	200

Food exchanges per serving: 1 Starch plus 1 Fat
Low-sodium diets: Omit salt.

Whole-Wheat Pita Bread

1 package active dry yeast
1 teaspoon honey
1 cup plus 2 tablespoons warm
(110–115°F) water

2¼ cups all-purpose flour
½ cup whole-wheat flour
1 teaspoon salt

*A*dd yeast and honey to warm water in a medium-sized bowl; let stand until foamy, about 5 minutes. Combine flours and salt in a large mixing bowl. Pour yeast mixture into center, and stir until dough can be gathered into a ball. Knead dough on a floured board until smooth. Place in a large, lightly oiled bowl. Cover with a damp towel, and place in a dry, draft-free place until dough has doubled, 1–2 hours.

Punch down dough; place on a lightly floured board. Divide dough into 12 equal pieces. Shape into circles and place on nonstick cookie sheets. Allow to rest, covered with damp towel, 30 minutes. On lightly floured board, roll out each piece of dough to a circle, about 5 inches in diameter. Place on cookie sheets; let stand 30 minutes.

Preheat oven to 500°F. Bake pitas on middle rack of oven 5 minutes. Remove from cookie sheets and let cool on rack. Store in airtight container in refrigerator.

To serve, reheat pitas wrapped in aluminum foil at 350°F for 10 minutes.

12 servings
1 serving = 1 pita

CAL.	CHO(g)	PRO.(g)	TOTAL FAT(g)	SAT. FAT(g)	CHOL.(mg)	FIBER(g)	SODIUM(mg)
110	23	3	0	0	0	1.5	185

Food exchanges per serving: 1½ Starches
Low-sodium diets: Omit salt.

Buttermilk Corn Bread

1 cup sifted all-purpose flour
½ teaspoon baking soda
2 teaspoons baking powder
½ teaspoon salt
1 tablespoon sugar
1 cup yellow cornmeal

1 egg, beaten
1 cup cultured buttermilk, made
     from skim milk, or low-fat
     (1½% milk fat) buttermilk
3 tablespoons margarine, melted

Preheat oven to 425°F. Prepare an 8-inch square pan with nonstick cooking spray. Sift together dry ingredients in a large bowl. In a medium-sized bowl, combine egg, buttermilk, and margarine; add to dry ingredients, stirring until well mixed. With a mixer or rotary beater, beat 1 minute. Turn into prepared pan.

Bake 20–25 minutes. Cool slightly. Cut into 16 2-inch squares. Serve warm.

16 servings
1 serving = 1 2-inch square

CAL.	CHO(g)	PRO.(g)	TOTAL FAT(g)	SAT. FAT(g)	CHOL.(mg)	FIBER(g)	SODIUM(mg)
90	14	2	3	0.5	15	0.5	215

Food exchange per serving: 1 Starch
Low-sodium diets: Omit salt. Substitute unsalted margarine.

Muffins and Biscuits

Southwestern Corn Muffins

To make blueberry corn muffins, omit the corn and chilies and add ¾ cup blueberries.

1 cup yellow cornmeal	1 cup cultured low-fat (1½% milk fat) buttermilk
¾ cup sifted all-purpose flour	
1½ teaspoons baking powder	2 tablespoons margarine, melted
½ teaspoon salt	½ cup canned or frozen corn, drained if canned
½ teaspoon baking soda	
1 tablespoon sugar	2 tablespoons canned, peeled green chilies
1 egg, beaten	

Preheat oven to 375°F. Prepare a 12-muffin pan (2½-inch cups) with nonstick cooking spray, or line with paper baking cups.

In a large bowl, sift together all dry ingredients; mix lightly with a fork. In a medium-sized bowl, combine egg, buttermilk, and melted margarine; mix well. Add all at once to dry ingredients. Stir vigorously to mix well, then beat gently 1–2 minutes. Stir in corn and chilies. Fill cups of prepared muffin pans half full.

Bake 25–30 minutes. Serve hot.

12 servings
1 serving = 1 muffin

CAL.	CHO(g)	PRO.(g)	TOTAL FAT(g)	SAT. FAT(g)	CHOL.(mg)	FIBER(g)	SODIUM(mg)
115	18	3	3	0.5	20	1	285

Food exchanges per serving: 1 Starch plus 1 Vegetable
Low-sodium diets: Omit salt.

Bran Muffins

1 cup All-Bran cereal	½ teaspoon salt
2/3 cup skim milk	¼ cup sugar
½ cup sifted all-purpose flour	1 egg, beaten
1½ teaspoons baking powder	2 tablespoons canola or corn oil

Preheat oven to 400°F. Prepare nine 2-inch muffin cups with nonstick cooking spray or line with paper baking cups.

In a large mixing bowl, combine bran cereal and milk. In a medium-sized bowl, sift together flour, baking powder, salt, and sugar. In a small bowl, combine egg and oil. Add to bran and milk; mix well. Add dry ingredients all at once, and stir (do not beat) just enough to mix.

Measure 3 scant tablespoonfuls batter into each prepared muffin cup. Bake 25–30 minutes. Cool 5 minutes, then turn out of pans.

9 servings
1 serving = 1 muffin

CAL.	CHO(g)	PRO.(g)	TOTAL FAT(g)	SAT. FAT(g)	CHOL.(mg)	FIBER(g)	SODIUM(mg)
105	16	3	4	0.5	25	2.5	280

Food exchanges per serving: 1 Starch plus ½ Fat
Low-sodium diets: Omit salt.

Variation: Raisin Bran Muffins
Add ¼ cup soaked and drained seedless raisins to the dry ingredients in the recipe for Bran Muffins.

CAL.	CHO(g)	PRO.(g)	TOTAL FAT(g)	SAT. FAT(g)	CHOL.(mg)	FIBER(g)	SODIUM(mg)
115	18	3	4	0.5	25	2.5	280

Food exchanges per serving: 1 Starch plus ½ Fat
Low-sodium diets: Omit salt.

Applesauce Cinnamon Muffins

Another favorite, adapted with the permission of the Quaker Oats Company.

1¼ cups oat bran cereal, uncooked
1 cup whole-wheat flour
2 teaspoons ground cinnamon
1 teaspoon baking powder
¾ teaspoon baking soda
½ teaspoon salt

¾ cup unsweetened applesauce
½ cup honey
¼ cup canola or corn oil
1 egg
1 teaspoon pure vanilla extract
¼ cup chopped walnuts

Preheat oven to 375°F. Coat 12 medium-sized muffin cups with nonstick cooking spray or line with paper baking cups.

In medium bowl combine oat bran cereal, flour, cinnamon, baking powder, baking soda, and salt. In large bowl combine applesauce, honey, oil, egg, and vanilla. Stir in dry ingredients; mix well. Stir in nuts. Fill prepared muffin cups almost full.

Bake 15–20 minutes or until golden brown. Serve warm.

12 servings
1 serving = 1 muffin

CAL.	CHO(g)	PRO.(g)	TOTAL FAT(g)	SAT. FAT(g)	CHOL.(mg)	FIBER(g)	SODIUM(mg)
180	27	4	7	0.5	20	3	215

Food exchanges per serving: 1 Starch plus 1 Fat plus 1 Fruit
Low-sodium diets: Omit salt.

Oat Bran Muffins

Oat bran is a good ingredient in foods for people with diabetes or anyone who wants to consume more soluble fiber. This recipe was adapted from one provided by the Quaker Oats Company.

2¼ cups oat bran cereal, uncooked
¼ cup chopped nuts
¼ cup raisins
2 teaspoons baking powder
½ teaspoon salt

¾ cup skim milk
⅓ cup honey
2 eggs, beaten
2 tablespoons canola or corn oil

Preheat oven to 425°F. Coat 12 medium-sized muffin cups with nonstick cooking spray or line with paper baking cups.

In a large bowl, combine oat bran cereal, nuts, raisins, baking powder, and salt. Add remaining ingredients; mix just until dry ingredients are moistened. Fill prepared muffin cups almost full.

Bake 15–17 minutes or until golden brown. Serve warm.

12 servings
1 serving = 1 muffin

CAL.	CHO(g)	PRO.(g)	TOTAL FAT(g)	SAT. FAT(g)	CHOL.(mg)	FIBER(g)	SODIUM(mg)
150	21	5	6	0.5	35	2.5	190

Food exchanges per serving: 1 Starch plus 1 Fat plus ½ Fruit
Low-sodium diets: Omit salt.

Baking Powder Biscuits

2 cups sifted all-purpose flour
4 teaspoons baking powder
½ teaspoon salt

5 tablespoons margarine
¾ cup skim milk

Preheat oven to 425°F. Sift together flour, baking powder, and salt. Cut margarine in with a blending fork or dough blender until fat is the size of small peas. Add milk all at once. Stir until dough is all mixed and forms a ball.

Roll out on a lightly floured board to a thickness of about ¼ inch. Cut with a 2½-inch round cutter, or roll thicker and cut with a 2-inch cutter. Place 1 inch apart on a baking sheet. Bake 12–14 minutes.

12 servings
1 serving = 1 biscuit

CAL.	CHO(g)	PRO.(g)	TOTAL FAT(g)	SAT. FAT(g)	CHOL.(mg)	FIBER(g)	SODIUM(mg)
120	16	3	5	1	0	0.5	320

Food exchanges per serving: 1 Starch plus 1 Fat
Low-sodium diets: Omit salt. Substitute unsalted margarine.

Popovers

If you want really puffed up, high popovers, heat the custard cups or muffin pans *before* you pour the batter in.

2 eggs, beaten slightly	*½ teaspoon salt*
1 cup whole milk	*2 teaspoons canola or corn oil*
1 cup sifted all-purpose flour	

*P*reheat oven to 475°F. Prepare eight custard cups or a muffin pan with 2½-inch cups with butter-flavored nonstick cooking spray and set aside.

In a medium-sized mixing bowl, combine eggs, milk, flour, and salt; beat until frothy, about 1½ minutes. Add oil; beat only 30 seconds, no more. Pour batter into the custard cups or muffin cups.

Bake 15 minutes; reduce heat to 350°F and bake another 30 minutes or until firm and browned. A few minutes before popovers are completely cooked, pierce top or side of each with a sharp knife to let the steam escape.

If you prefer drier popovers, leave them in the oven with the oven door wide open for 10–15 minutes after the heat has been turned off.

Serve popovers hot.

8 servings
1 serving = 1 popover

CAL.	CHO*(g)*	PRO.*(g)*	TOTAL FAT*(g)*	SAT. FAT*(g)*	CHOL.*(mg)*	FIBER*(g)*	SODIUM*(mg)*
99	13	4	4	1	50	0.5	165

Food exchanges per serving: 1 Starch plus 1 Fat
Low-sodium diets: Omit salt.

Cream Puff Shells

These shells are lovely with pudding but are also delightful stuffed with tuna or chicken salad.

½ cup water	½ cup sifted all-purpose flour
1/16 teaspoon salt	2 large eggs
¼ cup margarine, cut into pieces	

Preheat oven to 450°F. Prepare baking sheet with nonstick cooking spray.

Boil water and salt in a saucepan; add margarine and bring to a vigorous boil. Add flour all at once. Keeping heat low, stir rapidly to blend; then beat strenuously with a wooden spoon until the mixture forms a ball and pulls away from the sides of the pan. Remove from heat; allow to cool a few minutes. Add eggs, one at a time, beating vigorously after each addition.

Drop 2 level tablespoons of batter onto prepared sheet for each shell; place batter at least 2 inches apart. Bake 10 minutes. Reduce heat to 400°F and continue baking until puffs are firm and browned, about 25 minutes.

Transfer to a wire rack. Slit each puff with the tip of a sharp knife to allow steam to escape. Let cool before filling.

9 servings
1 serving = 1 puff shell

CAL.	CHO(g)	PRO.(g)	TOTAL FAT(g)	SAT. FAT(g)	CHOL.(mg)	FIBER(g)	SODIUM(mg)
85	5	2	6	1	45	0	90

Food exchanges per serving (unfilled shell): 1 Fat plus ½ Starch
Low-sodium diets: Omit salt. Substitute unsalted margarine.

Bread Stuffing

This recipe will fill a 5- to 8-pound roasting chicken or capon. Double the recipe to stuff a 12- to 16-pound turkey. Add sautéed mushrooms if you like. This stuffing is a good starch with roast pork or pork chops as well as poultry.

3 slices whole-grain bread
2 cups unsalted hot Chicken Stock
   (see Index) or chicken broth

1 6-ounce box herb stuffing mix
½ cup finely chopped celery
½ cup finely chopped onion

Tear bread into bite-sized pieces and put in a medium-sized mixing bowl. Add remaining ingredients and mix well.

Stuff and roast prepared bird, or bake stuffing in an ovenproof casserole sprayed with cooking spray at 350°F for 35–40 minutes.

6 servings (makes 3 cups)
1 serving = ½ cup

CAL.	CHO(g)	PRO.(g)	TOTAL FAT(g)	SAT. FAT(g)	CHOL.(mg)	FIBER(g)	SODIUM(mg)
165	29	7	2	0	0	1.5	635

Food exchanges per serving: 2 Starches
Low-sodium diets: This recipe is not suitable because stuffing mix is salted.

Crepes and Pancakes

Basic Crepes

Use the crepes as a wrapper for Rainbow Pepper Sauté, Ratatouille, or Crabmeat Mushroom Crepes (see Index), or fill them with Red Plum Spread (see Index). For savory crepes, you can add your favorite minced fresh herbs to the batter. Crepes can be made in advance and frozen, with waxed paper between them, for later use.

⅔ cup all-purpose flour	1 cup skim milk
⅛ teaspoon salt	1 tablespoon margarine, melted
2 eggs, beaten	½ teaspoon canola or corn oil

Combine flour and salt in a medium-sized mixing bowl. Gradually add eggs, milk, and margarine, beating until smooth. Refrigerate crepe batter for at least 2 hours.

Brush bottom of an 8-inch crepe pan or nonstick skillet with oil; place pan over medium heat until oil is hot but not smoking. Pour 3 tablespoons batter into pan; quickly tilt pan in all directions so batter covers pan in a thin film. Cook crepe 1 minute or until edge of crepe lifts easily from pan. Crepe is ready for flipping when it can be shaken loose from pan. Flip crepe and cook about 30 seconds on the other side.

Place on a towel to cool. Stack between layers of waxed paper to prevent sticking. Repeat procedure with remaining batter.

4 servings (makes 8 crepes)
1 serving = 2 crepes

CAL.	CHO(g)	PRO.(g)	TOTAL FAT(g)	SAT. FAT(g)	CHOL.(mg)	FIBER(g)	SODIUM(mg)
85	10	4	3	0.5	55	0.5	85

Food exchanges per serving: 1 Starch plus ½ Fat
Low-sodium diets: Omit salt.

Buckwheat Crepes

Serve these crepes wrapped around Sautéed Vegetable Filling (recipe follows) or Lox Spread (see Index).

1½ cups buckwheat flour	2 cups skim milk
½ cup all-purpose flour	2 teaspoons margarine, melted
¼ teaspoon salt	½ teaspoon corn oil
3 eggs, beaten slightly	

*I*n a medium-sized mixing bowl, combine the flours and salt. Blend in eggs, milk, and melted margarine. Whisk until smooth. Let batter stand at room temperature for 30 minutes. If batter is too thick, add water by the tablespoonful until batter is pouring consistency.

Brush an 8-inch nonstick skillet with corn oil, and place over medium heat until warm. Pour 3 tablespoons of batter into pan; rotate pan to cover with a thin coating of batter. Cook about 45 seconds or until crepe is cooked and beginning to brown on the bottom. Turn crepe using a spatula coated with cooking spray, and continue cooking for about 20–30 seconds or until crepe is cooked.

Place cooked crepe on a clean dish towel or paper towel on the kitchen counter to absorb excess moisture. Repeat procedure until all the batter has been used.

Crepes can be placed between sheets of waxed paper or aluminum foil for easy handling and refrigerated for 3 days or frozen until ready to use.

8 servings (makes 16 crepes)
1 serving = 2 crepes

CAL.	CHO(g)	PRO.(g)	TOTAL FAT(g)	SAT. FAT(g)	CHOL.(mg)	FIBER(g)	SODIUM(mg)
165	25	8	4	1	80	3	135

Food exchanges per serving: 1½ Starches plus ½ Skim Milk
Low-sodium diets: Omit salt.

Sautéed Vegetable Filling for Buckwheat Crepes

This sautéed vegetable mixture can also be served as a vegetable.

1 tablespoon margarine	½ teaspoon dried oregano or
1 cup thinly sliced red onion	2 teaspoons chopped fresh
1 cup zucchini or other summer	oregano
squash strips	½ teaspoon dried tarragon or
1 cup red or green bell pepper	2 teaspoons chopped fresh
strips	tarragon
½ teaspoon dried basil or	2 tablespoons beef broth
2 teaspoons chopped fresh	
basil	

*M*elt margarine in a large nonstick skillet over medium heat. Add onion; sauté, stirring often, until tender. Mix in remaining ingredients except beef broth, and cook until vegetables are crisp but tender, stirring often. Add beef broth during cooking. Cool vegetable filling before placing in crepes.

4–8 servings (makes 2 cups)
1 serving = ¼ cup as filling *or* ½ cup as vegetable

Per ¼-cup serving:

CAL.	CHO(g)	PRO.(g)	TOTAL FAT(g)	SAT. FAT(g)	CHOL.(mg)	FIBER(g)	SODIUM(mg)
27	3	1	2	0	0	0.5	45

Food exchange per serving: 1 Vegetable

Per ½-cup serving:

CAL.	CHO(g)	PRO.(g)	TOTAL FAT(g)	SAT. FAT(g)	CHOL.(mg)	FIBER(g)	SODIUM(mg)
55	7	1	3	0.5	0	1	90

Food exchanges per serving: 1 Vegetable plus ½ Fat
Low-sodium diets: This recipe is excellent.

Leningrad Special Buckwheat Pancakes

These blinis can be served many ways. Try them with fruited yogurt, Pear Butter (see following recipe), or Granny Smith Applesauce (see Index).

½ cup all-purpose flour
¾ cup buckwheat flour
1 teaspoon baking powder
Sugar substitute equivalent to
    2 teaspoons sugar or
    2 teaspoons sugar

1 egg, beaten slightly
1 cup water
1 tablespoon margarine, melted
1 teaspoon margarine (for cooking)

Blend flours, baking powder, and sugar substitute in a bowl. Mix in egg, water, and melted margarine. Let batter stand 10 minutes.

Melt 1 teaspoon margarine in a 10-inch nonstick skillet over medium heat. Drop batter by the tablespoonful onto hot skillet. Cook until bubbles form around edges of pancakes. Thin remaining batter with additional water if necessary. Turn pancakes over with a spatula. Continue cooking until pancakes are done. Place pancakes on a heated dish and continue cooking in batches until all the pancakes have been prepared.

6 servings (makes 24 pancakes)
1 serving = 4 small pancakes

CAL.	CHO(g)	PRO.(g)	TOTAL FAT(g)	SAT. FAT(g)	CHOL.(mg)	FIBER(g)	SODIUM(mg)
125	19	4	4	0.5	35	2	120

Food exchanges per serving: 1 Starch plus 1 Fat
Low-sodium diets: This recipe is suitable.

Pear Butter

Pears vary considerably in sweetness. You can add sweetener to taste after cooking if desired. Use Pear Butter as a topping or on toast, as you would use regular butter or margarine. For a special taste treat, spread Pear Butter over chicken breasts or a pork chop before grilling or after cooking.

2½ pounds firm, ripe pears	*1 teaspoon ground cinnamon*
⅔ cup water	*¼ teaspoon ground nutmeg*
2 tablespoons fresh lemon juice	*1 teaspoon grated lemon zest*

*W*ash, core, and cut pears into quarters. Place pieces in a large saucepan. Add water and lemon juice, and bring mixture to boil over medium heat. Cover pot and simmer 35 minutes or until pears are tender. Puree pears using a food processor fitted with a steel blade or a food mill.

Return the puree to pot, including cooking liquid, and add cinnamon, nutmeg, and lemon zest. Simmer pear mixture over very low heat, uncovered, 40–50 minutes, stirring occasionally until mixture thickens.

Store in refrigerator no longer than 2 weeks.

72 servings (makes 3 cups)
1 serving = 2 teaspoons

CAL.	CHO(g)	PRO.(g)	TOTAL FAT(g)	SAT. FAT(g)	CHOL.(mg)	FIBER(g)	SODIUM(mg)
10	2	0	0	0	0	0.5	0

Food exchange per serving: a Free Food (up to 4 teaspoons)
Low-sodium diets: This recipe is excellent.

Pizza

Whole-Wheat Pizza Crust

Barbara Grunes shares this recipe from her book *Skinny Pizzas*. She recommends variations that include adding mustard, lemon zest, curry powder, pesto sauce, and/or dried rosemary for an extra-special flavor. Don't try to use a sugar substitute for the honey. The yeast action requires the honey or real sugar.

½ teaspoon honey	¾ cup whole-wheat flour
1 cup (scant) warm water (110°F or warm to the touch)	2 cups all-purpose flour
	½ teaspoon salt
1 package active dry yeast	1 tablespoon virgin olive oil

Proof yeast by stirring honey into warm water in a measuring cup or small bowl. Sprinkle yeast over water; stir until yeast dissolves. Let mixture stand in a draft-free area about 5 minutes or until yeast begins to bubble.

Meanwhile, mix flours with salt and oil in a food processor fitted with a steel blade, or in an electric mixer with a dough hook. Pour in yeast mixture and process until a soft, almost sticky dough is formed, about 5–10 seconds. If using an electric mixer, mix 3 minutes or until smooth dough is formed.

Knead dough by hand on a lightly floured surface or pastry cloth until smooth. If dough is too sticky, add flour by the tablespoon until it reaches the desired consistency. Put dough in a bowl and cover lightly with oiled plastic wrap and aluminum foil or a kitchen towel. Let dough rise until it doubles in bulk, about 45 minutes to 1 hour. Punch dough down and let stand 5 minutes. Knead for a few minutes more on a lightly floured board or pastry cloth. Dough is now ready to use or freeze for later use.

24 servings (makes 2 12″ round crusts or 2 9″ × 12″ rectangular crusts or 12 6″–7″ round crusts)
1 serving = ¹⁄₁₂ of a 12″ crust *or* ¹⁄₁₂ of a rectangular crust *or* ½ of a 6″–7″ crust

CAL.	CHO(g)	PRO.(g)	TOTAL FAT(g)	SAT. FAT(g)	CHOL.(mg)	FIBER(g)	SODIUM(mg)
60	11	2	1	0	0	1	45

Food exchange per serving: 1 Starch
Low-sodium diets: This recipe is suitable.

Sausage Mini Pizzas

If you can find hot Italian turkey sausage, substitute it and count this recipe as 2 Starch Exchanges plus 2 Medium-Fat Meat Exchanges plus 1 Vegetable Exchange, and deduct 40 calories.

2 links (8 ounces total) hot Italian sausage
4 English muffins, split
1 15-ounce can pizza sauce
1¼ cups shredded light or part-skim Mozzarella cheese

½ teaspoon dried oregano or 2 teaspoons chopped fresh oregano

*P*reheat oven to 375°F. Squeeze sausage from links and sauté in a nonstick skillet. Crumble sausage; put in colander and rinse to remove fat.

Arrange muffin halves on cookie sheet. Spoon equal portions of pizza sauce on each muffin half. Put small pieces of sausage on top of sauce, then top with cheese. Sprinkle with oregano.

Bake 8–10 minutes until cheese is melted and slightly browned.

4 servings
1 serving = 2 mini pizzas

CAL.	CHO(g)	PRO.(g)	TOTAL FAT(g)	SAT. FAT(g)	CHOL.(mg)	FIBER(g)	SODIUM(mg)
360	35	24	15	4.5	40	2.5	1,390

Food exchanges per serving: 2 Starches plus 2 High-Fat Meats plus 1 Vegetable
Low-sodium diets: This recipe is not suitable.

Chicken, Tomato, and Shallot Pizza

This recipe is adapted from Barbara Grunes's *Skinny Pizzas*. You can use prepared pizza or pasta sauce instead of the Chunky Tomato Sauce if you wish.

12 large shallots, peeled and
  minced

1 teaspoon sugar

1 Whole-Wheat Pizza Crust (see
  Index)

2 cups Chunky Tomato Sauce (see
  Index)

1½ cups chicken breast, cooked and
  slivered

¼ teaspoon dried basil

¼ teaspoon dried oregano

Preheat oven to 425°F. Glaze shallots by sautéing them in a small nonstick skillet until cooked, then sprinkling with sugar and cooking until they begin to shimmer.

Coat a 9″ × 12″ baking pan with nonstick cooking spray. Shape and stretch Pizza Crust dough by hand or with a rolling pin on a lightly floured pastry board until large enough to line baking pan. Fit pizza crust into pan, and spread with tomato sauce. Sprinkle chicken and glazed shallots evenly over sauce. Sprinkle with basil and oregano.

Bake 20 minutes or until crust is cooked and topping is hot. Serve immediately.

6 servings
1 serving = 2 3-inch-square pieces

CAL.	CHO(g)	PRO.(g)	TOTAL FAT(g)	SAT. FAT(g)	CHOL.(mg)	FIBER(g)	SODIUM(mg)
250	39	17	3	0.5	30	4	540

Food exchanges per serving: 2 Starches plus 1 Vegetable plus 1 Lean Meat
Low-sodium diets: Use unsalted pasta sauce or prepare Chunky Tomato Sauce without salt.

Zucchini and Wild Mushroom Cracker Pizza

This recipe first appeared in *Skinny Pizzas* by Barbara Grunes and is one of her favorites. Lahvosh is thin Armenian cracker bread. This recipe calls for the baked crisp type.

2 tablespoons margarine, divided
2 shallots, minced
1 zucchini, sliced thin horizontally
1½ pounds mixed brown
    mushrooms such as shiitake
    and chanterelles, sliced thin
¼ teaspoon freshly ground pepper

¼ teaspoon ground nutmeg
2 cups low-fat, small-curd cottage
    cheese
2 cups plain nonfat yogurt
¼ teaspoon mace
1 large (15-inch diameter) lahvosh
    cracker

*H*eat 1 tablespoon margarine with shallots in a nonstick skillet. Add zucchini; sauté on both sides until beginning to brown. Remove zucchini and reserve. Add remaining 1 tablespoon margarine and mushrooms; sauté, covered, until glazed and tender. Season with pepper and nutmeg. Set aside.

Puree cottage cheese in a food processor fitted with a steel blade. Mix in yogurt and mace.

Preheat oven to 375°F. Place lahvosh cracker on a nonstick or foil-covered cookie sheet. Spread cheese mixture on crust. Distribute mushroom mixture evenly over cheese. Arrange zucchini slices in a design over mushrooms.

Bake pizza on lowest rack in oven 20 minutes or until hot.

Cut with pizza wheel or a pair of kitchen shears.

8 servings
1 serving = 1 slice (⅛ of pizza)

CAL.	CHO*(g)*	PRO.*(g)*	TOTAL FAT*(g)*	SAT. FAT*(g)*	CHOL.*(mg)*	FIBER*(g)*	SODIUM*(mg)*
190	23	14	5	1	5	1.5	380

Food exchanges per serving: 1 Starch plus 1 Low-Fat Meat plus 1 Vegetable
Low-sodium diets: Use unsalted cottage cheese.

Focaccia with Red Onions and Poppy Seeds

Another gift from Barbara Grunes is this use of the basic Whole-Wheat Pizza Crust. Focaccia is a pan bread made from pizza dough. It is usually made with lots of oil, but this recipe is not. It can be baked in a cast-iron frying pan from which it can be served directly. Focaccia can be wrapped, frozen, and reheated before serving.

2 tablespoons good-quality olive
    oil, divided
1 Whole-Wheat Pizza Crust
    (see Index)
2 cups red sliced onions

3 cloves garlic, sliced horizontally
¼ teaspoon salt
¼ teaspoon freshly ground pepper
3 tablespoons poppy seeds

Preheat oven to 425°F. Brush a 9-inch cast-iron skillet or baking pan with 1½ teaspoons of the olive oil.

With lightly floured hands, place pizza crust dough in pan and push it from the center to the edge, using knuckles or fingers. Using your fingers or a fork, press about 10 indentations around the dough's rim. Brush the rim of dough with 1½ teaspoons of the olive oil.

To prepare topping, heat remaining 1 tablespoon olive oil in a nonstick skillet. Add onions and garlic; sauté over medium heat about 5 minutes, stirring occasionally. Season with salt and pepper. Stir in poppy seeds. Remove from heat. Cool slightly.

Spread onion mixture over dough, leaving ½ inch of plain dough around rim of pan. Bake on lowest rack of oven 20 minutes or until golden brown around the rim and cooked through. Cool slightly in pan. Serve hot or warm.

10 servings
1 serving = 1 slice (¹⁄₁₀ of focaccia)

CAL.	CHO(g)	PRO.(g)	TOTAL FAT(g)	SAT. FAT(g)	CHOL.(mg)	FIBER(g)	SODIUM(mg)
125	18	3	5	0.5	0	1.5	115

Food exchanges per serving: 1 Starch plus 1 Fat
Low-sodium diets: This recipe is excellent.

Sandwiches

Dilled Lamb in Pita Pockets

I love this sandwich. You can make the Lamb Meatballs and the Yogurt Dill Dip in advance. Let family or guests stuff the pitas at the table. They and you will enjoy the meal and get lots of vitamin A, fiber, potassium, and iron as a bonus.

½ recipe (6 pitas) Whole-Wheat Pita Bread (see Index) or 12-ounce package of 6 whole-wheat or onion pita pockets

1 recipe Lamb Meatballs (see Index)

1 recipe Yogurt Dill Dip (see Index)

3 carrots, peeled and shredded (about 2 cups)

12 small sprigs fresh dill

*C*ut pita pockets in half and warm them in the oven or microwave. Fill each half pocket with 2–3 meatballs. Top with Yogurt Dill Dip and shredded carrots. Garnish pockets with dill sprigs.

6 servings
1 serving = 2 stuffed pita halves

CAL.	CHO(g)	PRO.(g)	TOTAL FAT(g)	SAT. FAT(g)	CHOL.(mg)	FIBER(g)	SODIUM(mg)
360	45	22	10	3.5	110	6	890

Food exchanges per serving: 2½ Starches plus 2 Medium-Fat Meats plus 1 Vegetable
Low-sodium diets: Omit salt in recipes for meatballs and dip.

Chicken Salad Baked in Nests

Students at Mundelein College, now part of Chicago's Loyola University, tested this recipe, and they judged it a prize-winner.

4 hard rolls
½ cup fat-free mayonnaise
1 tablespoon fresh lemon juice
1 teaspoon grated lemon zest
1½ teaspoons curry powder
1½ cups lightly packed diced cooked
    chicken

½ cup diced tomato
¼ cup finely chopped scallions
2 1-ounce slices American cheese,
    halved

Preheat oven to 350°F. Cut top off each roll and scoop out soft bread from inside to make a nest. Discard scooped-out portions. In a medium bowl, mix mayonnaise, lemon juice, zest, and curry powder. Add chicken, tomato, and scallions, and mix again. Spoon chicken mixture into the nests (each nest will hold ½ cup).

Place nests in a shallow baking pan and cover with foil. Bake 20 minutes; remove foil and put ½ slice of American cheese on top of each nest. Continue baking, uncovered, about 8 minutes, until cheese melts.

4 servings
1 serving = 1 nest

CAL.	CHO(g)	PRO.(g)	TOTAL FAT(g)	SAT. FAT(g)	CHOL.(mg)	FIBER(g)	SODIUM(mg)
340	29	28	11	4	75	1.5	710

Food exchanges per serving: 2 Starches plus 3 Lean Meats
Low-sodium diets: Use reduced-sodium cheese.

Rainbow Pepper Boats with Herbed Cheese

Everyone who tries these loves them, and they make a quick and easy meal. If the rolls are larger than 2 ounces each, scoop out some of the soft bread inside before filling with the pepper mixture.

4 (2-ounce each) crusty hard rolls, long style
1 recipe Rainbow Pepper Sauté (see Index)

6 ounces herbed goat cheese
4 leaves fresh basil or *sprigs of other fresh herb*

Preheat oven to 350°F. Cut rolls almost through lengthwise.

With cut side up, stuff rolls with Rainbow Pepper Sauté. Top peppers with thinly sliced or crumbled goat cheese. Put sandwiches on baking pan; heat 6–8 minutes until sandwiches are warm and cheese begins to melt. Garnish with herb sprigs; serve warm.

4 servings
1 serving = 1 sandwich

CAL.	CHO*(g)*	PRO.*(g)*	TOTAL FAT*(g)*	SAT. FAT*(g)*	CHOL.*(mg)*	FIBER*(g)*	SODIUM*(mg)*
350	40	15	15	7	20	3	605

Food exchanges per serving: 2 Starches plus 1½ Medium-Fat Meats plus 2 Vegetables plus 1 Fat
Low-sodium diets: This recipe is acceptable for occasional use. Omit salt from Rainbow Pepper Sauté.

Veggie Roll-Ups

Lahvosh is a delicious Armenian cracker bread that comes in several sizes and shapes. If you can find refrigerated, soft, unbaked lahvosh, preferably whole-wheat, skip the first steps of this recipe and just arrange and roll the sandwich. You can make other rolled sandwiches with the same technique using thinly sliced ham or turkey or tuna salad.

1 15-inch-diameter (about 5 ounces) lahvosh cracker
¼ cup light or reduced-calorie mayonnaise
4 ounces shaved Lorraine Swiss or light Jarlsberg or Swiss cheese
¼ teaspoon salt
⅛ teaspoon freshly ground pepper

1 red bell pepper, roasted and sliced
1 4½-ounce jar quartered marinated artichoke hearts, drained
½ red onion, sliced very thin
1 small ripe avocado, sliced thin
1½ cups (2 ounces total) alfalfa sprouts

If using crisp baked lahvosh, wet lahvosh under cold running water and put wet cracker between damp cloth kitchen towels for 45–60 minutes to soften. Sprinkle towel with more water if it starts to dry.

Put softened or unbaked lahvosh, sesame side down, on a damp towel. Brush top with mayonnaise. Cover with slices of cheese; season with salt and pepper. Arrange roasted pepper, artichoke hearts, onion, and avocado in rows across center of lahvosh. Distribute sprouts over top.

Gently roll lahvosh, jelly roll style, as tightly as possible into one long roll. Wrap roll tightly in plastic wrap and refrigerate at least 3 hours. Slice when ready to serve.

6 servings
1 serving = 2 1-inch slices

CAL.	CHO(g)	PRO.(g)	TOTAL FAT(g)	SAT. FAT(g)	CHOL.(mg)	FIBER(g)	SODIUM(mg)
240	25	10	12	3	15	1.5	440

Food exchanges per serving: 1 Starch plus 1 Medium-Fat Meat plus 1 Vegetable plus 1 Fat
Low-sodium diets: Omit salt.

Cajun Catfish Sandwiches

1 tablespoon light or reduced-
    calorie mayonnaise
1 teaspoon lemon juice
½ teaspoon drained capers
    (optional)

4 onion rolls or sandwich buns
4 fillets of Cajun Catfish (see
    Index), hot or warm
4 lettuce leaves
4 slices tomato

Make sandwich sauce by mixing mayonnaise, lemon juice, and capers.

Toast buns and spread with sandwich sauce. Stack buns with fish, lettuce, and tomatoes.

4 servings
1 serving = 1 sandwich

CAL.	CHO(g)	PRO.(g)	TOTAL FAT(g)	SAT. FAT(g)	CHOL.(mg)	FIBER(g)	SODIUM(mg)
380	31	27	16	2.5	50	0.5	945

Food exchanges per serving: 2 Starches plus 3 Medium-Fat Meats
Low-sodium diets: Prepare catfish using low-sodium instructions on recipe; omit capers.

Cold Turkey Reuben Sandwich

4 teaspoons plain low-fat yogurt
8 slices rye bread
8 ounces thinly sliced cooked turkey
    breast

1⅓ cups Sweet and Sour Red
    Cabbage (see Index), drained

Spread 1 teaspoon yogurt on each of 4 slices rye bread. Divide sliced turkey among tops of bread slices. Spoon ⅓ cup Sweet and Sour Red Cabbage on each sandwich; top with remaining bread.

4 servings
1 serving = 1 sandwich

CAL.	CHO(g)	PRO.(g)	TOTAL FAT(g)	SAT. FAT(g)	CHOL.(mg)	FIBER(g)	SODIUM(mg)
260	33	23	3	0.5	45	4.5	495

Food exchanges per serving: 2 Starches plus 2 Very Lean Meats
Low-sodium diets: Omit salt from Sweet and Sour Red Cabbage.

16
Meat

Carne Asada

1 lime
2 (1¼ pounds total) ½-inch-thick
    beef rib-eye steaks
⅓ cup shredded Co-Jack or
    Monterey Jack cheese

4 6-inch-diameter flour tortillas
½ cup prepared salsa

Squeeze lime juice over all surfaces of meat. Place steaks on a grill over a hot charcoal fire or under broiler. Grill 4 minutes; turn meat and cook another 3–4 minutes to medium rare.

While steaks are cooking, warm tortillas and salsa.

Divide cheese evenly on top of steaks. Cut each steak in half. Serve each portion of steak with a tortilla and salsa.

4 servings
1 serving = 1 4-ounce steak plus 1 tortilla plus 2 tablespoons salsa

CAL.	CHO(g)	PRO.(g)	TOTAL FAT(g)	SAT. FAT(g)	CHOL.(mg)	FIBER(g)	SODIUM(mg)
400	14	28	25	10	90	0.5	485

Food exchanges per serving: 4 Medium-Fat Meats plus 1 Starch plus 1 Fat
Low-sodium diets: Use unsalted salsa.

London Broil with Sautéed Mushrooms

London broil is from the top round of beef, a very lean but not tender cut. It needs to be marinated before cooking. To maximize tenderness, slice it thinly across the grain before serving. It is best cooked quickly to medium rare or medium. The meat can go from delectable to overcooked and tough in just a few minutes.

1 tablespoon Dijon or spicy mustard
2 tablespoons teriyaki marinade
2 cloves garlic, crushed
1½ pounds 1-inch-thick London broil

2 teaspoons margarine or butter
½ pound large mushrooms, sliced
¼ teaspoon salt
⅛ teaspoon freshly ground pepper

*M*ix mustard, teriyaki marinade, and garlic; brush mixture on meat. Cover and refrigerate at least 1 hour.

Broil or charbroil meat 5 minutes on each side until it is medium rare. While meat is cooking, heat margarine in a nonstick skillet. Add mushrooms and sauté; add salt and pepper when mushrooms are cooked.

Remove meat from broiler and allow it to rest 5 minutes. Slice it thinly across the grain, on the diagonal. Serve beef slices topped with sautéed mushrooms.

6 servings
1 serving = 3 ounces meat plus ⅓ cup mushrooms

CAL.	CHO(g)	PRO.(g)	TOTAL FAT(g)	SAT. FAT(g)	CHOL.(mg)	FIBER(g)	SODIUM(mg)
195	3	26	8	2.5	65	0.5	450

Food exchanges per serving: 3 Lean Meats plus 1 Vegetable
Low-sodium diets: Substitute light (reduced-sodium) soy sauce for teriyaki marinade; omit salt.

Bulgogi

This marinated steak is a popular Korean entree. Grill the steak and slice it, or cut the raw marinated steak into very thin strips and thread them onto skewers and grill. Try this with Spicy Orange Noodle Salad (see Index) or steamed rice, along with Fennel and Red Grapefruit Salad or Thai Cucumber Salad (see Index).

4 scallions, cut in pieces
1-inch cube peeled gingerroot or 2
*   tablespoons grated gingerroot*
2 tablespoons light (reduced-
*   sodium) soy sauce*
1 tablespoon rice or cider vinegar
1 tablespoon toasted sesame seeds

2 teaspoons Oriental dark-roasted
*   sesame oil*
1½ teaspoons honey or sugar
¼ teaspoon freshly ground pepper
1½ pounds boneless sirloin steak,
*   well trimmed*

*P*lace all ingredients except meat in the bowl of a food processor or blender. Process 1 minute to form a rough paste marinade.

Put meat on a cutting board. Score steak with ½-inch deep cuts in a 1-inch crisscross pattern on both sides of the meat. Pound meat with a meat mallet or heavy pan to tenderize.

Transfer meat to a shallow nonmetallic dish. Brush surfaces with marinade; pour remaining marinade over meat. Cover and refrigerate 2–8 hours, turning occasionally.

Prepare a hot charcoal fire or grill. Wipe off most of marinade. Grill steak until medium rare, about 4 minutes per side. Slice into thin strips and serve hot.

6 servings
1 serving = 3½ ounces sliced steak

CAL.	CHO(g)	PRO.(g)	TOTAL FAT(g)	SAT. FAT(g)	CHOL.(mg)	FIBER(g)	SODIUM(mg)
185	2	26	7	2.5	75	0	155

Food exchanges per serving: 3½ Lean Meats
Low-sodium diets: This recipe is excellent.

Pronto Spicy Beef with Black Bean Salsa

This recipe is the 1993 National Beef Cook-Off "Best of Beef" recipe and is used with permission of the American National CattleWomen, Inc. You can also make it with a 1½-inch-thick boneless sirloin steak.

1½- to 2-pound beef tri-top (bottom sirloin) roast

Seasoning

1 tablespoon chili powder
1 teaspoon ground cumin
1 teaspoon salt
½ teaspoon ground red pepper

Black Bean Salsa

1 15-ounce can black beans, rinsed and drained
1 medium tomato, chopped
1 small red onion, chopped fine
3 tablespoons chopped fresh cilantro

Combine chili powder, cumin, salt, and red pepper. Reserve 2 teaspoons for salsa.

Trim fat from beef roast. Press remaining seasoning mixture evenly onto surface of roast. Grill over medium coals to desired doneness, or use a prepared stovetop grill.

Meanwhile, in a medium bowl, combine beans, tomato, onion, cilantro, and reserved seasoning mixture; mix until blended.

Carve roast across the grain into thin slices. Arrange beef and bean salsa on serving platter.

6–8 servings (meat plus 2½ cups salsa)
1 serving = 3–4 ounces beef plus ⅓ cup salsa

CAL.	CHO(g)	PRO.(g)	TOTAL FAT(g)	SAT. FAT(g)	CHOL.(mg)	FIBER(g)	SODIUM(mg)
205	9	27	6	2.5	70	2.5	480

Food exchanges per serving: 3½ Lean Meats plus 1 Vegetable *or* 3½ Lean Meats plus 1 Starch
Low-sodium diets: Omit salt.

Beef Stroganoff

Beef stroganoff is traditionally served over noodles. Try it over curly noodles for a more festive look.

1¼ pounds beef tenderloin tips, well trimmed

2 teaspoons margarine, divided

2 medium sweet Spanish onions, sliced thin

8 ounces mushrooms, sliced thin

1 teaspoon minced garlic

1 cup beef broth

½ cup dry red wine or ½ cup additional beef broth

⅔ cup fat-free sour cream

⅓ cup sour half-and-half

½ teaspoon salt

¼ teaspoon freshly ground pepper

1 tablespoon minced fresh parsley

Cut tenderloin into ½-inch-wide strips. Heat 1 teaspoon of the margarine in a large nonstick skillet over high heat. Add meat strips and quickly sauté, about 1 minute, to brown edges of meat. Remove meat from pan.

Lower heat, add remaining 1 teaspoon margarine and the onions; sauté about 5 minutes until onions are translucent. Add mushrooms and garlic and continue cooking until mushrooms and onions are lightly browned.

Add broth and wine, and bring to a boil. Reduce heat, add fat-free sour cream, sour half-and-half, salt, and pepper. Stir in meat strips and heat only until meat is heated through. Top with minced parsley.

6 servings (makes 6 cups)
1 serving = 1 cup

CAL.	CHO(g)	PRO.(g)	TOTAL FAT(g)	SAT. FAT(g)	CHOL.(mg)	FIBER(g)	SODIUM(mg)
250	10	24	11	4	65	1.5	555

Food exchanges per serving: 3 Lean Meats plus 1 Vegetable
Low-sodium diets: Omit salt; substitute unsalted beef broth.

Hoisin Beef and Peppers

This recipe is also good with bok choy in place of the onions and green peppers. Beef is easier to slice thinly if it is well chilled.

¾ pound beef skirt steak, well
    trimmed
¼ cup Hoisin sauce
¾ teaspoon freshly ground black
    pepper, divided
1 tablespoon peanut or corn oil

1 large onion, sliced
2 medium green bell peppers,
    seeded and cut in rings
½ teaspoon salt
2 tablespoons dry roasted peanuts

Slice beef across the grain in ½-inch-wide strips. Toss steak strips with Hoisin sauce; season with ½ teaspoon of the black pepper.

Heat oil in a large nonstick skillet. Add onion and sauté about 5 minutes until translucent. Add green peppers and cook just until peppers begin to soften. Season vegetables with salt and remaining black pepper. Remove vegetables from pan.

Raise heat and add beef to the same skillet, turning to brown all sides but with inside of beef remaining rare. Return vegetables to pan, add peanuts, and stir to heat through.

4 servings (makes 5 cups)
1 serving = 1¼ cups

CAL.	CHO(g)	PRO.(g)	TOTAL FAT(g)	SAT. FAT(g)	CHOL.(mg)	FIBER(g)	SODIUM(mg)
265	17	19	12	3.5	45	2	655

Food exchanges per serving: 2½ Medium-Fat Meats plus 1 Other Carbohydrate
Low-sodium diets: This dish can be used occasionally unless sodium is severely restricted. Omit salt. Hoisin sauce has a lot of sodium, but there is no unsalted version available, and it is a primary flavor of this dish.

Sesame-Ginger Beef Steak

This recipe is a favorite from the Meat Board Test Kitchens. Make enough steak and peppers to turn leftovers into Spicy Sesame Beef Salad (see Index). Cook the meat to no more than medium so that it stays tender.

½ cup dry red wine	*2 teaspoons grated fresh gingerroot*
2 tablespoons dry sherry	*2 garlic cloves, minced*
1 tablespoon Oriental dark-roasted sesame oil	*1½ pounds beef flank, boneless sirloin, or top round steak*
1 tablespoon light (reduced-sodium) soy sauce	*1 medium green bell pepper*
	1 medium red bell pepper
1 tablespoon vinegar	*1 medium yellow bell pepper*

*I*n a small bowl or jar, combine wine, sherry, sesame oil, soy sauce, vinegar, ginger, and garlic. Refrigerate ¼ cup of this marinade.

Place steak in plastic bag; add remaining marinade, turning to coat. Close bag securely and marinate in refrigerator 6–8 hours (or overnight, if desired), turning occasionally.

Cut peppers in half lengthwise; remove seeds. Remove steak from marinade and place with pepper halves on grid over medium coals. Grill 12–15 minutes, turning once and brushing with marinade from beef before turning.

Cook steak to rare (140°F) or medium (160°F).

Carve steak diagonally across the grain into thin slices. Serve with grilled peppers and reserved marinade as sauce.

4 servings
1 serving = 3 ounces meat plus 1 pepper

CAL.	CHO*(g)*	PRO.*(g)*	TOTAL FAT*(g)*	SAT. FAT*(g)*	CHOL.*(mg)*	FIBER*(g)*	SODIUM*(mg)*
210	4	24	10	4	55	1	110

Food exchanges per serving: 3 Lean Meats plus 1 Vegetable
Low-sodium diets: This recipe is excellent.

Sukiyaki

Sukiyaki can be arranged decoratively on a large platter and cooked at the table using an electric skillet, a wok, or a chafing dish. This dish is traditionally served with steamed rice.

1 pound boneless lean skirt steak, sirloin, or tenderloin, partially frozen

6 scallions, cut into 1½-inch slivers

1 cup sliced onion

1 cup sliced celery

1 cup sliced mushrooms

5 ounces bean threads or other transparent noodles suitable for sukiyaki

2 ounces soft tofu, cut into ½-inch cubes

½ pound fresh spinach, trimmed, washed, and dried with paper towels

¼ cup beef broth

Sauce

¼ cup light (reduced-sodium) soy sauce

¼ cup dry white wine

¼ cup beef broth

Sugar substitute equivalent to 2 tablespoons sugar

*M*eat is partially frozen to aid in slicing; cut against the grain in paper-thin (¹⁄₁₆-inch) slices. Arrange meat on platter. Arrange scallions, onion, celery, and mushrooms on platter decoratively.

Heat 1 quart of water to boiling point in a 2-quart saucepan over high heat. Add noodles. Cook 2 minutes. Drain. For easy handling, use kitchen scissors and cut noodles into 2- to 3-inch pieces; add to platter along with tofu and spinach. Combine soy sauce, white wine, beef broth, and sugar substitute in a small bowl to make a sauce.

Heat wok to high. Add beef broth and beef slices; cook, stirring quickly with chopsticks until beef begins to brown. Add one-third of the sauce. Stir in scallions, onions, celery, and mushrooms; continue cooking and stirring as they cook. Stir in noodles and one-third of the sauce and mix well. Add tofu, spinach, and the remaining sauce. Serve immediately.

6 servings (makes 6 cups)

1 serving = 1 cup

CAL.	CHO(g)	PRO.(g)	TOTAL FAT(g)	SAT. FAT(g)	CHOL.(mg)	FIBER(g)	SODIUM(mg)
230	28	19	4	1	45	2	625

Food exchanges per serving: 2 Starches plus 1½ Lean Meats
Low-sodium diets: This recipe can be used occasionally if sodium restriction is mild or moderate.

Japanese Steak and Pea Pods

If the steak is partially frozen, it will be much easier to slice. After cutting, thaw to room temperature before cooking. This is a stir-fry recipe with a total cooking time of only about 7–8 minutes.

1¼ pounds boneless sirloin,
   partially frozen
2 tablespoons light (reduced-
   sodium) soy sauce
2 tablespoons dry sherry
1 tablespoon corn or peanut oil
1 cup diagonally sliced celery

¾ cup diagonally sliced scallions
   with tops
1 6-ounce package frozen Chinese
   pea pods, thawed, or 6 ounces
   cleaned fresh snow peas
¾ cup tomato juice

Cut meat into strips 1″ × 2″ × ½″. Mix the soy sauce and sherry together and pour over the steak strips; marinate 10 minutes.

Meanwhile, heat oil in a large nonstick skillet over high heat. Brown edges of meat quickly while stirring vigorously. Add celery and scallions. Cover, lower heat to medium, and cook 3 minutes. Add snow peas and tomato juice; cook, stirring, until snow peas are hot but still crisp. To keep meat tender and flavorful, do not overcook.

4 servings (makes 4 cups)
1 serving = 1 cup

CAL.	CHO(g)	PRO.(g)	TOTAL FAT(g)	SAT. FAT(g)	CHOL.(mg)	FIBER(g)	SODIUM(mg)
265	9	33	10	2.5	85	1	580

Food exchanges per serving: 4 Lean Meats plus 1 Vegetable
Low-sodium diets: Substitute unsalted tomato juice. This recipe is acceptable for occasional use.

Creole Steak

2 pounds lean round steak
¼ cup all-purpose flour
2 teaspoons salt
2 teaspoons paprika
½ teaspoon freshly ground black
    pepper
3 tablespoons corn or canola oil

1 cup chopped onion
⅓ cup chopped green bell pepper
1 16-ounce can tomatoes
½ cup uncooked rice
1 cup condensed beef broth
1 cup water

Cut steak into seven equal serving pieces. In a medium bowl, mix flour, salt, paprika, and black pepper; dredge meat in mixture.

Heat oil in a large nonstick skillet. Lightly brown onion and green pepper. Remove vegetables from oil. Brown meat in remaining oil. Cover meat with onion and green pepper. Cut up tomatoes and add with their liquid to meat.

Sprinkle rice into pan; add broth and water. Mix thoroughly; bring to a boil. Lower heat, and cover tightly. Simmer 1½ hours or until meat is tender, stirring occasionally.

7 servings
1 serving = 3 ounces meat plus ½ cup rice mixture

CAL.	CHO(g)	PRO.(g)	TOTAL FAT(g)	SAT. FAT(g)	CHOL.(mg)	FIBER(g)	SODIUM(mg)
325	20	32	13	3	75	1	1,045

Food exchanges per serving: 4 Lean Meats plus 1 Starch plus 1 Vegetable
Low-sodium diets: Omit salt. Use unsalted canned tomatoes and beef broth.

Roast Beef with Caraway Seeds

¾ cup chopped onion, divided
1 teaspoon salt
1 tablespoon caraway seeds
2½ pounds boneless rolled rump or
    chuck roast, well trimmed

1 tablespoon canola or corn oil
⅓ cup vinegar
1 cup unsweetened apple juice

Preheat oven to 325°F. In a small bowl, combine ¼ cup of the onion with salt and caraway seeds. Press this mixture into the roast.

In a roasting pan, heat the oil and add remaining onion; stir over medium heat for 5 minutes, until onions are translucent. Put roast in pan; add vinegar, apple juice, and enough water to cover the bottom of the pan with ½ inch liquid.

Bake, uncovered, about 1½ hours for medium rare or longer if you prefer. Baste with liquid several times during cooking. Trim away extra fat, and discard drippings.

7 servings (makes 1¾ pounds cooked before final trimming; about 22 ounces edible lean meat)
1 serving = 3-ounce slice lean beef

CAL.	CHO*(g)*	PRO.*(g)*	TOTAL FAT*(g)*	SAT. FAT*(g)*	CHOL.*(mg)*	FIBER*(g)*	SODIUM*(mg)*
215	7	26	9	2.5	70	0.5	375

Food exchanges per serving: 3 Lean Meats plus 1 Vegetable
Low-sodium diets: Substitute 2 cloves garlic, crushed, for the salt.

Roast Beef with Anchovies

Garlic lovers should insert thin slices of garlic into the beef along with the anchovies.

4 pounds eye of round of beef, well trimmed

2 tablespoons olive oil

1 2-ounce can flat anchovies, packed in oil

2 teaspoons coarsely ground pepper

Preheat oven to 300°F. Rub beef with olive oil and oil from anchovy can. Cut slits into beef, and insert half the anchovies into the slits; spread remaining anchovies on top of meat. Sprinkle roast with pepper. Put roast in a shallow roasting pan; cover tightly with foil.

Roast 1 hour for medium-rare. Meat thermometer should read 150°F. Cook longer if you prefer your meat more well done. Let roast rest 10 minutes before carving.

12 servings
1 serving = 4 ounces lean meat (Hearty eaters may have larger portions, so plan accordingly.)

CAL.	CHO(g)	PRO.(g)	TOTAL FAT(g)	SAT. FAT(g)	CHOL.(mg)	FIBER(g)	SODIUM(mg)
220	0	34	8	2.5	80	0	245

Food exchanges per serving: 4 Lean Meats
Low-sodium diets: Substitute 4 cloves of garlic, cut in slivers, for the anchovies.

Party Beef Tenderloin

A whole beef tenderloin, when trimmed, weighs approximately 4 pounds (raw). Have your meat cutter trim a whole or a half tenderloin. He or she will lard it or put strips of fat across the top because it is a very lean cut. This exterior fat will keep the meat juicy, and you discard it before eating the meat. This cut is wonderful cooked on a barbecue. Season the meat, and cook it over coals with white ash. The cooking time depends on the heat of the fire, so watch it carefully and use an instant-read thermometer to avoid overcooking.

1 whole beef tenderloin, trimmed   *1 teaspoon cracked pepper*
2 teaspoons minced fresh garlic   *½ teaspoon salt*

*P*reheat oven to 450°F or prepare grill. Season roast with garlic, cracked pepper, and salt or your favorite seasonings. Put tenderloin on grill or on a rack in an uncovered roasting pan.

Roast or grill 40 minutes for rare to medium-rare beef. A meat thermometer will register 140°F. Let meat rest for 10 minutes before slicing so that the juices remain in the meat.

10 servings
1 serving = 3 ounces (Hearty eaters will want more, so plan accordingly.)

CAL.	CHO*(g)*	PRO.*(g)*	TOTAL FAT*(g)*	SAT. FAT*(g)*	CHOL.*(mg)*	FIBER*(g)*	SODIUM*(mg)*
190	0	24	10	3.5	70	0	160

Food exchanges per serving: 3 Lean Meats
Low-sodium diets: Omit salt.

Classic Beef Bourguignon

This slow-cooking (2½ hours), delicious, fragrant dish is nice to make on a Sunday afternoon. It can be prepared ahead and for a crowd. Serve it over noodles with crusty bread and a simple salad.

2 pounds lean boneless beef, cut into 1½-inch cubes	*1 teaspoon minced garlic*
¾ teaspoon herbes de Provence or other herb mixture	*12 ounces carrots, peeled and cut into 1-inch lengths*
¾ teaspoon coarsely ground pepper	*1½ cups peeled pearl onions or frozen small whole onions*
2 tablespoons canola or corn oil	*12 ounces small mushrooms, whole*
1 14-ounce can beef broth	*2 tablespoons cornstarch*
1⅓ cups Burgundy wine, divided	*¼ cup minced fresh parsley*

Sprinkle herbs and pepper over beef pieces. Heat oil in a Dutch oven or deep pan; add meat and brown about 10 minutes. Pour off drippings. Add broth, 1 cup wine, and garlic. Reduce heat to low, cover pan tightly, and simmer 1 hour.

Add carrots, cook for 30 minutes, covered. Add onions and mushrooms. Cook another 30 minutes, covered.

Mix cornstarch with remaining ⅓ cup wine. Add this mixture to stew, stirring until sauce has thickened. Add parsley and serve.

6 servings (makes 6 cups)
1 serving = 1 cup

CAL.	CHO*(g)*	PRO.*(g)*	TOTAL FAT*(g)*	SAT. FAT*(g)*	CHOL.*(mg)*	FIBER*(g)*	SODIUM*(mg)*
310	16	36	10	2.5	90	2.5	575

Food exchanges per serving: 4 Lean Meats plus 1 Starch *or* 4 Lean Meats plus 3 Vegetables
Low-sodium diets: Substitute unsalted beef broth.

Autumn Beef Stew

This recipe may be simmered in a large covered pot on top of the stove. The oven method saves pot watching.

¼ cup all-purpose flour	1 teaspoon Worcestershire sauce
1¼ teaspoons salt	2 cups pared, quartered, and sliced potato
½ teaspoon freshly ground pepper	
½ teaspoon dry mustard	1 cup sliced onion
1¼ pounds top round steak, 1 inch thick	1 cup sliced carrot
	2 teaspoons snipped fresh dill or ½ teaspoon dried dill (optional)
1 tablespoon canola or corn oil	
2½ cups water	

Preheat oven to 350°F. Combine flour, salt, pepper, and mustard in a paper bag. Trim off all fat around outside of round steak; cut meat into 1-inch cubes. Shake meat cubes in paper bag with flour, a few at a time, until well coated.

Heat oil in a large skillet; brown meat over medium heat, turning with tongs until evenly browned. Transfer meat to a 2½-quart casserole; set aside.

Sprinkle seasoned flour remaining in paper bag into the fat remaining in skillet; stir vigorously until smooth and mixed. Add water and Worcestershire sauce. Cook and stir until smooth; pour on top of meat in casserole. Cover and cook in the oven 2 hours.

Mix vegetables and dill into meat; cover and cook in oven 1 more hour or until meat and vegetables are tender.

4 servings (makes 5 cups)
1 serving = 1¼ cups

CAL.	CHO(g)	PRO.(g)	TOTAL FAT(g)	SAT. FAT(g)	CHOL.(mg)	FIBER(g)	SODIUM(mg)
330	26	35	8	2	80	3	790

Food exchanges per serving: 4 Lean Meats plus 1 Starch plus 2 Vegetables
Low-sodium diets: Omit salt.

Variation: Old-Fashioned Lamb Stew
Substitute lean lamb cubes, and add extra dill to taste.

Old-Fashioned Meat Loaf

This recipe was a favorite of Kay Middleton, coauthor of the first edition of this book. We enjoyed it together in meat loaf sandwiches. The molded method, rather than filling a loaf pan, allows more fat to drain away.

1½ pounds 90% lean ground beef
2 slices whole-grain bread, finely crumbled
½ cup chopped onion
½ cup finely chopped celery

½ cup beef broth
½ cup egg substitute or 2 eggs
1 tablespoon Worcestershire sauce
¼ cup catsup or chili sauce

Preheat oven to 350°F. Line a shallow baking pan with foil.

In a large bowl, combine all ingredients except catsup, and mix well with your hands. Turn meat mixture onto foil in pan, and shape it into a loaf 4½ inches wide, 2½ inches high, and 8 inches long. With a knife, make a crisscross pattern across the top. Drizzle catsup across the top.

Cover meat loaf with a tent of foil that does not touch the top. Bake 45 minutes. Remove foil cover and bake uncovered another 30 minutes.

Remove meat loaf from pan and cool 5 minutes before slicing. If serving hot, slice into ¾-inch slices. If chilled, cut half as thick and double the number of slices per serving.

10 servings (makes 1 loaf weighing 1 pound 12 ounces cooked)
1 serving = 1 ¾-inch slice (almost 3 ounces)

CAL.	CHO(g)	PRO.(g)	TOTAL FAT(g)	SAT. FAT(g)	CHOL.(mg)	FIBER(g)	SODIUM(mg)
155	6	16	7	2.5	40	0.5	275

Food exchanges per serving: 2 Lean Meats plus 1 Vegetable *or* 2 Lean Meats plus ½ Starch
Low-sodium diets: Substitute unsalted beef broth and unsalted catsup.

Polpettone

This is a variation of my friend Clara Coen's family recipe brought with her from Italy. This firm and very tasty meat loaf is delicious hot and even better served cold or in sandwiches.

1 pound 90% lean ground round or sirloin	3 tablespoons chopped fresh parsley
½ pound turkey or chicken Italian sausage	1 egg
1 tablespoon dried basil	¾ teaspoon crushed dried rosemary
⅔ cup bread crumbs	½ teaspoon crushed red pepper flakes
¼ cup grated Parmesan cheese	2 hard-boiled eggs

Preheat oven to 400°F. Combine all ingredients except hard-boiled eggs in a large bowl. Mix by hand until crumbs are well distributed through meat.

Line an 8½″ × 4½″ × 2½″ loaf pan with foil. Spray foil with cooking spray. Pack half of meat mixture into bottom of pan. Cut each egg into six wedges, and arrange wedges in strips running the length of the loaf. Cover egg layer with remaining meat mixture; press together firmly to form well-shaped loaf. Push loaf to one side of pan to create a gap for fat drippings to flow into.

Bake 30 minutes. Reduce heat to 325°F and bake 30 minutes more.

Turn meat loaf out of pan and drain well. Allow to sit 10 minutes before cutting into thin (2-ounce) slices.

7 servings (makes 1 loaf weighing 1 pound 12 ounces cooked)
1 serving = 2 2-ounce (about ½-inch) slices

CAL.	CHO(g)	PRO.(g)	TOTAL FAT(g)	SAT. FAT(g)	CHOL.(mg)	FIBER(g)	SODIUM(mg)
255	9	24	14	5	150	0.5	430

Food exchanges per serving: 3 Medium-Fat Meats plus ½ Starch
Low-sodium diets: This recipe is not suitable.

Szechwan Bean Curd

Hot oil is an infused chili oil used in Asian cooking. If you don't have it and want a spicier flavor, increase the red pepper flakes to ½ teaspoon.

4 ounces 85% lean ground beef
1 cup chopped scallions with tops
1 clove garlic, minced
¾ cup Chicken Stock (see Index) or chicken broth
2 tablespoons light (reduced-sodium) soy sauce
1 tablespoon chili sauce

1 teaspoon sesame oil
¼ teaspoon hot oil (optional)
¼ teaspoon crushed red pepper flakes
2 tablespoons cornstarch
2 tablespoons cold water
1 cup bean curd (tofu), cut into ½-inch cubes

Place ground beef, scallions, and garlic in a nonstick skillet; cook over medium heat, stirring quickly, until beef is browned. Stir in Chicken Stock, soy sauce, chili sauce, oils, and red pepper flakes.

Mix cornstarch with cold water. Add to skillet. Cook, stirring constantly, until sauce thickens. Gently stir in bean curd. Continue cooking over medium heat 3 minutes.

4 servings (makes 4 cups)
1 serving = 1 cup

CAL.	CHO(g)	PRO.(g)	TOTAL FAT(g)	SAT. FAT(g)	CHOL.(mg)	FIBER(g)	SODIUM(mg)
160	9	12	9	2.5	20	1.5	405

Food exchanges per serving: 2 Medium-Fat Meats plus ½ Starch
Low-sodium diets: This recipe is acceptable.

Lemony Beef, Vegetables, and Barley

From the Meat Board Test Kitchen, here's one-pan cooking at its nutrient-rich best! Be sure to purchase quick-cooking barley—it cooks in 15 minutes. I like a bit more lemon, so I added an extra teaspoon of grated lemon zest to the original recipe.

1 pound 90% lean ground beef	½ teaspoon salt
8 ounces mushrooms, sliced	¼ teaspoon freshly ground pepper
1 medium onion, chopped	1 10-ounce package frozen peas
1 clove garlic, crushed	and carrots, defrosted
1 14-ounce can beef broth	2 teaspoons grated lemon zest
½ cup quick-cooking barley	

*I*n a large nonstick skillet, cook and stir ground beef, mushrooms, onion, and garlic over medium heat 8–10 minutes or until beef is no longer pink, breaking beef up into ¾-inch crumbles. Pour off drippings.

Stir in broth, barley, salt, and pepper; bring to a boil. Reduce heat to medium-low. Cover tightly, and simmer 10 minutes. Add peas and carrots; continue cooking 2–5 minutes or until barley is tender. Stir in lemon zest.

6 servings (makes 6 cups)
1 serving = 1 cup

CAL.	CHO(g)	PRO.(g)	TOTAL FAT(g)	SAT. FAT(g)	CHOL.(mg)	FIBER(g)	SODIUM(mg)
245	19	17	11	4	45	2	725

Food exchanges per serving: 2 Medium-Fat Meats plus 1 Starch plus 1 Vegetable
Low-sodium diets: Substitute unsalted broth; omit salt.

Hungarian Cabbage Rolls

12 (about 1 pound) large green
   cabbage leaves
1 cup diced cooked carrot
¾ pound 90% lean ground beef
¼ cup uncooked brown rice
1 egg, beaten slightly
1½ cups tomato juice

1 16-ounce can stewed tomatoes,
   with liquid
1 medium onion, sliced
¼ teaspoon salt
¼ teaspoon freshly ground pepper
2 cloves garlic, crushed

Preheat oven to 325°F. Boil 2 quarts water in a large saucepan or Dutch oven. Arrange cabbage leaves loosely in pan. Cover and cook over medium heat until cabbage is limp but not soft, about 8 minutes. Drain and cool leaves.

Puree carrot in a blender or a food processor fitted with steel blade. In a medium bowl, mix carrot with ground beef, rice, and egg. Spoon 2 tablespoons meat mixture onto each cabbage leaf. Tuck ends in and roll up jelly roll style.

Place seam side down in a 9″ × 13″ baking pan. Pour tomato juice, tomatoes and liquid, onion slices, and seasonings over cabbage rolls. Cover and bake 1 hour; uncover and cook an additional 30 minutes.

6 servings (makes 12 cabbage rolls)
1 serving = 2 cabbage rolls

CAL.	CHO(g)	PRO.(g)	TOTAL FAT(g)	SAT. FAT(g)	CHOL.(mg)	FIBER(g)	SODIUM(mg)
210	23	16	7	2.5	70	5	585

Food exchanges per serving: 2 Lean Meats plus 1 Starch plus 1 Vegetable
Low-sodium diets: Omit salt. Substitute unsalted tomato juice and unsalted canned tomatoes.

Easy Beef and Salsa Burrito

This recipe is adapted from a 1993 National Beef Cook-Off finalist. Use mild, medium, or hot salsa as you prefer. My husband, Peter, comments: "*This is delicious!*"

1 pound 90% lean ground beef
1 tablespoon chili powder
¼ teaspoon ground cumin
¼ teaspoon salt
¼ teaspoon freshly ground pepper
1 10-ounce package frozen chopped
     spinach, defrosted and well
     drained

1 cup prepared chunky salsa
¾ cup shredded Co-Jack cheese
1 package (10 small) 6-inch-
     diameter tortillas, warmed

In a large nonstick skillet, brown ground beef over medium heat 8–10 minutes or until no longer pink, stirring occasionally. Put ground beef in a colander and rinse to remove fat.

Return beef to skillet; season with chili powder, cumin, salt, and pepper. Stir in spinach and salsa; heat through. Remove from heat; stir in cheese.

Warm tortillas in the oven.

To serve, spoon ⅓ cup beef mixture into center of each tortilla. Fold bottom edge up over filling; fold sides to center, overlapping edges.

10 servings
1 serving = 1 burrito

CAL.	CHO(g)	PRO.(g)	TOTAL FAT(g)	SAT. FAT(g)	CHOL.(mg)	FIBER(g)	SODIUM(mg)
190	14	14	8	3.5	35	1.5	515

Food exchanges per serving: 2 Lean Meats plus 1 Starch
Low-sodium diets: Use unsalted salsa.

Chili con Carne

If you break crackers on top of chili, count 6 saltines or 24 oyster crackers as one Starch Exchange.

1 pound 85% lean ground beef
1 cup chopped onion
1 cup finely chopped celery
½ cup finely chopped green bell pepper
1 16-ounce can tomatoes, cut up, with liquid
1¼ teaspoons salt

2 cloves garlic, minced
½ teaspoon dried oregano
1 tablespoon chili powder (more if desired)
1 16-ounce can kidney beans, with liquid
1 cup water

Sauté beef in a medium-sized nonstick pot until no pink remains. Drain meat in colander to remove fat; return meat to pot. Add onion, celery, and green pepper; mix well. Cover and cook over medium heat 2–3 minutes.

Add all remaining ingredients; mix well. Bring to a boil; cover, reduce heat to low, and simmer gently 25 minutes, stirring occasionally.

6 servings (makes 6 cups)
1 serving = 1 cup

CAL.	CHO(g)	PRO.(g)	TOTAL FAT(g)	SAT. FAT(g)	CHOL.(mg)	FIBER(g)	SODIUM(mg)
250	19	19	11	4	45	6.5	915

Food exchanges per serving: 2 Medium-Fat Meats plus 1 Starch plus 1 Vegetable
Low-sodium diets: Omit salt. Use unsalted canned vegetables and unsalted crackers for topping.

Sloppy Joes

This recipe is among the best known of Kay Middleton's (coauthor of the first edition of this book). Kids love it.

1 pound 85% lean ground beef
¼ cup finely chopped onion
¾ cup finely chopped celery with
    leaves
¼ cup chopped green bell pepper
½ teaspoon grated lemon zest

¼ cup catsup
¾ cup beef broth
1 teaspoon salt
½ teaspoon dry mustard
1 teaspoon Worcestershire sauce

Cook meat in a large nonstick skillet. Drain to remove fat and return meat to skillet. Add onion, celery, and green pepper. Stir and cook 1–2 minutes.

Combine all remaining ingredients in a small bowl; add to meat. Mix well and bring to a boil. Cover, reduce heat to low, and let simmer gently 15 minutes, stirring frequently, until cooked and well mixed.

6 servings (makes 3 cups)
1 serving = ½ cup

CAL.	CHO(g)	PRO.(g)	TOTAL FAT(g)	SAT. FAT(g)	CHOL.(mg)	FIBER(g)	SODIUM(mg)
170	4	14	11	4	45	0.5	570

Food exchanges per serving: 2 Medium-Fat Meats plus 1 Vegetable (When served on a whole hamburger bun, add 2 Starch Exchanges.)
Low-sodium diets: Omit salt. Use low-sodium catsup and unsalted beef broth.

Beef Porcupines in Tomato Sauce

1 pound 90% lean ground beef

¼ cup uncooked long-grain rice

¼ cup dry bread crumbs

1 teaspoon salt

2 tablespoons minced fresh parsley

2 tablespoons water

1 tablespoon canola or corn oil

1 10½-ounce can condensed tomato
    soup

2 cloves garlic, minced

2 teaspoons Worcestershire sauce

2 cups water

Combine ground beef, rice, bread crumbs, salt, parsley, and 2 tablespoons water. Roll beef mixture into 20 meatballs, each about 1¼ inch in diameter.

Heat oil in a large nonstick skillet. Add meatballs and brown over medium heat, turning frequently. Add remaining ingredients; cover and simmer gently 1 hour or until rice is tender. Serve meatballs with tomato sauce from pan.

4 servings
1 serving = 5 meatballs plus ⅓ cup sauce

CAL.	CHO(g)	PRO.(g)	TOTAL FAT(g)	SAT. FAT(g)	CHOL.(mg)	FIBER(g)	SODIUM(mg)
350	25	26	16	5	70	0.5	1,235

Food exchanges per serving: 3 Medium-Fat Meats plus 1 Starch plus 1 Other Carbohydrate *or* 3 Medium-Fat Meats plus 1 Starch plus 1 Vegetable
Low-sodium diets: Omit salt; use unsalted tomato soup.

Roast Veal with Mushrooms

Select very light-colored veal, which is younger and more tender than dark-colored veal.

1 3-pound boneless veal rump roast, boned and tied	*2 teaspoons snipped fresh rosemary or ½ teaspoon dried rosemary*
1 teaspoon salt	*8 slices bacon*
½ teaspoon cracked pepper	*½ pound fresh mushrooms, sliced*

*P*reheat oven to 325°F. Season roast with salt, pepper, and rosemary. Arrange bacon slices across top of roast. Roast meat, uncovered, about 40 minutes per pound, until a meat thermometer registers 165°F (medium-well done). During last half hour of cooking, add sliced mushrooms to roasting pan.

Pour pan drippings and mushrooms into a gravy separator or small bowl. Remove separable fat with gravy separator or turkey baster. Discard separable fat and serve remaining liquid with mushrooms as gravy.

8 servings
1 serving = 3 ounces veal plus ½–1 slice bacon plus 2 tablespoons mushroom gravy.

CAL.	CHO*(g)*	PRO.*(g)*	TOTAL FAT*(g)*	SAT. FAT*(g)*	CHOL.*(mg)*	FIBER*(g)*	SODIUM*(mg)*
330	1	35	20	7.5	195	0.5	460

Food exchanges per serving: 4 Medium-Fat Meats
Low-sodium diets: Omit salt; use only 4 slices bacon.

Baked Veal Chops

½ cup skim milk
1 teaspoon salt
¼ teaspoon freshly ground pepper
Dash hot-pepper sauce
¼ cup crushed cornflakes
1 tablespoon snipped fresh basil or
　　2 teaspoons dried basil

4 (about 1½ pounds total) lean loin
　　or shoulder veal chops
2 teaspoons canola or corn oil
1 tablespoon fresh lemon juice
2 teaspoons chopped fresh parsley
1 teaspoon freshly grated lemon
　　zest

In a shallow dish, combine milk, salt, pepper, and hot-pepper sauce. In another shallow dish, mix cornflakes and basil. Dip veal chops first in milk mixture, then in seasoned cornflake crumbs to coat on all sides. Place on a plate, cover, and refrigerate for at least 30 minutes.

Preheat oven to 375°F. Prepare a shallow baking pan with nonstick cooking spray. Place chops in pan; drizzle oil on top. Bake 45–60 minutes or until tender.

In a small bowl, mix lemon juice, parsley, and lemon zest. Sprinkle on chops 2 minutes before removing from the oven.

4 servings
1 serving = 1 chop

CAL.	CHO(g)	PRO.(g)	TOTAL FAT(g)	SAT. FAT(g)	CHOL.(mg)	FIBER(g)	SODIUM(mg)
170	8	21	6	1	80	0	460

Food exchanges per serving: 3 Lean Meats plus ½ Starch
Low-sodium diets: Omit salt.

Grilled Veal Chops with Fruit Salsa

This recipe was adapted from the 1993 Grand Prize Winner of the Favorite Veal Recipe Contest.

Fruit Salsa

1 small ripe papaya, peeled, seeded, and cut into ½-inch pieces

1 ripe nectarine, pitted and chopped

2 tablespoons finely chopped red bell pepper

1 jalapeño pepper, seeded and chopped fine

2 tablespoons chopped cilantro

1 small green scallion, sliced thin

Veal Chops

6 (6 ounces each) veal loin or rib chops, cut ¾ inch thick

1 tablespoon olive oil

¼ teaspoon salt

⅛ teaspoon white pepper

2 tablespoons chopped cilantro

Cilantro sprigs for garnish

*I*n a medium bowl, combine salsa ingredients. Cover and set aside.

Lightly brush veal chops with olive oil; season with salt and white pepper. Sprinkle cilantro on both sides of each chop. Place veal on grid over medium coals. Grill 12–14 minutes uncovered (10–12 minutes covered) for medium, or to desired doneness; turn once. Garnish chops with cilantro sprigs and serve with salsa.

6 servings
1 serving = 1 chop plus ¼ cup salsa

CAL.	CHO(g)	PRO.(g)	TOTAL FAT(g)	SAT. FAT(g)	CHOL.(mg)	FIBER(g)	SODIUM(mg)
265	7	25	15	5.5	105	1	185

Food exchanges per serving: 3 Medium-Fat Meats plus ½ Fruit
Low-sodium diets: This recipe is excellent.

Veal Piccata

Veal scallops are very thin slices of veal from the round or loin. They should have no visible fat or tendon, and are sometimes cut and sold frozen. Turkey breast slices may be substituted to make Turkey Piccata.

2 tablespoons all-purpose flour
½ teaspoon salt
¼ teaspoon freshly ground pepper
1¼ pounds veal scallops, sliced very thin
3 tablespoons margarine, divided

1 lemon with rind, sliced very thin crosswise
⅓ cup dry white wine
⅓ cup fresh lemon juice
2 tablespoons chopped fresh parsley

Combine flour, salt, and pepper: sprinkle on both sides of veal scallops. Heat half of the margarine over medium heat in a large nonstick skillet, and quickly sauté half the veal 2–3 minutes, until the edges brown slightly; repeat process with remaining margarine and veal. Remove meat from pan and set it aside.

To the pan drippings add three-quarters of the lemon slices, all of the wine, and the lemon juice; scrape drippings into this liquid, mix well, and bring mixture to a boil. Return veal to pan and cook gently 2–3 minutes to blend flavors.

Serve immediately on a warmed platter. Garnish with remaining lemon slices and chopped parsley.

4 servings
1 serving = 3½ ounces cooked veal plus 2 tablespoons lemon sauce

CAL.	CHO(g)	PRO.(g)	TOTAL FAT(g)	SAT. FAT(g)	CHOL.(mg)	FIBER(g)	SODIUM(mg)
265	8	31	11	2	110	0	465

Food exchanges per serving: 4 Lean Meats plus ½ Fruit
Low-sodium diets: Omit salt. Use unsalted margarine.

Honey-Dijon Veal and Zucchini Stir-Fry

This recipe, adapted from one developed in the Test Kitchens of the National Live Stock and Meat Board, uses lean, tender veal leg cutlets, ideal for stir-frying—just cut into strips and cook. Using a nonstick skillet means less oil is needed; constant stirring of veal and vegetables ensures fast, even cooking. A prepared honey-Dijon barbecue sauce is a quick, one-step way to make a no-fail sauce for the stir-fry. You can make the recipe with 3 zucchinis if you want to add a Vegetable Exchange to this one-dish meal.

4 ounces uncooked spaghetti

1 pound veal leg cutlets, cut ⅛- to ¼-inch thick

1 tablespoon corn or canola oil, divided

1 medium onion, cut into thin wedges

1 medium zucchini, cut lengthwise in half and then crosswise into thin slices

¼ cup prepared honey-Dijon barbecue sauce

1 tablespoon water

Cook spaghetti according to package directions; keep warm. If veal cutlets are thicker, pound into ⅛-inch thickness. Stack veal; cut into 1″ × 3″ strips.

In a large nonstick skillet, heat 1 teaspoon of the oil over medium-high heat. Add half the veal and stir-fry 1–2 minutes or until outside surface is no longer pink. (Do not overcook.) Remove veal. Repeat with remaining veal and additional 1 teaspoon oil.

In same skillet, heat the remaining 1 teaspoon oil. Add onions and stir-fry 2 minutes. Add zucchini and stir-fry 3 minutes or until crisp-tender. Add barbecue sauce, water, and veal; stir to combine. Heat through.

Serve over the spaghetti.

4 servings
1 serving = ½ cup spaghetti plus 1 cup stir-fry

CAL.	CHO(g)	PRO.(g)	TOTAL FAT(g)	SAT. FAT(g)	CHOL.(mg)	FIBER(g)	SODIUM(mg)
310	33	29	6	1	90	1.5	210

Food exchanges per serving: 3 Lean Meats plus 2 Starches plus 1 Vegetable
Low-sodium diets: This recipe is acceptable.

Tex-Mex Veal Burgers

This wonderful recipe was the 1993 Third Place Winner in the Favorite Veal Recipe Contest Sponsored by the National Live Stock and Meat Board. The burgers can also be made with ground turkey. I make the veal patties ¾ inch thick because I like the extra moistness of the meat. I have also cooked them indoors on a stovetop grill. The generous amount of bell peppers not only adds flavor but really boosts levels of protective antioxidant vitamins.

1 teaspoon olive oil	2 tablespoons dry bread crumbs
⅔ cup finely chopped red or green bell pepper	1 tablespoon finely chopped cilantro
½ cup finely chopped onion	½ teaspoon salt
1 egg, lightly beaten	1 pound ground veal
	1 cup prepared or home-style salsa

In a small nonstick skillet, heat oil over medium heat until hot. Add bell pepper and onion; cook and stir 5 minutes or until tender. Cool.

In a large bowl, combine pepper mixture, egg, bread crumbs, cilantro, and salt. Add veal; mix lightly but thoroughly. Shape into 4 ½-inch patties.

Place patties on grid over medium coals. Grill 10–12 minutes uncovered (8–10 minutes covered) for medium, or to desired doneness; turn once.

Serve with salsa.

4 servings
1 serving = 1 burger plus ¼ cup salsa

CAL.	CHO(g)	PRO.(g)	TOTAL FAT(g)	SAT. FAT(g)	CHOL.(mg)	FIBER(g)	SODIUM(mg)
220	9	22	9	3.5	140	0.5	1,035

Food exchanges per serving: 3 Lean Meats plus 2 Vegetables
Low-sodium diets: Omit salt; use unsalted salsa.

Rack of Lamb

This recipe is an easy but elegant entree. Have the meat cutter remove the flat bone at the back of the rack so that you can carve the chops easily.

1 tablespoon Dijon mustard
1 tablespoon lemon juice
2 cloves garlic, crushed
¼ teaspoon salt
½ teaspoon dried rosemary, thyme,
  or mint leaves, crushed

1–1½-pound rack of lamb (7–8
  ribs), well trimmed
6 sprigs watercress

Preheat oven to 500°F. In a small bowl, combine all ingredients except lamb and watercress. Make shallow crisscross marks on the fat side of the meat. Brush all surfaces of lamb with mustard mixture.

Put lamb in a small roasting pan lined with foil or in a disposable pan. Fold a piece of foil around exposed rib ends of chops to protect against burning. Roast meat 10 minutes. Reduce heat to 400°F; roast another 20–30 minutes until medium rare. A meat thermometer should reach 145°F.

To serve, cut into single-rib portions. Garnish chops with watercress.

3 servings
1 serving = 2–3 small chops

CAL.	CHO(g)	PRO.(g)	TOTAL FAT(g)	SAT. FAT(g)	CHOL.(mg)	FIBER(g)	SODIUM(mg)
205	1	22	11	4	75	0	370

Food exchanges per serving: 3 Lean Meats
Low-sodium diets: Omit salt.

Roast Leg of Lamb

Boned cuts are easier to carve, but they take longer to cook. Traditional accompaniments include potatoes and peas, green beans, tomatoes, or Ratatouille (see Index).

1 5- to 8-pound whole leg of lamb
    or *1 boned and rolled 4- to 6-pound leg of lamb*
2 large cloves of garlic, cut in slivers

1½ teaspoons light (reduced-sodium) soy sauce
1 teaspoon coarsely ground pepper
1 teaspoon dried rosemary, thyme, or dill

Preheat oven to 350°F. Make small, deep slits in surface of roast and insert slivers of garlic. Rub surface of meat with soy sauce. Sprinkle with coarsely ground pepper and rosemary, thyme, or dill.

Place lamb, fat side up, on a rack in a roasting pan. Set in middle of the oven. Roast for 1½ hours, basting with fat from bottom of pan every 30 minutes. Roast 45 minutes more. Test with an instant-read meat thermometer every 15 minutes. Lamb will be medium and juicy at 140°F. A leg with bone will take about 1½ hours to cook; a boned and rolled leg about 2¼–2½ hours.

When lamb is done, remove from oven and place on a board or platter to rest so juices will stay in the meat. Remove and discard strings if roast is rolled.

Carve roast in long, thin slices parallel to the bone. Trim fat before eating.

Number of servings depends on size of roast
1 serving = 3 ounces lean lamb

CAL.	CHO(g)	PRO.(g)	TOTAL FAT(g)	SAT. FAT(g)	CHOL.(mg)	FIBER(g)	SODIUM(mg)
175	0	24	8	3	80	0	120

Food exchanges per serving: 3 Lean Meats
Low-sodium diets: Season meat generously with salt-free herb blend; omit soy sauce.

Shish Kebab

You can substitute or add green bell pepper, cherry tomatoes, or other quick-cooking vegetables. You will also enjoy this recipe using cubes of boneless chicken breasts or thighs instead of the lamb. Chicken marinates faster than lamb.

3 tablespoons virgin olive oil
2 tablespoons balsamic vinegar
2 teaspoons dried oregano
½ teaspoon salt
¼ teaspoon freshly ground pepper

1 large sweet Spanish onion
1 pound lean lamb, cut into 1-inch
* cubes*
8 ounces whole mushrooms, washed

Soak eight bamboo skewers in water for 10 minutes so they won't burn, or use metal skewers. Meanwhile make marinade by combining oil, vinegar, oregano, salt and pepper. Cut onion into eight wedges; cut each wedge in half crosswise.

Thread meat and vegetables on skewers, alternating meat and vegetables. Baste all surfaces with marinade, and allow to marinate at least 1 hour (2–8 hours is better).

Broil or charbroil 8–10 minutes, turning skewers often until vegetables are tender and lamb has browned on outside but remains pink inside.

4 servings
1 serving = 2 skewers

CAL.	CHO(g)	PRO.(g)	TOTAL FAT(g)	SAT. FAT(g)	CHOL.(mg)	FIBER(g)	SODIUM(mg)
250	11	26	11	3	75	2	210

Food exchanges per serving: 3 Lean Meats plus 2 Vegetables *or* 3 Lean Meats plus 1 Starch
Low-sodium diets: Omit salt.

Lamb Curry

If you serve this delicious, traditional Lamb Curry with rice, don't forget to add the Starch Exchanges. Try it over Rizzi Bizzi (see Index).

2 tablespoons margarine
2 cups coarsely chopped onion
1 large clove garlic, minced
1½ pounds boneless lean lamb, cut into 1-inch cubes
3 tablespoons all-purpose flour
1 tablespoon curry powder (or more to taste)

¼ teaspoon ground ginger
1 teaspoon salt
1½ cups hot Chicken Stock (see Index) or chicken broth
1 16-ounce can tomatoes, including liquid
1 cup cubed, pared apple

Heat margarine in a large deep skillet. Add onion, garlic, and lamb; cook over medium heat until meat is browned all over. Remove lamb and onion; set aside.

Combine flour, curry powder, ginger, and salt; stir into remaining fat in skillet. Blend well. Add hot Chicken Stock slowly, stirring constantly, until smooth and beginning to bubble. Cut tomatoes into bite-sized pieces; add tomatoes with tomato liquid, lamb, onion, and apple to mixture in pan. Stir to blend; bring to a simmer.

Cover and cook over low heat, stirring occasionally, about 45 minutes or until meat is tender.

6 servings (makes 4½ cups)
1 serving = ¾ cup

CAL.	CHO(g)	PRO.(g)	TOTAL FAT(g)	SAT. FAT(g)	CHOL.(mg)	FIBER(g)	SODIUM(mg)
270	15	25	12	3.5	75	2	865

Food exchanges per serving: 3 Lean Meats plus 1 Starch
Low-sodium diets: Omit salt. Use unsalted chicken broth and unsalted canned tomatoes.

Lamb Meatballs

Try these meatballs with Brown Rice Pilaf and Indian Carrot Salad. They are also used in Dilled Lamb in Pita Pockets (see Index for all three of these recipes). You may want to save some for a very good second meal.

12 ounces ground lean lamb
½ cup seasoned bread crumbs,
    divided
1 zucchini, shredded
2 eggs

2 tablespoons tomato paste
2 cloves garlic, minced
1 tablespoon chopped fresh parsley
1 teaspoon dried oregano

Preheat oven to 425°F. Prepare a jelly roll pan or roasting pan with nonstick cooking spray.

In a bowl, combine all ingredients except ¼ cup of the bread crumbs. Form meat mixture into 1-inch balls. Roll meatballs in remaining ¼ cup bread crumbs.

Arrange meatballs on pan. Bake 10 minutes. Turn; bake 5 minutes more. Do not overcook.

6 servings
1 serving = 5 meatballs

CAL.	CHO(g)	PRO.(g)	TOTAL FAT(g)	SAT. FAT(g)	CHOL.(mg)	FIBER(g)	SODIUM(mg)
170	10	14	8	3	110	1	365

Food exchanges per serving: 2 Lean Meats plus ½ Starch
Low-sodium diets: Use plain bread crumbs and add ½ teaspoon dried oregano, basil, or mint to the bread crumbs.

Garlicky Lamb and Eggplant Rolls

2 medium (2 pounds total)
    eggplants
1½ teaspoons salt
1 pound lean ground lamb
1 medium onion, chopped
4 large cloves garlic, minced

2 tablespoons chopped fresh mint
    leaves or 2 teaspoons dried
    mint
1 teaspoon coarsely ground pepper
Mint sprigs for garnish

Peel eggplants and cut lengthwise into ⅓-inch-thick slices. There will be about 16 slices. Spread slices on a cooling rack; sprinkle with salt. Set aside about 15 minutes.

Meanwhile, sauté lamb and onion in a large nonstick skillet until lamb is no longer pink. Add garlic, mint, and pepper. Cook 2 minutes longer. Pour mixture into a colander to drain fat.

With a paper towel, pat liquid released from eggplant and wipe off most of the salt. Put 3 slices eggplant in the large nonstick skillet, add ¼ cup water. Cover and cook over low heat 3 minutes. Turn eggplant over and continue cooking until eggplant is tender. Repeat process with remaining batches of eggplant.

Preheat oven to 400°F. Spray ovenproof flat casserole with nonstick cooking spray. Spread eggplant strips with equal parts lamb mixture. Roll up jelly roll style, and place rolls in prepared pan. If eggplant strips do not hold together well, pat rolls together. If extra lamb remains, sprinkle it around the rolls.

Bake 20–25 minutes until tops of eggplant rolls are lightly browned. Garnish with mint sprigs.

4 servings
1 serving = 4 rolls

CAL.	CHO(g)	PRO.(g)	TOTAL FAT(g)	SAT. FAT(g)	CHOL.(mg)	FIBER(g)	SODIUM(mg)
265	17	23	12	4.5	75	3.5	490

Food exchanges per serving: 3 Lean Meats plus 1 Starch *or* 3 Lean Meats plus 3 Vegetables
Low-sodium diets: Omit salt.

Rio Grande Pork Roast

You can use a larger or smaller roast, but adjust cooking time accordingly. Cook the roast to an internal temperature of 160°F. The amount of seasonings and glaze in the recipe can be used for a roast of 2–4 pounds. Each 4-ounce cooked portion will provide about the same nutrient profile regardless of the size of the roast. Leftovers make great sandwiches.

1 teaspoon salt
1 teaspoon finely minced garlic
1½ teaspoons chili powder, divided
1 3-pound rolled pork loin, well trimmed

2 tablespoons cider vinegar
½ cup low-sugar orange marmalade

Preheat oven to 325°F. In a small bowl, mix salt, garlic, and 1 teaspoon chili powder; rub pork with the mixture. Put meat rack in roasting pan and roast 1¼ hours.

Meanwhile, mix vinegar, remaining ½ teaspoon chili powder, and marmalade; pour mixture over meat, covering all surfaces. Roast 10 more minutes until glaze browns.

Remove roast from oven; let stand 10 minutes before slicing. Add enough hot water to drippings to make 1 cup gravy; stir to blend.

2-pound roast: 6 servings
3-pound roast: 9 servings
1 serving = 4 ounces roast plus 2 tablespoons gravy

CAL.	CHO(g)	PRO.(g)	TOTAL FAT(g)	SAT. FAT(g)	CHOL.(mg)	FIBER(g)	SODIUM(mg)
260	6	33	11	4	90	0	310

Food exchanges per serving: 4 Lean Meats plus ½ Fruit
Low-sodium diets: Omit salt; increase garlic to 1½ teaspoons and chili powder to 2½ teaspoons.

Roast Pork Loin

You can use either boneless rolled pork loin or the center loin on a rack of bones. Seasoning the meat 8–24 hours in advance enhances the flavor, but you can season the roast just before cooking.

1 3- to 3½-pound center loin or   *¼ teaspoon ground thyme*
    rolled double pork loin   *¼ teaspoon ground nutmeg or*
1 teaspoon salt   *cinnamon*
½ teaspoon freshly ground pepper

Preheat oven to 350°F. Lightly score surface of meat to allow seasoning to permeate meat. In a small bowl, mix salt, pepper, thyme, and nutmeg or cinnamon. Rub all surfaces of meat with this mixture.

Roast meat, fattest side up, in a roasting pan on the middle rack of the oven. Baste every half hour with fat drippings. Test after 1¼ hours with a meat thermometer; it will read 160°F when pork is cooked and juicy. A roast with bones should take 1½–2 hours. A 3- to 3½-pound rolled tied pork roast will take about 2–2½ hours. (The timing of a roast depends more on diameter than weight.)

When thermometer reaches 160°F, remove roast from oven. Place on a board and let rest for 10 minutes to set juices. Carve meat straight down in 1/4-inch slices like a loaf of bread. Trim fat from meat before eating.

Number of servings depends on size of roast.
1 serving = 3 ounces lean pork roast

CAL.	CHO(g)	PRO.(g)	TOTAL FAT(g)	SAT. FAT(g)	CHOL.(mg)	FIBER(g)	SODIUM(mg)
165	0	26	6	2	65	0	100

Food exchanges per serving: 3 Lean Meats
Low-sodium diets: Omit salt; add 1 teaspoon minced fresh garlic and 1 teaspoon grated gingerroot.

Hungarian-Style Pork and Sauerkraut

Josephine Anderson, who cooked for our family when I was a child, made this dish with pork spareribs and sour cream and served it with mashed potatoes or stuffed baked potatoes. I've lightened it up by using lean pork chops and yogurt. It still tastes great!

1 tablespoon margarine
1 large onion, sliced thin
1 14-ounce can sauerkraut, rinsed
   and drained
1 cup apple juice

1 tablespoon Hungarian paprika
4 (1¼ pounds total) ½-inch-thick
   center-cut pork chops
½ teaspoon freshly ground pepper
1 cup plain low-fat yogurt

*H*eat margarine in a large nonstick skillet. Add onion; sauté until lightly browned. Remove onion to bowl; mix in sauerkraut, apple juice, and paprika.

Season pork chops with pepper. Brown on both sides in the skillet. Add sauerkraut mixture; cover tightly and simmer 30 minutes over low heat. Turn chops occasionally and baste with pan liquids.

Remove chops to warmed serving platter or dishes. Stir yogurt into sauerkraut and heat through. Do not allow sauce to boil, or it may curdle. Top meat with sauerkraut mixture.

4 servings
1 serving = 1 pork chop plus ½ cup sauerkraut

CAL.	CHO*(g)*	PRO.*(g)*	TOTAL FAT*(g)*	SAT. FAT*(g)*	CHOL.*(mg)*	FIBER*(g)*	SODIUM*(mg)*
255	19	26	9	2.5	60	2.5	360

Food exchanges per serving: 3 Lean Meats plus 1 Starch *or* 3 Lean Meats plus 1 Other Carbohydrate
Low-sodium diets: This recipe is suitable for occasional use.

Pork Chops with Apples

2 teaspoons margarine   ¼ teaspoon salt
1 cup sliced apples   ¼ teaspoon freshly ground pepper
½ teaspoon ground cinnamon
2 ½-inch-thick center-cut pork
   chops, well trimmed

Heat margarine in a large nonstick skillet. Add apples; sauté until tender but not mushy. Sprinkle with cinnamon. Remove apples to serving plate.

Season pork chops with salt and pepper. Sauté in liquid from apples until almost cooked, turning to brown both sides. Cook until chops are done, about 10 minutes. Don't overcook, as chops will become rubbery.

Serve apples over chops.

2 servings
1 serving = 1 pork chop plus ½ cup apples

CAL.	CHO(g)	PRO.(g)	TOTAL FAT(g)	SAT. FAT(g)	CHOL.(mg)	FIBER(g)	SODIUM(mg)
185	9	17	9	2.5	50	1.5	350

Food exchanges per serving: 3 Lean Meats plus ½ Fruit
Low-sodium diets: Omit salt.

Herbed Pork Chops

If you season the pork chops and refrigerate them several hours to absorb flavor, they will be even tastier. This dry marinade is one of my favorites, but you can also use the same method with other seasonings—like lemon zest and garlic, or orange zest, Chinese five-spice seasoning, or teriyaki sauce.

1 teaspoon herbes de Provence or 1 teaspoon finely chopped fresh tarragon, 1 teaspoon snipped fresh thyme, and 1 teaspoon snipped fresh parsley

1 clove garlic, chopped fine
½ teaspoon salt
¼ teaspoon freshly ground pepper
6 (about 2 pounds total) boneless pork loin chops, well trimmed

*C*ombine herbs, garlic, salt, and pepper in a small bowl. Sprinkle seasoning mixture over pork chops. Refrigerate several hours if time permits.

Preheat oven to 400°F. Heat a heavy ovenproof skillet over high heat. Spray with nonstick cooking spray. Add pork chops; sear 2 minutes on each side to slightly brown the chops and seal in the juices. Transfer pan to oven and bake 10 minutes.

Remove separable fat before eating chops.

6 servings
1 serving = 1 pork chop

CAL.	CHO*(g)*	PRO.*(g)*	TOTAL FAT*(g)*	SAT. FAT*(g)*	CHOL.*(mg)*	FIBER*(g)*	SODIUM*(mg)*
200	0	27	9	3.5	80	0	250

Food exchanges per serving: 4 Lean Meats
Low-sodium diets: Omit salt.

Baked Pork Chops with Stuffing

6 (about 2 pounds total) ½-inch-
    thick center-cut pork chops,
    well trimmed

½ teaspoon salt
¼ teaspoon freshly ground pepper
1 recipe Bread Stuffing (see Index)

Preheat oven to 350°F. Season pork chops with salt and pepper. Spray a nonstick skillet with cooking spray and heat. Add pork chops; brown lightly on both sides.

Prepare a small roasting pan with nonstick cooking spray.

Lean 1 chop against edge of pan, put ½ cup stuffing against first chop, then place second chop against stuffing. Continue alternating chops with stuffing, concluding with stuffing at end.

Bake 40–45 minutes, uncovered, until chops are tender and stuffing is baked and crusty. Remove separable fat before eating chops.

6 servings
1 serving = 1 pork chop plus ½ cup stuffing

CAL.	CHO(g)	PRO.(g)	TOTAL FAT(g)	SAT. FAT(g)	CHOL.(mg)	FIBER(g)	SODIUM(mg)
305	29	29	7	2	2	1.5	885

Food exchanges per serving: 3 Lean Meats plus 2 Starches
Low-sodium diets: This recipe is not suitable.

Pork Medallions with Cranberry Raisin Sauce

Cranberry Raisin Sauce

2 tablespoons corn oil, divided
¼ cup finely chopped onion
¼ cup orange juice
⅓ cup golden raisins
½ cup cranberries, washed
½ teaspoon ground ginger

Pork Medallions

1 pound pork tenderloin, trimmed
of fat and membrane (about
13 ounces trimmed)
½ teaspoon salt
¼ teaspoon freshly ground pepper

Heat 1 tablespoon of the oil in a medium-sized saucepan. Add onion and sauté about 5 minutes until translucent. Add orange juice, raisins, cranberries, and ginger. Simmer, stirring frequently, about 10 minutes until cranberries have popped and sauce has slightly thickened. Remove from heat.

Cut pork tenderloin into 1-inch-thick slices. Pound slices to ½ inch thick. Season these pork medallions with salt and pepper. Heat remaining 1 tablespoon oil in a large nonstick skillet. Sauté meat until lightly brown, about 2 minutes each side.

Serve pork topped with sauce.

4 servings
1 serving = 2 pork medallions plus ¼ cup fruit sauce

CAL.	CHO(g)	PRO.(g)	TOTAL FAT(g)	SAT. FAT(g)	CHOL.(mg)	FIBER(g)	SODIUM(mg)
290	24	25	11	2	75	2	335

Food exchanges per serving: 3 Lean Meats plus 2 Fruits *or* 3 Lean Meats plus 1 Fruit plus 1 Vegetable
Low-sodium diets: Omit salt.

Sesame Pork Coins

Try this quick and easy entree with stir-fried vegetables or with Spicy Orange Noodle Salad (see Index).

½ pound well-trimmed pork
    tenderloin
1 tablespoon teriyaki sauce

2 teaspoons sesame seeds
1 teaspoon Oriental dark-roasted
    sesame oil

Cut tenderloin into ½-inch slices. Brush meat on both sides with teriyaki sauce; allow to marinate 10 minutes. Sprinkle seasoned pork with sesame seeds.

Brush a nonstick skillet with sesame oil. Heat skillet until hot. Quickly sauté pork coins 1–2 minutes on each side until lightly browned.

3 servings
1 serving = 4 coins

CAL.	CHO(g)	PRO.(g)	TOTAL FAT(g)	SAT. FAT(g)	CHOL.(mg)	FIBER(g)	SODIUM(mg)
115	1	16	5	1	50	0	270

Food exchanges per serving: 2 Lean Meats
Low-sodium diets: Substitute light (reduced-sodium) soy sauce for the teriyaki sauce.

Stir-Fried Pork and Asparagus

1 pound pork tenderloin, well
    trimmed, chilled
3 tablespoons light (reduced-
    sodium) soy sauce
2 tablespoons sherry vinegar
1 tablespoon grated gingerroot
2–3 cloves garlic, minced fine
1 tablespoon peanut oil

1 pound asparagus, washed,
    trimmed, and cut into 3-inch
    pieces (about 12 ounces
    cleaned)
1 red bell pepper, sliced thin
1½ teaspoons cornstarch
2 tablespoons slivered almonds,
    toasted

Slice pork into ¼-inch-thick medallions. Cut medallions into thin strips.

In a small bowl or jar, combine soy sauce, vinegar, gingerroot, and garlic, to make marinade. Put pork and marinade into a plastic bag; seal bag and mix well. Refrigerate 1 hour.

Heat oil in a large, nonstick skillet. Remove pork from bag, reserving marinade. Stir-fry pork strips, then remove from pan. In pan juices, stir-fry asparagus and pepper strips about 4–5 minutes until crisp and tender.

Add cornstarch to reserved marinade. Mix to dissolve cornstarch, and add marinade to vegetables in skillet. Cook over medium-high heat and stir until sauce thickens. Reduce heat, add pork, and heat through.

Serve garnished with toasted almonds.

5 servings (makes 5 cups)
1 serving = 1 cup

CAL.	CHO(g)	PRO.(g)	TOTAL FAT(g)	SAT. FAT(g)	CHOL.(mg)	FIBER(g)	SODIUM(mg)
180	6	22	8	1.5	60	1	410

Food exchanges per serving: 3 Lean Meats plus 1 Vegetable
Low-sodium diets: Reduce amount of light soy sauce to 1½ tablespoons.

Stir-Fried Pork with Napa Cabbage

This spicy entree is delicious served with rice or noodles.

¼ cup beef broth
½ teaspoon minced garlic
½ teaspoon minced fresh gingerroot
8 scallions, chopped
1 pound pork tenderloin, cut into
    1½″ × ½″ strips

4 cups shredded Napa cabbage
½ teaspoon salt
½ teaspoon crushed red pepper
    flakes

Heat broth in a large nonstick skillet or in a wok. Add garlic, ginger, and scallions; stir-fry 1 minute. Add pork, stir-fry until pink color is nearly gone, about 1 minute. Mix in cabbage; cover and continue cooking 3–5 minutes or until cabbage is tender, stirring once.

Season with salt and red pepper flakes to taste.

4 servings
1 serving = 1 cup

CAL.	CHO(g)	PRO.(g)	TOTAL FAT(g)	SAT. FAT(g)	CHOL.(mg)	FIBER(g)	SODIUM(mg)
160	5	25	4	1.5	75	1.5	445

Food exchanges per serving: 3 Very Lean Meats plus 1 Vegetable
Low-sodium diets: Omit salt; substitute unsalted beef broth.

Broiled Ham Steak

You can grill this ham steak in a nonstick pan or on a griddle sprayed with nonstick cooking spray.

1 pound center-cut lean ham slice,   *2 teaspoons spicy or Dijon mustard*
       ½ inch thick

Preheat broiler. Cut small ridges in fat surrounding edge of ham so that edges will not curl. Brush each side of ham slice with mustard.

    Put ham on a broiler pan; broil 3 inches from heat about 3 minutes on each side. Cut ham into 3-ounce portions.

5 servings
1 serving = 3 ounces lean ham steak

CAL.	CHO*(g)*	PRO.*(g)*	TOTAL FAT*(g)*	SAT. FAT*(g)*	CHOL.*(mg)*	FIBER*(g)*	SODIUM*(mg)*
120	1	18	5	1.5	45	0	1,320

Food exchanges per serving: 2½ Lean Meats
Low-sodium diets: This recipe is not suitable.

Baked Ham

Precooked hams are available both in cans and in the meat case of your grocery store. Hams should reach a temperature of 140°F when they are reheated for serving hot. Most hams these days are quite lean. They differ in the type of smoke, cure, and seasoning. I like to serve the ham with Mustard Sauce (recipe follows).

1 precooked ham (any size)	*1 teaspoon whole cloves*
1–2 teaspoons dry mustard	

*P*reheat oven to 325°F. Place ham in a roasting pan. Score surface of ham and season with mustard. Stud with cloves.

Bake ham 10–15 minutes per pound.

Trim ham of separable fat before serving.

Number of servings depends on size of ham
1 serving = 3 ounces lean sliced ham

CAL.	CHO(g)	PRO.(g)	TOTAL FAT(g)	SAT. FAT(g)	CHOL.(mg)	FIBER(g)	SODIUM(mg)
125	1	18	5	1.5	45	0	1,025

Food exchanges per serving: 2½ Lean Meats
Low-sodium diets: This recipe is not suitable.

Mustard Sauce

This sauce is delicious served with ham, pork, or Canadian bacon.

2 egg yolks	*1 tablespoon prepared mustard*
½ teaspoon dry mustard	*1 tablespoon fresh lemon juice*
3 tablespoons white vinegar	*Sugar substitute equivalent to*
3 tablespoons skim milk	*2 teaspoons sugar*

*B*eat egg yolks with dry mustard in the top of a double boiler until blended. Add vinegar gradually, beating after each addition.

Cook over simmering water, stirring constantly until thick and smooth. Add milk gradually, beating it in with a fork or wire whip. Cook 5 more minutes over simmering water.

Remove from heat. Let cool 10 minutes. Add remaining ingredients and blend well.

12 servings (makes ¾ cup)
1 serving = 1 tablespoon

CAL.	CHO(g)	PRO.(g)	TOTAL FAT(g)	SAT. FAT(g)	CHOL.(mg)	FIBER(g)	SODIUM(mg)
14	1	1	1	0.5	35	0	20

Food exchanges per serving: a Free Food
Low-sodium diets: This recipe is excellent.

Ham Rosettes

Here is a decorative way to serve only 1 ounce of meat! Rosettes can be served as a breakfast meat or at room temperature with Green Bean and Romano Salad (see Index) or a pasta salad.

1 tablespoon spicy mustard   *6 ounces shaved smoked ham*
1 tablespoon water

Preheat oven to 350°F. Spray a six-cup muffin tin with butter-flavored cooking spray.

In a small bowl, mix mustard with water.

Separate ham slices and arrange in soft folds (like a flower with edges up) in the muffin cups. Each cup should hold one or two slices of ham. Drizzle 1 teaspoon mustard sauce over each flower.

Bake 10 minutes until ham is hot and edges browned.

Allow to cool 5 minutes to set shape. Remove from mold.

6 servings
1 serving = 1 ham flower

CAL.	CHO(g)	PRO.(g)	TOTAL FAT(g)	SAT. FAT(g)	CHOL.(mg)	FIBER(g)	SODIUM(mg)
40	0	5	2	0.5	15	0	435

Food exchange per serving: 1 Very Lean Meat
Low-sodium diets: This recipe is not suitable.

17

Poultry

Chicken

In the United States, raw poultry, particularly chicken, often carries salmonella, a potentially harmful bacteria, and should always be rinsed under running water before use. Also, cooking the chicken to an internal temperature of at least 140°F destroys the bacteria in the chicken.

It's important to avoid letting juices from raw poultry contaminate any kitchen surface, including cutting boards, knives, or dish towels, that could touch other food you may eat uncooked. Also, whenever you handle raw poultry, wash your hands with hot soapy water before touching other food.

Be sure you do not put cooked chicken on any pan or platter that has held raw chicken, and never pour marinades that have touched raw chicken over the cooked bird. Marinades that cook on the bird are safe, as are marinades added to sauces that are heated to a boil.

Roast Chicken

For this recipe, you can use any size chicken, roasting chicken, or capon. Using a larger bird provides a greater percentage of lean meat, and leftovers are both versatile and delicious.

The recipe calls for 2 tablespoons oil. Don't be concerned about the added fat. It seasons the bird and crisps the skin to keep the bird moist, but if you remove the skin and don't eat the drippings, the added fat doesn't count. Try serving the bird with Lean Gravy (recipe follows), one of our chutneys, or Granny Smith Applesauce (see Index).

1 4- to 5-pound roasting chicken or capon	2 tablespoons olive oil
6 cloves garlic, divided	1 teaspoon salt
1 lemon, cut in half	½ teaspoon freshly ground pepper
	½ cup fresh parsley sprigs

Preheat oven to 425°F. Wash chicken under running water. Pat dry with paper towels. Trim and discard extra fat.

Crush 2 cloves garlic. In a small bowl, combine juice of ½ of the lemon, crushed garlic, olive oil, salt, and pepper.

Brush inside cavity of the bird with some of the lemon oil mixture. Cut remaining lemon half in pieces; put lemon pieces, remaining 4 garlic cloves, and parsley sprigs in cavity of chicken. Tie legs together with cotton string, or tuck legs in cavity of bird.

Set chicken, breast side up, on a rack in a roasting pan. Brush all outside surfaces of the bird with remaining lemon oil mixture. Roast on the lower or middle rack of oven, turning over every 30 minutes and basting with pan juices at each turn. Allow 25 minutes per pound; an instant-read meat thermometer should register 165°F.

Remove chicken from oven; let rest about 15 minutes to set juices. While chicken is resting, cover lightly with foil to keep it hot.

Carve the chicken or cut into pieces. Remove skin before eating.

Number of servings depends on weight of the bird
1 serving = 3 ounces cooked, boneless, skinless chicken

Light meat per 3 ounces:

CAL.	CHO(g)	PRO.(g)	TOTAL FAT(g)	SAT. FAT(g)	CHOL.(mg)	FIBER(g)	SODIUM(mg)
120	0	21	3	1	60	0	150

Food exchanges per serving: 3 Very Lean Meats
Low-sodium diets: Omit salt.

Dark meat per 3 ounces:

CAL.	CHO(g)	PRO.(g)	TOTAL FAT(g)	SAT. FAT(g)	CHOL.(mg)	FIBER(g)	SODIUM(mg)
140	0	18	7	2	55	0	150

Food exchanges per serving: 3 Lean Meats
Low-sodium diets: Omit salt.

Lean Gravy

Canned reduced-sodium broth can be substituted for the homemade Chicken Stock, which is unsalted and has fat removed. You may also want to try fat-free chicken, pork, or beef gravy in a can or jar. These gravies are quite good, and the nutrient values are on the label.

1½ cups Chicken Stock (see Index)   2 teaspoons cornstarch
    or beef stock, divided, chilled   ⅛ teaspoon salt
    or at room temperature   2 dashes freshly ground pepper
1 tablespoon finely minced onion

In a small saucepan, combine 1 cup of the stock and the onion. Simmer gently until liquid is reduced by one-half.

Combine cornstarch with remaining ½ cup stock, stirring with a whisk until smooth and well blended. Add mixture gradually to the concentrated stock, stirring constantly. Cook and whisk over medium heat until thickened and smooth. Stir in salt and pepper.

4 servings (makes 1 cup)
1 serving = ¼ cup

CAL.	CHO(g)	PRO.(g)	TOTAL FAT(g)	SAT. FAT(g)	CHOL.(mg)	FIBER(g)	SODIUM(mg)
15	3	1	1	0.5	0	0	110

Food exchanges per serving: a Free Food
Low-sodium diets: Omit salt.

Chicken and Shrimp Paella

A wonderful and nutrient-rich one-dish meal.

6 chicken pieces (2 legs, 2 thighs, 2 breasts), well rinsed
1 tablespoon olive oil
4 cloves garlic, minced
½ cup chopped scallion with top
2 cups cooked brown or saffron rice
3 medium tomatoes, cut into wedges (2 cups total)
½ cup sliced red onion

2 cups frozen green peas, defrosted
1 2-ounce jar chopped pimiento with juice
½ teaspoon salt
½ teaspoon freshly ground pepper
3 large bay leaves
12 (10 ounces total), shelled and cleaned large, raw shrimp

Preheat oven to 375°F. Arrange chicken in a baking pan on a rack; bake 45 minutes or until chicken is tender. Remove and discard chicken skin. Set chicken pieces aside.

Heat oil in a large nonstick skillet or wok. Add garlic and scallion; sauté until tender, stirring occasionally. Add reserved chicken pieces and remaining ingredients. Cover and continue cooking 15 minutes, adding shrimp during last 5 minutes.

Remove bay leaves. Serve hot.

6 servings
1 serving = 1 chicken piece plus ⅔ cup rice/vegetable mixture

CAL.	CHO*(g)*	PRO.*(g)*	TOTAL FAT*(g)*	SAT. FAT*(g)*	CHOL.*(mg)*	FIBER*(g)*	SODIUM*(mg)*
305	28	31	8	1.5	115	4	355

Food exchanges per serving: 3 Lean Meats plus 2 Starches plus 1 Vegetable
Low-sodium diets: Omit salt.

Chicken Cacciatore

1 2½- to 3-pound chicken, cut into
    pieces, skin removed, well
    rinsed
1 tablespoon olive oil
½ cup chopped onion
½ cup finely sliced strips green bell
    pepper
1 16-ounce can tomatoes, cut up,
    with liquid

⅓ cup tomato paste
¾ teaspoon salt
1 clove garlic, crushed
½ teaspoon crushed dried oregano
⅛ teaspoon ground allspice
¼ cup fresh lemon juice
½ cup water

Preheat oven to 400°F. Prepare a large casserole with nonstick cooking spray. Wipe chicken pieces with a damp cloth.

Heat olive oil in a large nonstick skillet. Add chicken pieces and brown on both sides; transfer to casserole. Cook onion and pepper strips in skillet over medium heat 3–4 minutes, stirring frequently. Combine all remaining ingredients in a medium bowl. Mix well; add to onion and green pepper. Bring to a boil. Pour mixture on top of chicken.

Bake 30 minutes. Turn chicken over and baste with sauce; bake 20–30 minutes more, until chicken is tender.

4 servings
1 serving = ¼ chicken (breast and wing or leg and thigh) plus ½ cup tomato mixture

CAL.	CHO(g)	PRO.(g)	TOTAL FAT(g)	SAT. FAT(g)	CHOL.(mg)	FIBER(g)	SODIUM(mg)
285	13	37	9	2	115	2.5	895

Food exchanges per serving: 4 Lean Meats plus 2 Vegetables
Low-sodium diets: Omit salt. Use unsalted canned tomatoes and unsalted tomato paste.

Grilled Chicken Breasts with Spicy Thai Dipping Sauce

Terrific for parties, the colorful, tasty Thai sauce has quite a lot of sugar. You won't use all of the sauce but will need extra so you can dip. I calculated the values based on eating half of the sauce.

4 chicken breast halves, well rinsed, wing section removed
¼ cup fresh lemon juice
2 cloves garlic, crushed
½ teaspoon salt
½ fresh lime, cut into thin slices

Thai Dipping Sauce

½ small red bell pepper, chopped (about ⅓ cup)
½ cup white vinegar
⅓ cup sugar
½ teaspoon crushed red pepper flakes

Marinate the chicken pieces in lemon juice. Refrigerate for several hours.

In a blender or food processor, puree red bell pepper with vinegar. In a small saucepan, combine vinegar, sugar, and red pepper flakes. Simmer sauce 8–10 minutes. Remove from heat and let cool. Pour sauce through a strainer or sieve. It will be a clear, beautiful deep orange color.

Preheat broiler. Drain chicken; rub with garlic, and sprinkle with salt. Broil chicken on rack of broiler pan about 6 inches away from heat, turning every 5 minutes, about 20 minutes total.

Garnish chicken with lime slices. Serve with individual ramekins of dipping sauce. Remove chicken skin before dipping chicken.

4 servings
1 serving = 1 breast half plus 2 tablespoons sauce

CAL.	CHO(g)	PRO.(g)	TOTAL FAT(g)	SAT. FAT(g)	CHOL.(mg)	FIBER(g)	SODIUM(mg)
260	11	33	9	2.5	90	0	215

Food exchanges per serving: 4 Lean Meats plus 1 Other Carbohydrate
Low-sodium diets: Omit salt.

Tandoori Chicken Breasts

Delicious hot or chilled. Try these with rice or couscous and Thai Cucumber Salad (see Index). Sliced fresh mangoes or mango chutney are a traditional accompaniment, or stuff the chicken in pita pockets and add Cucumber Riata (see Index) and shredded carrots. If you want to cook this recipe indoors, use a well-seasoned grill pan (a skillet with a ridged inner surface), an indoor barbecue, or a stovetop grill.

4 (about 1 pound total) boneless, skinless chicken breasts	½ teaspoon turmeric
¼ cup plain low-fat yogurt	½ teaspoon cumin
1 clove garlic, crushed	½ teaspoon ground ginger
½ teaspoon paprika	Dash cayenne
	Dash freshly ground pepper

Wash chicken and pat dry. Cut breasts in half crosswise, and put between pieces of wax paper or plastic wrap. Pound chicken gently with side of a meat mallet or bottom of a heavy glass to flatten each piece until ¼ to ½ inch thick.

Make tandoori paste by combining yogurt and all seasonings in a small bowl. Brush chicken pieces with seasoned paste, wrap in plastic wrap, and refrigerate at least 2 hours or overnight.

Prepare a charcoal grill, letting coals burn until ashen. Oil rack or prepare with a nonstick cooking spray. Grill 2–4 minutes on each side, just until chicken is cooked through.

4 servings
1 serving = 3½ ounces chicken

CAL.	CHO(g)	PRO.(g)	TOTAL FAT(g)	SAT. FAT(g)	CHOL.(mg)	FIBER(g)	SODIUM(mg)
140	2	27	2	0.5	65	0	85

Food exchanges per serving: 4 Very Lean Meats
Low-sodium diets: This recipe is excellent.

Chicken Breasts with Raspberry Sauce

Cooking chicken breasts with their skin on keeps them moist, but remove the skin before eating the chicken. About half of the fat in chicken is in the skin. These nutrient calculations are based on the chicken eaten without the skin.

1 tablespoon olive oil
1 red onion, thinly sliced
4 (about 1½ pounds total) chicken breast halves, wing section removed

½ teaspoon salt
¼ teaspoon freshly ground pepper
1 cup cran-raspberry or raspberry-apple juice
¾ cup fresh raspberries

*H*eat oil in a large nonstick skillet. Add onion; sauté 2 minutes until translucent. Remove onion from pan and set aside.

Season chicken breasts with salt and pepper; add to pan and cook over medium heat only until surface is slightly browned. Add juice to pan and continue cooking until chicken is cooked through, about 12 minutes.

Remove chicken from pan.

Add onions to skillet; cook until liquid has a syrupy consistency. Add raspberries; heat through. Serve chicken breasts topped with raspberry sauce.

4 servings
1 serving = 1 breast half plus ⅓ cup sauce

CAL.	CHO(g)	PRO.(g)	TOTAL FAT(g)	SAT. FAT(g)	CHOL.(mg)	FIBER(g)	SODIUM(mg)
340	16	34	15	4	95	2	360

Food exchanges per serving: 5 Lean Meats plus 1 Fruit
Low-sodium diets: Omit salt.

Chicken Breasts on a Bed of Mushrooms

1 ounce dried shiitake mushrooms
⅓ cup flour, divided
¼ teaspoon salt
⅛ teaspoon freshly ground pepper
4 (about 1 pound total) boneless, skinless chicken breast halves

2 tablespoons olive oil
1 large shallot, minced
8 ounces fresh mushrooms, washed and sliced
¾ cup dry white wine
1 tablespoon chopped fresh parsley

Soak dried mushrooms in 1 cup warm water for 30 minutes to soften before cooking. Combine ¼ cup of the flour with salt and pepper on a small flat dish. Dredge chicken breasts in flour mixture.

Heat 1 tablespoon olive oil in a large nonstick skillet over medium heat. Add chicken and sauté 3–4 minutes on each side until lightly browned. Remove chicken from pan.

Add remaining oil to skillet. Add shallots and fresh mushrooms; sauté until mushrooms are softened and slightly browned. Add the remaining 2 tablespoons flour, stirring to blend flour into pan juices.

Remove shiitake mushrooms from soaking liquid and cut into very thin strips. Add shiitake mushrooms, soaking liquid, and wine to skillet. Bring to a boil and cook 5 minutes, stirring often, until mushroom sauce is slightly thickened.

Return chicken to sauce and cook about 2 minutes until chicken is heated through. Stir in parsley just before serving.

Remove chicken breasts from pan. Arrange mushrooms on plates or a platter; top with chicken. Remove chicken skin before eating chicken.

4 servings
1 serving = 1 3½-ounce breast plus ½ cup mushrooms

CAL.	CHO(g)	PRO.(g)	TOTAL FAT(g)	SAT. FAT(g)	CHOL.(mg)	FIBER(g)	SODIUM(mg)
290	17	29	9	1.5	65	1	215

Food exchanges per serving: 4 Lean Meats plus 1 Vegetable plus ½ Starch *or* 4 Lean Meats plus 1 Other Carbohydrate
Low-sodium diets: This recipe is suitable; omit salt if desired.

Gingered Chicken Breasts

1 recipe Pickled Ginger (see Index)
2 teaspoons light (reduced-sodium) soy sauce

1 clove garlic, crushed
2 whole chicken breasts, cut in half, skin removed

Preheat oven to 325°F. Chop Pickled Ginger in a food processor fitted with a steel blade. Add soy sauce and garlic: process 10 seconds more.

Arrange chicken breasts on a nonstick cookie sheet or a shallow nonstick casserole. Brush with ginger mixture. Bake 25–30 minutes or until chicken is done.

4 servings
1 serving = ½ breast

CAL.	CHO(g)	PRO.(g)	TOTAL FAT(g)	SAT. FAT(g)	CHOL.(mg)	FIBER(g)	SODIUM(mg)
145	3	28	1.5	0.5	70	0	250

Food exchanges per serving: 4 Very Lean Meats
Low-sodium diets: This recipe is fine.

Dijon Chicken

2 whole boneless, skinless chicken
   breasts
2 tablespoons margarine
2 cloves garlic, crushed
½ cup dry white wine
¼ cup water

2 tablespoons Dijon mustard
½ teaspoon dried dill
½ teaspoon salt
¼ teaspoon coarsely ground pepper
⅓ cup chopped fresh parsley

Preheat oven to 325°F. Cut each boned breast into 2 pieces. Put pieces on a wooden cutting board and pound them with a meat mallet or the side of a rolling pin until ½ inch thick.

Melt margarine in a large nonstick skillet; add garlic and cook 2 minutes over medium heat. Add chicken pieces; brown 3 minutes on each side. Transfer chicken to a 1½-quart shallow casserole.

Put wine, water, mustard, dill, salt, and pepper into the skillet; stir to mix with the chicken drippings. Bring to a boil and cook 1 minute. Pour over chicken in casserole.

Cover and bake 30 minutes. Add parsley. Baste chicken with sauce and cook 5 more minutes.

4 servings
1 serving = ½ breast plus 2 tablespoons sauce

CAL.	CHO(g)	PRO.(g)	TOTAL FAT(g)	SAT. FAT(g)	CHOL.(mg)	FIBER(g)	SODIUM(mg)
195	1	28	7	1.5	70	0.5	600

Food exchanges per serving: 4 Very Lean Meats
Low-sodium diets: Omit salt.

Spicy Szechwan Chicken

This recipe is my family's favorite! Be sure to have all ingredients sliced or diced and measured before you start stir-frying. Warning: This recipe is delicious but hot!

1 pound boneless, skinless chicken breasts
4 teaspoons cornstarch, divided
1 egg white
2 tablespoons canola or corn oil
¾ cup thinly sliced, canned bamboo shoots, drained
¼ cup diced green chilies, drained
½ cup shelled, roasted, skinned peanuts

1 clove garlic, minced fine
1 teaspoon sugar
2 tablespoons soy sauce
3 tablespoons dry sherry
1 teaspoon peeled, grated fresh gingerroot
2 tablespoons finely chopped scallion

Cut chicken into 2″ × ½″ strips. Place in a large pie plate. Sprinkle 2 teaspoons of the cornstarch over chicken; mix well to coat chicken. Add egg white and mix again.

Heat oil in a 12-inch skillet or wok. Add chicken and bamboo shoots, and stir-fry about 3 minutes, stirring often. Add chilies and peanuts; stir-fry 2 minutes.

In a small bowl, combine garlic, sugar, soy sauce, sherry, gingerroot, and remaining 2 teaspoons cornstarch; add to skillet. Stir-fry and simmer until sauce is thick and smooth and mixture is well blended. Add scallion; stir-fry 30 seconds to warm scallions. Serve immediately.

6 servings (makes 4 cups)
1 serving = ⅔ cup

CAL.	CHO(g)	PRO.(g)	TOTAL FAT(g)	SAT. FAT(g)	CHOL.(mg)	FIBER(g)	SODIUM(mg)
225	7	22	11	2	45	1	440

Food exchanges per serving: 3 Lean Meats plus 1 Vegetable
Low-sodium diets: Substitute light (reduced-sodium) soy sauce.

Chicken Cantonese

1½ pounds boneless, skinless chicken breasts, well rinsed
1 tablespoon peanut or corn oil
½ cup diagonally sliced celery
½ cup sliced scallion
1 clove garlic, minced
1¼ cups Chicken Stock (see Index) or chicken broth
1 teaspoon salt
½ teaspoon ground ginger or ¾ teaspoon grated gingerroot

2 dashes freshly ground black pepper
1 cup coarsely chopped green bell pepper (2-inch squares)
6 ounces frozen snow peas or fresh snow peas, trimmed
1 tablespoon cornstarch
¼ cup cold water

Cut chicken breasts into 2″ × ½″ strips. Heat oil in a large deep skillet or wok. Add celery, scallion, garlic, and chicken strips; stir-fry over medium heat 3–4 minutes, turning the ingredients frequently with a large wooden spoon or fork.

Add Chicken Stock, salt, ginger, and black pepper; cover and bring to a boil. Add green pepper and snow peas; cover and cook over medium heat 5 minutes or until green pepper and snow peas are crisp-tender.

Meanwhile, dissolve cornstarch in cold water; stir cornstarch mixture into skillet. Cook over medium heat until sauce is thick and clear, stirring constantly.

6 servings (makes 4½ cups)
1 serving = ¾ cup

CAL.	CHO(g)	PRO.(g)	TOTAL FAT(g)	SAT. FAT(g)	CHOL.(mg)	FIBER(g)	SODIUM(mg)
180	6	28	4	1	65	0.5	475

Food exchanges per serving: 4 Very Lean Meats plus 1 Vegetable
Low-sodium diets: Omit salt. Use unsalted chicken broth.

Chicken and White Bean Chili

Use medium or hot chili powder and green chilies to make this chili as spicy as you like. Whether it's hot or mild, you'll get lots of fiber, vitamins A and C, and niacin.

1 pound boneless, skinless chicken (breasts and thighs), well rinsed

1 quart Chicken Stock (see Index) or chicken broth

1 medium onion, chopped

1 15-ounce can cannellini beans (white kidney beans), with liquid

1 16-ounce can diced tomatoes, with liquid

1 4½-ounce can chopped, peeled green chilies

1 green bell pepper, diced

1 tablespoon chili powder

1 teaspoon minced garlic

*C*ut chicken into ½-inch cubes. Put Chicken Stock in a large pot; add chicken and onion. Simmer 20 minutes.

Add remaining ingredients; simmer another 40 minutes, stirring occasionally.

6 servings (makes 6 cups)
1 serving = 1 cup

CAL.	CHO*(g)*	PRO.*(g)*	TOTAL FAT*(g)*	SAT. FAT*(g)*	CHOL.*(mg)*	FIBER*(g)*	SODIUM*(mg)*
200	21	24	4	1	55	6.5	645

Food exchanges per serving: 3 Very Lean Meats plus 1 Starch plus 1 Vegetable
Low-sodium diets: Use unsalted canned beans and tomatoes. If unsalted beans aren't available, rinse beans and discard liquid from can. Add ½ cup water.

Chicken Tetrazzini

Serve this casserole with a green vegetable and a crisp green or fruit salad. You can make it ahead and heat it right before dinner. If the casserole is chilled, add a few minutes to the baking time. If you are in a hurry or are cooking for one or two, put the tetrazzini in individual single-serve casseroles, which cook more quickly.

2 teaspoons margarine

½ sweet Spanish onion, chopped

4 ounces mushrooms, washed and sliced

1 tablespoon + 1 teaspoon cornstarch

¾ cup Chicken Stock (see Index) or chicken broth

¾ cup skim milk

½ teaspoon salt

¼ teaspoon freshly ground black pepper

2 cups cooked spaghettini, cappellini, or other thin pasta

1 cup chopped cooked skinless chicken

2 tablespoons chopped pimiento or roasted red pepper

2 tablespoons seasoned bread crumbs

1 tablespoon grated Parmesan cheese

Preheat oven to 350°F. Melt margarine in a large nonstick skillet. Add onion and mushrooms; stir-fry until vegetables are slightly browned. Remove from pan and reserve.

In a small bowl, dissolve cornstarch in Chicken Stock. Put stock and milk in the skillet. Simmer, stirring constantly, until mixture thickens. Season sauce with salt and pepper. Add spaghettini, mushrooms and onion, chicken, and pimiento. Stir to combine. Transfer mixture to a casserole sprayed with cooking spray.

In a small bowl, mix bread crumbs and Parmesan. Top casserole with crumbs. Cover lightly with foil, and bake 25–30 minutes.

4 servings (makes 4 cups)
1 serving = 1 cup

CAL.	CHO(g)	PRO.(g)	TOTAL FAT(g)	SAT. FAT(g)	CHOL.(mg)	FIBER(g)	SODIUM(mg)
255	32	18	6	1.5	35	2	475

Food exchanges per serving: 2 Lean Meats plus 2 Starches
Low-sodium diets: Omit salt. Substitute plain bread crumbs for seasoned crumbs.

Broiled Garlic Chicken

The calculated values below are based on chicken eaten with skin. If you remove the skin, count chicken as 5 Lean Meat Exchanges.

1 2¾- to 3-pound chicken,	*1 tablespoon minced fresh garlic*
quartered or cut into 8 pieces	*1 teaspoon salt*
1 lemon	*¼ teaspoon freshly ground pepper*

*P*reheat broiler. Rinse chicken pieces under running water and pat pieces dry with a paper towel. Squeeze juice of lemon over all surfaces of chicken. Season chicken on both sides with garlic, salt, and pepper.

Put chicken on a broiler pan; broil 4 inches from heat about 20 minutes, turning every 5 minutes and basting at each turn. Discard pan drippings.

Serve hot or chilled.

4 servings
1 serving = ¼ chicken

CAL.	CHO(g)	PRO.(g)	TOTAL FAT(g)	SAT. FAT(g)	CHOL.(mg)	FIBER(g)	SODIUM(mg)
350	1	39	20	5.5	125	0	670

Food exchanges per serving: 5 Medium-Fat Meats
Low-sodium diets: Omit salt.

Chicken Livers with Onions, Peppers, and Mushrooms

If you have leftovers of this dish, create a lovely pâté. Just coarsely puree the mixture in a food processor with a steel blade—not too long, because you want flecks of red pepper to show. Chill the mixture in a small bowl or mold. One cup of the original mixture yields ¾ cup pâté.

¼ cup flour
1 teaspoon salt, divided
¾ teaspoon freshly ground black pepper, divided
1 pound chicken livers, rinsed and drained
3 tablespoons margarine, divided
1 large Spanish onion, cut into 1-inch cubes

12 ounces fresh large mushrooms, washed and cut into thick slices
1 large red bell pepper, cut into 1-inch cubes
1 tablespoon chopped fresh parsley

In a medium bowl, mix flour with ½ teaspoon of the salt and ½ teaspoon of the black pepper. Toss livers with flour mixture to coat.

Melt 2 tablespoons margarine in a large nonstick skillet. Add onion; sauté about 5 minutes, until translucent, stirring often. Add mushrooms and red pepper; sauté about 8 minutes more until mushrooms and pepper soften. Gently remove vegetables from pan, leaving any liquid.

Melt remaining 1 tablespoon margarine in the skillet. Add chicken livers. Sauté over medium-high heat until outsides have been browned but insides are still pink. Add vegetables and heat through. Season with remaining ½ teaspoon salt and ¼ teaspoon black pepper. Serve immediately, topped with parsley.

5 servings (makes 5 cups)
1 serving = 1 cup

CAL.	CHO*(g)*	PRO.*(g)*	TOTAL FAT*(g)*	SAT. FAT*(g)*	CHOL.*(mg)*	FIBER*(g)*	SODIUM*(mg)*
250	19	20	11	2.5	400	2.5	600

Food exchanges per serving: 2 Medium-Fat Meats plus 2 Vegetables plus ½ Starch *or* 2 Medium-Fat Meats plus 1 Starch
Low-sodium diets: Omit salt.

Barbecued Chicken—Inside or Out

Great on the outdoor grill; delicious oven-baked, too!

2⅓- to 3-pound chicken, cut up and rinsed   *¾ cup barbecue sauce, hickory or other flavor*

To oven-bake: Preheat oven to 400°F. Line bottom and sides of a shallow baking pan with foil or prepare pan with nonstick cooking spray.

Baste each chicken piece with sauce. Arrange chicken pieces in pan with skin sides up; pour remaining sauce evenly on top. Cover pan with foil; bake 45 minutes. Uncover pan, baste again, and bake another 20 minutes.

To outdoor-grill: Prepare outdoor grill. When coals are hot and ashen, baste chicken with sauce. Put chicken on grill; cook about 30 minutes, turning and basting several times during the cooking process.

4 servings
1 serving = ½ breast and wing plus 2 tablespoons sauce *or* 1 leg and 1 thigh plus 2 tablespoons sauce

CAL.	CHO*(g)*	PRO.*(g)*	TOTAL FAT*(g)*	SAT. FAT*(g)*	CHOL.*(mg)*	FIBER*(g)*	SODIUM*(mg)*
350	4	38	19	5	120	0	365

Food exchanges per serving: 5 Lean Meats plus 1 Vegetable
Low-sodium diets: Substitute a reduced-sodium barbecue sauce.

Rock Cornish Game Hens

Spiced Game Hens

Serve these game hens surrounded by stir-fried or roasted vegetables. Remove most of the skin when you eat the hen.

2 (20 ounces each) Rock Cornish
    game hens
1 teaspoon Chinese five-spice
    powder
2 teaspoons Oriental dark-roasted
    sesame oil

2 teaspoons light (reduced-sodium)
    soy sauce
6–8 drops hot pepper sauce

Split hens in half lengthwise; rinse them and discard giblets. In a small bowl, combine five-spice powder, sesame oil, soy sauce, and pepper sauce. Brush all surfaces of hens with seasoning mixture; set aside 15 minutes.

Preheat broiler. Line a broiler pan with foil, or use a disposable foil broiler pan. Arrange hens on pan skin side up. Broil 3 inches from heat 15 minutes, turning every 5 minutes, until cooked through but moist.

4 servings
1 serving = ½ hen

CAL.	CHO(g)	PRO.(g)	TOTAL FAT(g)	SAT. FAT(g)	CHOL.(mg)	FIBER(g)	SODIUM(mg)
250	1	31	13	3.5	95	0	195

Food exchanges per serving: 4 Lean Meats
Low-sodium diets: This recipe is acceptable.

Rock Cornish Hens with Tart Cherry Sauce

Try these hens on a bed of Brown Rice Pilaf (see Index) with Sesame Sugar Snaps (see Index). Remove most of the skin when you eat the hen.

*3 (20–22 ounces each) Rock
    Cornish game hens*
1 teaspoon seasoned salt
¾ teaspoon freshly ground pepper
*1 16-ounce can tart pitted cherries,
    packed in water*
1 tablespoon cornstarch

*⅔ cup Chicken Stock (see Index),
    chicken broth, or dry white
    wine*
1 teaspoon grated orange zest
*Sugar substitute equivalent to
    2 tablespoons sugar*

Split hens in half lengthwise; rinse them and discard giblets. Season hens with seasoned salt and pepper.

Preheat broiler. Line a broiler pan with foil, or use a disposable foil pan. Arrange hens on pan with skin side up. Broil 3 inches from heat 15 minutes, turning every 5 minutes until cooked through but moist.

While hens are cooking, drain liquid from cherries into a small saucepan. Add cornstarch to liquid and stir until dissolved; add Chicken Stock or wine. Cook over low heat, stirring often until liquid has thickened to the consistency of a sauce. Add cherries and orange zest; remove from heat. Stir in sugar substitute. Taste and add more sugar substitute if desired.

6 servings
1 serving = ½ game hen plus ⅓ cup cherry sauce

CAL.	CHO*(g)*	PRO.*(g)*	TOTAL FAT*(g)*	SAT. FAT*(g)*	CHOL.*(mg)*	FIBER*(g)*	SODIUM*(mg)*
330	16	40	12	3	100	0	325

Food exchanges per serving: 5 Lean Meats plus 1 Fruit
Low-sodium diets: Substitute light (reduced-sodium) seasoned salt.

Turkey

Today, markets offer whole fresh and frozen turkeys and turkey parts such as breasts, turkey quarters, and legs. Frozen turkeys and fresh turkeys packed by major packers give clear, easy-to-follow directions on the packages.

Roast Turkey

The size of the turkey determines cooking time. Stuffed birds take 20–30 minutes longer to cook than unstuffed ones. If you are short of time, use Julia Child's method of cutting the whole turkey into quarters and roasting the pieces. It will take about 2 hours to cook instead of 4.

You may want to use additional seasonings to enhance this basic recipe.

1 12- to 16-pound turkey   *2 teaspoons seasoned salt*
4 tablespoons margarine   *1 teaspoon freshly ground pepper*

Preheat oven to 325°F. Rinse turkey under running water. Pat dry with paper towels.

Melt margarine in a small bowl or saucepan; mix in seasoned salt and pepper. Brush turkey, inside and out, with seasoned margarine. Tie legs together with cotton string, or tuck ends of legs into cavity. Skewer neck end closed, and fasten wings to bird with wooden toothpicks or skewers.

Put turkey, breast side up, on a rack in a roasting pan. Place pan on lower rack of oven. Roast, basting turkey every 30 minutes with pan juices. Turn turkey over each hour for even browning and crisper skin. If turkey starts to brown too much, cover it loosely with foil, shiny side up.

Roast turkey about 4 hours or until an instant-read meat thermometer registers 165°F. The thickest part of the drumsticks should feel fairly tender when pressed, and the leg should move slightly in the hip socket.

Remove turkey from oven. Cover lightly with foil. To set juices, allow turkey to rest 20–30 minutes before carving.

Number of servings depends on size of turkey
1 serving = 3 ounces cooked boneless, skinless turkey

Light meat per 3 ounces:

CAL.	CHO(g)	PRO.(g)	TOTAL FAT(g)	SAT. FAT(g)	CHOL.(mg)	FIBER(g)	SODIUM(mg)
120	0	23	2.5	1	55	0	250

Food exchanges per serving: 3 Very Lean Meats
Low-sodium diets: Omit seasoned salt.

Dark meat per 3 ounces:

CAL.	CHO(g)	PRO.(g)	TOTAL FAT(g)	SAT. FAT(g)	CHOL.(mg)	FIBER(g)	SODIUM(mg)
145	0	22	6	2	65	0	250

Food exchanges per serving: 3 Lean Meats
Low-sodium diets: Omit seasoned salt.

Turkey Breast with Spinach Stuffing

This tasty dish is great hot or at room temperature. It can be made ahead and sliced for a beautiful buffet presentation.

2 (1¾ pounds total) boneless turkey breast tenderloins
½ teaspoon salt
¼ teaspoon freshly ground black pepper
2 cups (¼ pound total) fresh spinach, washed, stems removed

1 small onion, quartered
2 large cloves garlic, peeled
1 roasted red pepper, fresh or bottled
2 teaspoons olive oil
4 sprigs fresh rosemary or 1 teaspoon dried rosemary

Preheat oven to 325°F. Butterfly each tenderloin by slicing it crosswise in half. Season all surfaces of turkey with salt and pepper.

Put spinach, onion, and garlic in a food processor; process until vegetables are chopped. Spread each tenderloin with spinach mixture. Slice roasted pepper; arrange slices over spinach mixture. Roll turkey around filling. Tie rolls with cotton string every 2 inches, or firmly secure rolls with wooden toothpicks.

Prepare a roasting pan with nonstick cooking spray. Put turkey rolls in pan; brush with olive oil and top with rosemary. Roast 1 hour, basting several times with pan liquids, until turkey is golden brown.

Remove string and/or toothpicks. Cut into ½-inch slices and top with pan liquids.

6 servings
1 serving = 4 ½-inch slices

CAL.	CHO(g)	PRO.(g)	TOTAL FAT(g)	SAT. FAT(g)	CHOL.(mg)	FIBER(g)	SODIUM(mg)
180	4	33	3	0.5	80	1	260

Food exchanges per serving: 4 Very Lean Meats plus 1 Vegetable
Low-sodium diets: Omit salt.

Turkey Milanese

6 (1 pound total) fresh turkey
   breast slices
2 egg whites
2 tablespoons skim milk
½ cup seasoned bread crumbs

¼ cup flour
¼ teaspoon salt
2 tablespoons margarine or butter
2 tablespoons grated Parmesan
   cheese

Place each turkey breast slice between two pieces of plastic wrap. Using the side of a meat mallet or bottom of a heavy glass, pound to half of original thickness.

In a medium bowl, whisk together egg white and milk. In a shallow dish, mix bread crumbs, flour, and salt. Dip turkey slices into egg mixture, then dredge in crumbs to thoroughly coat. Double-dip turkey if there is extra egg or crumb mixture.

Preheat oven to 300°F. In a large nonstick skillet, melt 1 tablespoon margarine over medium heat. Cook 3 turkey cutlets about 2–3 minutes on each side until outside is lightly browned. Transfer cutlets to an ovenproof platter, and keep warm in oven. Repeat the process to cook remaining cutlets. Sprinkle each cutlet with 1 teaspoon grated cheese.

Bake 2–3 minutes until cheese begins to melt.

6 servings
1 serving = 1 3- to 3½-ounce cutlet

CAL.	CHO(g)	PRO.(g)	TOTAL FAT(g)	SAT. FAT(g)	CHOL.(mg)	FIBER(g)	SODIUM(mg)
190	11	23	5	1	50	0.5	490

Food exchanges per serving: 3 Very Lean Meats plus 1 Starch
Low-sodium diets: Omit salt; substitute plain bread crumbs.

Turkey Vegetable Stir-Fry

⅓ cup beef or chicken broth
½ cup chopped onion
½ cup chopped celery
½ cup chopped green bell pepper
1 cup chopped tomato, including
    liquid

3 tablespoons minced fresh parsley
½ teaspoon crumbled dried oregano
¼ teaspoon freshly ground black
    pepper
1 pound sliced turkey breast (8 thin
    scallops)

*H*eat broth in a large nonstick skillet. Add onion and celery; cook quickly over moderately high heat until soft. Add green pepper, tomato, parsley, oregano, and black pepper. Continue cooking until tender, stirring with a wooden spoon.

Remove vegetables, leaving some liquid in bottom of skillet. Quickly cook turkey scallops in pan juices, about 1 minute on each side or until cooked.

Arrange turkey slices on individual dishes, and spoon 3 tablespoons vegetables over each serving. Serve immediately.

4 servings
1 serving = 2 turkey scallops plus 3 tablespoons vegetables

CAL.	CHO(g)	PRO.(g)	TOTAL FAT(g)	SAT. FAT(g)	CHOL.(mg)	FIBER(g)	SODIUM(mg)
150	6	29	1	0	70	1.5	210

Food exchanges per serving: 4 Very Lean Meats plus 1 Vegetable
Low-sodium diets: This recipe is excellent.

Mideast Turkey Meatballs with Yogurt Dill Sauce

1 pound low-fat ground turkey
1 cup plain low-fat yogurt, divided
½ cup chopped onion
1 tablespoon lemon juice
¼ cup chopped fresh parsley
½ teaspoon minced fresh garlic
½ teaspoon salt

¼ teaspoon ground cinnamon
⅛ teaspoon ground cloves
¼ teaspoon chili powder
1½ teaspoons snipped fresh dill or
   ½ teaspoon dried dill
¼ teaspoon cracked pepper

Preheat oven to 400°F. Combine turkey, 3 tablespoons of the yogurt, onion, lemon juice, parsley, garlic, salt, cinnamon, cloves, and chili powder. Shape into 20 meatballs, each 1¼–1½ inches in diameter. Place on a shallow pan and bake 25 minutes turning balls once midway through cooking time.

While meatballs are cooking, mix remaining yogurt, dill, and pepper to make sauce. To serve, pour yogurt dill sauce over meatballs.

5 servings
1 serving = 4 meatballs plus 2 tablespoons sauce

CAL.	CHO(g)	PRO.(g)	TOTAL FAT(g)	SAT. FAT(g)	CHOL.(mg)	FIBER(g)	SODIUM(mg)
165	5	19	8	2.5	70	0.5	340

Food exchanges per serving: 2 Lean Meats plus ½ Milk
Low-sodium diets: Omit salt.

Dijon Turkey Burgers

2 teaspoons corn oil
1 cup chopped onion
1 pound low-fat ground turkey
3 tablespoons Dijon or brown spicy
　　mustard

2 tablespoons chopped fresh parsley
½ teaspoon salt
¼ teaspoon freshly ground pepper

*I*n a large skillet, heat oil. Add onion and sauté until lightly browned. In a bowl, combine turkey, onion, and seasonings. Shape mixture into five patties.

　　Place patties on skillet and cook over medium heat about 12 minutes, turning occasionally.

5 servings
1 serving = 1 burger

CAL.	CHO(g)	PRO.(g)	TOTAL FAT(g)	SAT. FAT(g)	CHOL.(mg)	FIBER(g)	SODIUM(mg)
170	3	16	9	2	65	0.5	520

Food exchanges per serving: 2 Medium-Fat Meats
Low-sodium diets: Omit salt.

Cajun Sausage in Acorn Squash

In New Orleans, they use a very spicy sausage called andouille for this dish. If you can find it and like very spicy foods, substitute andouille for half of the lean smoked turkey sausage.

2 (2 pounds total) small acorn
   squash
2 tablespoons reduced-sugar maple-
   flavored syrup
2 teaspoons margarine
1 medium onion, sliced thin
1 medium green bell pepper, cored
   and sliced

1 clove garlic, crushed
8 ounces lean smoked turkey
   sausage
⅓ cup water
2 teaspoons Cajun seasoning

Preheat oven to 375°F. Cut each squash in half; remove core and seeds. Brush all orange surfaces of squash with maple syrup; pour remaining syrup in cavity of squash.

Put ½ inch hot water in a shallow roasting pan. Put squash halves in pan, cut side up. Cover tightly with foil and bake about 45 minutes until squash is tender when tested with a fork. Remove foil, baste squash with syrup, and bake 10–15 more minutes.

While squash is baking, melt margarine in a large nonstick skillet. Add onion, green pepper, and garlic; sauté until onions are lightly browned. Cut sausage into thin slices on the diagonal. Add sausage, water, and Cajun seasoning; stir to mix well. Cover and simmer 10 minutes, stirring occasionally. Taste and add more Cajun seasoning if desired.

To serve, fill each squash half with sausage mixture.

4 servings
1 serving = ½ squash plus 1 cup sausage/vegetables

CAL.	CHO(g)	PRO.(g)	TOTAL FAT(g)	SAT. FAT(g)	CHOL.(mg)	FIBER(g)	SODIUM(mg)
220	30	10	7	3	30	7	1,075

Food exchanges per serving: 2 Starches plus 1 Medium-Fat Meat
Low-sodium diets: This recipe is not suitable.

Duck

Although duck has been considered very high in fat, the meat of duck, without skin and visible fat, is actually quite lean. The trick is to prepare duck so that most of the fat cooks off or is trimmed off. Duck retains more moisture and flavor cooked with some of its skin on, but remove the skin, which is fatty, before you eat the duck. Muscovy ducks are more expensive than most other ducklings but have more lean meat and less fat.

Sometimes you can buy boned duck breasts, but it's often more economical to buy a 4½- to 5-pound duckling and have the meat cutter bone it. That way you'll have a duck breast plus meat from the leg and thigh. Before cooking, trim off any skin and fat that does not have meat attached to it. From a 5-pound duck you will get about 2¼ pounds raw duck meat with skin attached, which will yield about 1¼ pounds roasted duck with skin or almost 1 pound of cooked duck meat with skin removed.

Roast Duckling with Mango Chutney

If you can get only whole ducks, quarter each bird and increase cooking time to 1½–1¾ hours. Serve duck quarters, and remove separable fat and skin before eating the duck. The nutritional values will be about the same.

2¼ pounds boneless duck (light and dark meat) with skin attached
¾ teaspoon seasoned salt

¼ teaspoon freshly ground pepper
1 cup Mango Chutney (see Index)

Heat oven to 425°F. Trim off any skin and fat not attached to duck meat. Prick duck through skin side with fork every few inches. This allows fat to drain from duck. Season duck with seasoned salt and pepper.

Arrange a wire cooling rack over a roasting pan; place duck, skin side up, on rack. Roast 25 minutes. Remove from oven; drain fat from bottom of roasting pan. Reduce heat to 350°F, roast 35 minutes more.

Warm Mango Chutney in a small saucepan. Brush surfaces of duck with some of the chutney. Return duck to oven for 15 minutes until duck surfaces are glazed. Serve duckling pieces topped with remaining Mango Chutney. Remove and discard skin before eating the duck.

4 servings
1 serving = 3½ ounces skinless, boneless duck plus scant ¼ cup Mango Chutney

CAL.	CHO*(g)*	PRO.*(g)*	TOTAL FAT*(g)*	SAT. FAT*(g)*	CHOL.*(mg)*	FIBER*(g)*	SODIUM*(mg)*
300	18	27	13	4.5	100	1	235

Food exchanges per serving: 4 Lean Meats plus 1 Fruit
Low-sodium diets: Substitute light (reduced-sodium) seasoned salt.

Duck Breast with Seville Sauce

This piquant preparation is a change from duckling with fruit sauce. Seville Sauce, which includes onions, olives, and sherry, is served throughout Spain—although I first tasted it at a ski lodge in France. This recipe uses duck breast. You can also use a whole duck, quartered and trimmed, but increase roasting time to 1½–1¾ hours.

1 large or 2 small (1¼–1½ pounds total) boneless duck breasts
½ teaspoon seasoned salt
¼ teaspoon freshly ground pepper
1 teaspoon olive oil
1 small onion, sliced thin
¾ cup orange juice

1 medium carrot, grated
¼ cup pimiento-stuffed olives, chopped coarse
¾ teaspoon chopped fresh thyme or ¼ teaspoon dried thyme
1 teaspoon cornstarch
¼ cup dry sherry or dry red wine

Preheat oven to 425°F. Prick duck through skin with a fork every few inches. Season duck on all surfaces with seasoned salt and pepper.

Arrange a wire cooking rack over a roasting pan. Place duck, skin side up, on rack, allowing heat to circulate around the duck and the fat to drain. Roast duck 25 minutes. Remove from oven; drain fat from roasting pan. Reduce heat to 350°F, and roast 35 minutes more.

Toward the end of the cooking time for the duck, warm olive oil in a small skillet; sauté onion over low heat until translucent. Add orange juice, carrot, olives, and thyme; simmer 5 minutes.

Dissolve cornstarch in sherry. Add to the skillet and simmer about 3 minutes until sauce thickens.

Remove duck from oven, trim off fat and skin. Cut into thin slices and place on a warmed platter. Pour sauce over duck slices. Serve immediately.

4 servings
1 serving = 3 ounces duck meat plus ⅓ cup sauce

CAL.	CHO(g)	PRO.(g)	TOTAL FAT(g)	SAT. FAT(g)	CHOL.(mg)	FIBER(g)	SODIUM(mg)
255	12	21	12	4	75	1.5	345

Food exchanges per serving: 3 Lean Meats plus 1 Vegetable plus ½ Fruit *or* 3 Lean Meats plus 1 Other Carbohydrate
Low-sodium diets: Substitute light (reduced-sodium) seasoned salt.

18
Seafood

Grilled Salmon with Cilantro Spinach Sauce

You will find many salmon recipes in this book—because it is a heart-healthy fish and because almost everyone enjoys salmon, even many who don't like fish.

Sauce

2 cups fresh spinach, washed and
    trimmed
½ cup cilantro, washed and
    trimmed
½ cup light or reduced-calorie
    mayonnaise
½ cup sour half-and-half
½ teaspoon Dijon mustard
½ teaspoon salt
¼ teaspoon freshly ground pepper

Fish

6 (5 ounces each) salmon fillets
1 tablespoon margarine, melted
Additional cilantro for garnish

Prepare sauce: Pat greens dry with a paper towel. Puree spinach, cilantro, and mayonnaise in a food processor fitted with a steel blade. Add remaining sauce ingredients, and continue processing only until all ingredients are combined. Sauce may be prepared up to one day in advance and refrigerated until serving time.

    Brush salmon fillets with melted margarine; place on a prepared grill over ashen coals or on a broiler rack about 3–4 inches from heat source. Cook

321

salmon about 3 minutes, depending on the thickness of the fillets and the distance from the heat source. Turn fillets with a spatula and continue cooking for 2–3 minutes or until fish begins to flake when tested with a fork. Fish is best when slightly undercooked.

Drizzle sauce decoratively around and/or over salmon fillets. Garnish with cilantro and serve immediately.

6 servings
1 serving = 1 salmon fillet plus ¼ cup sauce

CAL.	CHO(g)	PRO.(g)	TOTAL FAT(g)	SAT. FAT(g)	CHOL.(mg)	FIBER(g)	SODIUM(mg)
305	3	29	19	4.5	90	0.5	410

Food exchanges per serving: 4 Lean Meats plus 1 Vegetable plus 1 Fat
Low-sodium diets: Omit salt.

Grilled Salmon Steaks with Rosemary

Salmon is a popular fish, rich in heart-healthy omega-3 fatty acids. If you prefer not to use a grill, these salmon steaks can also be prepared indoors in the broiler.

1 tablespoon crumbled dried sage	2 tablespoons fresh lemon juice
¼ teaspoon white pepper	2 tablespoons olive oil
3 tablespoons crumbled dried rosemary, divided	6 (5 ounces each) salmon steaks
	1 lemon, cut into 6 wedges

*I*n a small bowl, mix together sage, pepper, and 1½ tablespoons of the rosemary. Add lemon juice and olive oil. Brush both sides of each salmon steak with the mixture.

Prepare a wire grilling basket with nonstick cooking spray. Arrange salmon steaks securely in the basket. Sprinkle remaining 1½ tablespoons rosemary over hot coals for extra flavor.

Grill steaks about 6 minutes on each side, depending on the thickness of the fish and the distance from the coals. Fish is cooked when it flakes easily when tested with a fork. Be sure not to overcook the fish.

Serve with lemon wedges.

6 servings
1 serving = 1 fish steak

CAL.	CHO*(g)*	PRO.*(g)*	TOTAL FAT*(g)*	SAT. FAT*(g)*	CHOL.*(mg)*	FIBER*(g)*	SODIUM*(mg)*
230	4	25	13	2	70	0	60

Food exchanges per serving: 4 Lean Meats
Low-sodium diets: This recipe is excellent.

Simple Poached Salmon

Each ounce of salmon is considered a Lean Meat Exchange because it has a bit more fat than most other fish. If you poach a very low fat fish (see the list of Very Lean Meat Exchanges) count each ounce as a Very Lean Meat Exchange. Don't be concerned about the amount of salt used in this recipe. Because the poaching liquid with most of the salt is discarded, you eat only the salt that is absorbed into the fish. Try serving poached fish with Cucumber Dill Sauce (recipe follows), Cilantro Salsa, Yogurt Dill Dip, or Roasted Onion Confiture (see Index).

1 medium onion, sliced thin
1 thinly sliced lemon, or 2 tablespoons fresh lemon juice
½ cup chopped celery
1 teaspoon salt

1 teaspoon dried dill or 4–5 sprigs fresh dill
1 teaspoon cracked black pepper
4 (5 ounces each) salmon steaks

To make poaching liquid, fill a large skillet half full of water. Add all ingredients except fish; bring to a boil. Cover and simmer 5 minutes.

Add salmon, cover, and poach about 5 minutes. Turn salmon over and poach 3–5 minutes more until fish is cooked.

4 servings
1 serving = 1 salmon steak

CAL.	CHO(g)	PRO.(g)	TOTAL FAT(g)	SAT. FAT(g)	CHOL.(mg)	FIBER(g)	SODIUM(mg)
175	0	25	8	1	70	0	110

Food exchanges per serving: 3 Lean Meats
Low-sodium diets: This recipe is excellent.

Salmon Patties with Cucumber Dill Sauce

Canned salmon has far more calcium than fresh salmon because we can eat the soft bones of the fish. Enjoy the calcium advantage—don't discard the bones.

Salmon Patties

1 can (14¾ ounces) red or pink
  salmon
⅔ cup dry oatmeal
¼ cup skim milk
½ cup egg substitute or *2 eggs,*
  beaten
3 tablespoons finely chopped onion
1 tablespoon snipped fresh dill
½ teaspoon salt
¼ teaspoon freshly ground pepper
2 teaspoons margarine

Cucumber Dill Sauce

½ cup plain low-fat yogurt
¼ small cucumber, seeded and diced
½ small tomato, diced fine
1 tablespoon finely chopped onion
1 tablespoon snipped fresh dill or
  ¾ teaspoon dried dill

*D*rain salmon; mash soft bones into salmon. Add oatmeal, milk, egg substitute, onion, dill, salt, and pepper; mix well. Form into six round patties.

Melt margarine in a nonstick skillet. Add salmon patties and cook over medium heat about 4 minutes on each side until patties are browned and heated through.

To prepare sauce, combine yogurt, cucumber, tomato, onion and dill in a small bowl. Mix well. Serve with or over salmon patties.

6 servings
1 serving = 1 patty plus ¼ cup sauce

CAL.	CHO(g)	PRO.(g)	TOTAL FAT(g)	SAT. FAT(g)	CHOL.(mg)	FIBER(g)	SODIUM(mg)
165	10	17	7	2.5	25	1.5	555

Food exchanges per serving: 2 Lean Meats plus ½ Starch
Low-sodium diets: Omit salt.

Salmon-Wrapped Scallop Kabobs

¾ pound fresh salmon, cut into
   very thin strips
¾ pound large sea scallops

Marinade

3 tablespoons light (reduced-
   sodium) soy sauce
2 tablespoons dry white wine
1 tablespoon light brown sugar
¾ teaspoon grated fresh gingerroot

Arrange salmon slices and scallops in a shallow glass bowl. Combine marinade ingredients in a small bowl or jar. Pour over seafood and marinate 30 minutes.

Drain seafood and reserve marinade. Wrap scallops in salmon strips; put 3 wrapped scallops on short bamboo skewers that have been soaked in water or on metal skewers.

To oven broil: Preheat broiler. Place a sheet of aluminum foil over broiler rack. Arrange seafood on foil; broil about 4 inches from heat until lightly done, about 4 minutes. Baste with marinade during cooking. Serve immediately.

To charcoal broil: Arrange skewers on oiled grill in a single layer. Grill about 3 minutes on each side or until cooked. Baste once with marinade when skewers are turned.

6 servings
1 serving = 3 rolls salmon-wrapped scallops

CAL.	CHO(g)	PRO.(g)	TOTAL FAT(g)	SAT. FAT(g)	CHOL.(mg)	FIBER(g)	SODIUM(mg)
145	4	21	4	0.5	50	0	415

Food exchanges per serving: 3 Very Lean Meats plus 1 Vegetable
Low-sodium diets: Reduce soy sauce to 2 tablespoons.

Peppered Tuna Steaks

These tuna steaks are really nice served atop Gently Steamed Spinach and with Fennel and Red Grapefruit Salad (see Index). If you have leftovers, serve the tuna in slices on top of a tossed green salad, on pasta, or with Panzanella (see Index).

2 teaspoons black peppercorns
2 teaspoons green or red
*   peppercorns*
2 teaspoons mustard seeds

4 (about 1 pound total) yellowfin
*   tuna steaks*
1 tablespoon lemon juice

*P*reheat oven to 400°F. Crush peppercorns and mustard seeds in a mortar and pestle, or wrap them in plastic film and crush with a meat mallet or hammer. Brush tuna steaks with lemon juice. Press crushed pepper and mustard seeds into tuna.

Prepare a roasting pan with nonstick cooking spray. Put tuna steaks in pan. Bake 10 minutes. (If you prefer, sauté peppered steaks in a nonstick skillet, about 4 minutes each side.)

4 servings
1 serving = 1 tuna steak

CAL.	CHO*(g)*	PRO.*(g)*	TOTAL FAT*(g)*	SAT. FAT*(g)*	CHOL.*(mg)*	FIBER*(g)*	SODIUM*(mg)*
125	2	24	2	0.5	45	0.5	40

Food exchanges per serving: 3 Very Lean Meats
Low-sodium diets: This recipe is excellent.

Hearty Halibut

¾ cup thinly sliced onion

6 (1½ pounds total) fresh or frozen
    halibut steaks, thawed

1 cup fresh mushrooms, sliced

¾ cup chopped fresh or drained
    canned tomato

¼ cup chopped green bell pepper

¼ cup minced fresh parsley

3 tablespoons finely chopped
    pimiento

½ cup dry white wine

2 tablespoons white vinegar

1 teaspoon salt

⅛ teaspoon freshly ground black
    pepper

1 tablespoon olive oil

Lemon wedges for garnish

Preheat oven to 350°F. Prepare a large baking pan with nonstick cooking spray. Arrange onion in bottom of pan. Place fish on top of onion.

In a medium bowl, combine mushrooms, tomato, green pepper, parsley, pimiento, wine, vinegar, salt, and black pepper. Spread on top of fish. Drizzle oil on top of vegetable mixture. Bake 20 minutes or until fish flakes easily with a fork.

Serve with lemon wedges.

6 servings
1 serving = 3 ounces cooked fish

CAL.	CHO(g)	PRO.(g)	TOTAL FAT(g)	SAT. FAT(g)	CHOL.(mg)	FIBER(g)	SODIUM(mg)
155	4	20	5	0.5	30	1	425

Food exchanges per serving: 3 Lean Meats plus 1 Vegetable
Low-sodium diets: Omit salt.

Cod Southwestern Style

Fish

2 pounds fresh or frozen cod or
    other fish fillets, thawed
¼ teaspoon salt
⅛ teaspoon freshly ground black
    pepper
⅔ cup dry white wine
⅔ cup Chicken Stock (see Index) or
    chicken broth

Sauce

4 tablespoons margarine
½ cup chopped onion
1⅓ cups diced green bell pepper
3 large tomatoes, peeled and diced
2 tablespoons fresh lemon juice
1 teaspoon chili powder
½ teaspoon salt
⅛ teaspoon freshly ground pepper
1 clove garlic, crushed
¼ teaspoon ground thyme
¼ teaspoon dried oregano
3 ounces Monterey Jack cheese with
    peppers

Preheat oven to 350°F. Divide cod into 6 equal portions. Season with salt and pepper. Place cod in a large skillet; pour wine and Chicken Stock over it. Cover and bring to a boil; reduce heat to low, and poach fish 10 minutes.

Meanwhile, prepare the sauce. Melt margarine in a medium skillet. Add onion; sauté until translucent. Add green pepper and cook gently for 3 minutes. Add remaining sauce ingredients except cheese; simmer 10 minutes.

Place fish on an ovenproof serving platter. Cover entirely with sauce. Cut cheese into 6 thin slices. Place a slice of cheese over each portion of fish. Heat in oven for a few minutes, just long enough to melt cheese.

6 servings
1 serving = 4 ounces cooked fish plus ⅓ cup sauce

CAL.	CHO(g)	PRO.(g)	TOTAL FAT(g)	SAT. FAT(g)	CHOL.(mg)	FIBER(g)	SODIUM(mg)
300	8	32	14	4	80	1.5	565

Food exchanges per serving: 4 Lean Meats plus 1 Vegetable
Low-sodium diets: Omit salt.

Red Snapper Creole

2 pounds fresh or frozen red
    snapper fillets, thawed
2 tablespoons margarine, melted
½ cup finely chopped celery
½ cup finely diced carrot
¼ cup chopped black olives

½ cup finely chopped green bell
    pepper
1 cup chopped onion
1 16-ounce can tomatoes, cut up
½ cup tomato sauce
2 tablespoons margarine

Preheat oven to 350°F. Cut fish into 6 serving pieces. Pour melted margarine into a large baking pan and set aside.

In a medium bowl, combine celery, carrot, olives, green pepper, onion, tomatoes, and tomato sauce. Spread half of this mixture in bottom of baking pan. Place fish pieces on top; cover with remaining vegetable mixture. Dot with margarine.

Bake 20–25 minutes or until fish flakes with a fork.

6 servings
1 serving = 4 ounces cooked fish plus ½ cup sauce

CAL.	CHO(g)	PRO.(g)	TOTAL FAT(g)	SAT. FAT(g)	CHOL.(mg)	FIBER(g)	SODIUM(mg)
265	9	33	11	2	55	2	495

Food exchanges per serving: 4 Lean Meats plus 2 Vegetables
Low-sodium diets: Use unsalted margarine, unsalted canned tomatoes, and unsalted tomato sauce. Omit olives if sodium restriction is 1 gram (1,000 milligrams) per day or less.

Havana Red Snapper

Try this bold-flavored fish served with rice and a simple green salad.

4 fillets (1 pound total) red snapper   *2–3 cloves garlic, minced*
1 orange   *1 5-ounce jar Spanish salad olives*
1 lime   *with pimiento, drained and*
2 teaspoons cornstarch   *sliced*
1 tablespoon good-quality olive oil   *1 tablespoon finely chopped*
1 sweet Spanish onion, sliced thin   *cilantro, divided*

*P*reheat oven to 450°F. Spray an ovenproof pan with nonstick cooking spray, and place fish fillets in pan. Grate zest from orange and lime; reserve for garnish.

Squeeze juice from both fruits into a small bowl. There should be about ½ cup orange and ¼ cup lime juice. Stir in cornstarch until it dissolves.

Pour olive oil into a large nonstick skillet. Add onion and garlic; sauté about 10 minutes, stirring occasionally. Add juice mixture, olives, and 2 teaspoons cilantro. Heat until mixture simmers and sauce thickens.

Pour sauce over fish. Bake 8–10 minutes until fish is cooked through. Serve fish hot, garnished with reserved orange and lime zest and remaining 1 teaspoon cilantro.

4 servings
1 serving = 1 fish fillet plus ⅓ cup sauce

CAL.	CHO(g)	PRO.(g)	TOTAL FAT(g)	SAT. FAT(g)	CHOL.(mg)	FIBER(g)	SODIUM(mg)
240	13	25	10	1.5	40	2	930

Food exchanges per serving: 3 Lean Meats plus 1 Vegetable plus ½ Fruit *or* 3 Lean Meats plus 1 Other Carbohydrate
Low-sodium diets: This recipe is not suitable.

Swordfish and Peach Brochette

If you marinate the fish and peppers in the morning, you can prepare a very quick and interesting meal in the evening.

<u>Marinade</u>

1 tablespoon corn or peanut oil

1 tablespoon light (reduced-sodium) soy sauce

1 tablespoon lemon juice

1 clove garlic, crushed

½ teaspoon finely grated lemon zest

½ teaspoon Chinese five-spice powder or 1½ teaspoons snipped fresh rosemary

1 pound swordfish steaks, 1 inch thick

1 medium green bell pepper

4 juice-packed peach halves, drained, or 2 medium-sized fresh peaches, peeled and halved

*P*repare a marinade by mixing together the oil, soy sauce, lemon juice, garlic, lemon zest, and five-spice powder or rosemary in a small bowl. Cut swordfish into 1-inch cubes. Core green pepper and cut into 1¼-inch pieces. Put swordfish cubes and pieces of pepper in a nonmetallic dish, and brush with marinade.

Cover and refrigerate for at least 1 hour. If using bamboo skewers, soak them in water while fish is marinating so skewers won't burn as fish cooks.

Cut each peach half into 4 pieces. Thread four bamboo or metal skewers with a piece of fish, then green pepper, then peach. Repeating sequence until there are 4–5 pieces of each item per skewer.

Broil or grill over hot coals about 6 minutes, turning every 2 minutes and basting with the marinade at each turn.

4 servings
1 serving = 1 skewer

CAL.	CHO(g)	PRO.(g)	TOTAL FAT(g)	SAT. FAT(g)	CHOL.(mg)	FIBER(g)	SODIUM(mg)
175	11	21	5	1.5	40	0.5	145

Food exchanges per serving: 3 Very Lean Meats plus 1 Fruit
Low-sodium diets: This recipe is excellent.

Cajun Catfish

Try this hot-skillet method. It's a modification of blackened catfish. True blackening requires bringing the pan to the smoking point, but most home kitchens lack proper ventilation for that method. This method avoids filling the kitchen with smoke and setting off a smoke alarm.

1 tablespoon Cajun seasoning or blackening spice blend
4 (5 ounces each) catfish fillets

1 tablespoon margarine or butter
2 teaspoons chopped fresh parsley

Sprinkle seasoning on both sides of fish. Refrigerate 1 hour (if you have time).

Melt margarine in large heavy skillet or griddle over high heat. Add fish and cook about 8 minutes, turning fish two or three times.

Serve hot, garnished with chopped parsley.

4 servings
1 serving = 1 fish fillet

CAL.	CHO(g)	PRO.(g)	TOTAL FAT(g)	SAT. FAT(g)	CHOL.(mg)	FIBER(g)	SODIUM(mg)
205	2	22	12	2.5	45	0	700

Food exchanges per serving: 3 Lean Meats
Low-sodium diets: Cajun spice blends include salt. Substitute a mixture of ½ teaspoon chili powder, ½ teaspoon finely minced garlic, and ½ teaspoon salt-free herb blend.

Grilled Catfish with Creole Gumbo Sauce

If an outdoor grill is not available, this fish can be prepared on a sheet of aluminum foil or on a nonstick cookie sheet in the broiler.

6 (5 ounces each) catfish (or
   whitefish) fillets
1 teaspoon minced garlic
1 teaspoon paprika
1 teaspoon snipped fresh tarragon
   or ½ teaspoon crumbled dried
   tarragon

1½ cups Creole Gumbo Sauce (see
   Index)

Sprinkle fish fillets with garlic, paprika, and tarragon. Prepare a wire grilling basket with nonstick cooking spray, and secure fish in basket.

Grill fish over medium-hot coals 3–4 minutes on each side, depending on thickness of fish and distance from coals. Fish is done when it flakes easily when tested with a fork.

Warm sauce in a small saucepan. Arrange a piece of fish on each plate and serve with sauce.

6 servings
1 serving = 1 fish fillet plus ¼ cup sauce

CAL.	CHO(g)	PRO.(g)	TOTAL FAT(g)	SAT. FAT(g)	CHOL.(mg)	FIBER(g)	SODIUM(mg)
220	5	22	12	2.5	45	1	585

Food exchanges per serving: 3 Medium-Fat Meats plus 1 Vegetable
Low-sodium diets: Prepare grilled fish as directed, and top with chopped fresh tomatoes.

Grilled Mackerel with Chopped Tomatoes

This delicious barbecue entree can also be prepared indoors under a broiler. Mackerel is a strong-flavored fish particularly high in omega-3 fatty acids.

6 (5 ounces each) mackerel fillets	½ teaspoon crumbled dried oregano
1 tablespoon lemon juice	2 cups chopped fresh tomato
¼ teaspoon freshly ground pepper	½ cup chopped fresh parsley

*A*rrange mackerel fillets in a shallow baking pan. Combine lemon juice, pepper, and oregano; sprinkle over fish. Prepare a wire grilling basket with nonstick cooking spray, and secure fish in basket.

Grill fish over medium-hot coals about 3–4 minutes on each side, depending on thickness of fish. Fish is done when it flakes easily when tested with a fork. Place mackerel on individual serving dishes.

Combine tomato and parsley and spread decoratively around and over mackerel. Serve fish hot with tomato mixture at room temperature.

6 servings
1 serving = 1 mackerel fillet with tomato topping

CAL.	CHO(g)	PRO.(g)	TOTAL FAT(g)	SAT. FAT(g)	CHOL.(mg)	FIBER(g)	SODIUM(mg)
305	4	27	20	4.5	100	1	135

Food exchanges per serving: 4 Medium-Fat Meats plus 1 Vegetable
Low-sodium diets: This recipe is excellent.

Foil-Baked Fish Fillets

To make a more elegant version, cook the fish in parchment packets, and cut the tops of the parchment packets on the dinner plates.

1 pound fresh or thawed frozen
    fish fillets
1½ teaspoons lemon juice
1 tablespoon finely chopped onion
1 tablespoon finely chopped celery
    with leaves

⅛ teaspoon salt
Dash freshly ground pepper
1 tablespoon olive oil

Preheat oven to 400°F. Cut fresh or thawed fillets into three individual serving pieces. Tear or cut three separate pieces of heavy-duty foil about 12–14 inches square. Coat centers of each piece of foil with nonstick cooking spray.

Place fish on foil; sprinkle with lemon juice. On top of fish spread a layer of onion, then a layer of celery. Sprinkle with salt, pepper, and olive oil.

Lift foil up from opposite sides of fish to come together across top; fold over twice; then pinch together to seal tightly. Seal ends in same way. Place foil packages in a shallow pan. Bake 20 minutes.

To serve, lift each package onto a dinner plate, unwrap, and transfer cooked fish and sauce with a wide pancake turner.

3 servings
1 serving = 1 foil package of fish (about 4 ounces cooked)

CAL.	CHO(g)	PRO.(g)	TOTAL FAT(g)	SAT. FAT(g)	CHOL.(mg)	FIBER(g)	SODIUM(mg)
175	1	27	7	1	65	0	175

Food exchanges per serving: 4 Lean Meats
Low-sodium diets: Omit salt.

Unfried Fish Fillets

This very basic preparation of fish deserves serving with Dill Sauce, Creole Gumbo Sauce, or one of the salsas (see Index).

4 (1 pound total) fish fillets	*1 teaspoon seasoned salt*
(walleyed pike, perch, sole,	*24 soda crackers, crushed fine*
flounder, or whitefish)	*1 tablespoon olive or corn oil*
1 cup skim milk	*Lemon wedges*

*P*reheat oven to 500°F. Prepare baking pan with nonstick cooking spray. Cut fish fillets into four serving pieces.

Mix milk and salt together in a shallow dish. Put cracker crumbs into a large pie plate. Dip each piece of fish into milk, then crumbs, then milk, then crumbs again to coat thoroughly. Place fish pieces in the baking pan. Sprinkle oil over tops of fish pieces.

Bake 10 minutes or until fish flakes lightly with a fork. Serve with lemon wedges.

4 servings
1 serving = 3½ ounces cooked fish

CAL.	CHO*(g)*	PRO.*(g)*	TOTAL FAT*(g)*	SAT. FAT*(g)*	CHOL.*(mg)*	FIBER*(g)*	SODIUM*(mg)*
230	16	26	7	4.5	45	0.5	625

Food exchanges per serving: 3 Lean Meats plus 1 Starch
Low-sodium diets: Substitute light (reduced-sodium) seasoned salt.

Clambake

This recipe can be made outdoors on a charcoal grill or inside on the kitchen stove. It is great served with Buttermilk Corn Bread (see Index) and a green salad.

3 pounds clams (small cherrystones, littlenecks, or soft steamer clams)

Seaweed (traditional but optional)

6 small ears corn in husks

2 teaspoons fresh lemon juice

6 tablespoons margarine, melted

Cover clams with water and let stand 30 minutes, drain to remove sand.

Place 1 inch of water and a layer of wet seaweed (if available at fish market) in the bottom of a large heavy kettle. Bring water to simmer. Top seaweed with corn, still in husks, and clams. Arrange a layer of seaweed on top. Cover kettle and steam over high heat about 10 minutes or until clams have opened.

Discard any clams that do not open. Discard seaweed unless using it to decorate the platter. Arrange clams and corn on a large platter or in individual bowls.

Strain pan juices to serve with clams. Add lemon juice and melted margarine. Serve strained pan juices and lemon margarine as dips for clams and corn.

6 servings
1 serving = ½ pound clams (about 6–8) plus 1 ear corn plus 1 tablespoon margarine for dipping

CAL.	CHO(g)	PRO.(g)	TOTAL FAT(g)	SAT. FAT(g)	CHOL.(mg)	FIBER(g)	SODIUM(mg)
205	18	7	13	2	10	3	165

Food exchanges per serving: 1 Starch plus 1 Lean Meat plus 2 Fats
Low-sodium diets: This recipe is excellent, but don't use seaweed.

Crabmeat Mushroom Crepes

This recipe can be made with canned salmon or leftover cooked fish or shellfish instead of crabmeat.

1 teaspoon margarine	1 tablespoon chopped fresh parsley
1 cup sliced fresh mushrooms	1½ teaspoons lemon juice
⅓ cup chopped scallions	1 teaspoon Dijon mustard
½ teaspoon dried thyme	⅛ teaspoon salt
1½ teaspoons all-purpose flour	Pinch cayenne pepper
⅓ cup skim milk	8 Basic Crepes (see Index)
1 cup frozen, canned, or fresh lump crabmeat, drained and flaked	

Melt margarine in a large skillet. Add mushrooms, scallions, and thyme; sauté until vegetables are tender. Reduce heat to low and add flour. Cook 1 minute, stirring constantly. Gradually add milk, cooking over medium heat, stirring constantly, until thickened and bubbly. Remove from heat; stir in crabmeat, parsley, lemon juice, mustard, salt, and cayenne.

Preheat oven to 350°F. Spoon 2 tablespoons crabmeat mixture down center of each crepe; roll up crepes and arrange in a baking pan prepared with nonstick cooking spray. Cover and bake twenty minutes or until thoroughly heated.

Broil crepes 4–6 inches from heat 1 minute or until golden brown.

4 servings
1 serving = 2 filled crepes

CAL.	CHO(g)	PRO.(g)	TOTAL FAT(g)	SAT. FAT(g)	CHOL.(mg)	FIBER(g)	SODIUM(mg)
235	23	17	8	1.5	145	1	400

Food exchanges per serving: 2 Lean Meats plus 1½ Starches
Low-sodium diets: Omit salt; use fresh or frozen crab, as canned crab is packed with salt.

Mussels Dijonnaise

Mussels can also be prepared this way and topped with 1 cup pasta sauce or Chunky Tomato Sauce (see Index). If you are unsure about soaking and cleaning mussels, look for frozen ones from New Zealand that are ready to heat and serve.

2 pounds mussels, scrubbed and
    beards discarded
½ cup chopped fresh parsley
4 bay leaves
1 cup dry white wine

1 cup Mustard Dressing
    (see Index), warmed
Fresh parsley sprigs for garnish

Cover mussels with water and soak 45 minutes; drain. In a 6-quart pot place chopped parsley, bay leaves, and wine. Heat to a boil and add mussels. Cover pan and cook mussels over high heat 3–4 minutes or until mussels have opened. Shake pan or stir during the cooking time.

Drain and discard any unopened mussels. Arrange mussels in a large bowl or in 4 deep soup bowls. Pour Mustard Dressing over the mussels and garnish with parsley sprigs.

4 servings
1 serving = ½ pound mussels

CAL.	CHO(g)	PRO.(g)	TOTAL FAT(g)	SAT. FAT(g)	CHOL.(mg)	FIBER(g)	SODIUM(mg)
115	7	10	4	1	125	0.5	745

Food exchanges per serving: 1 Lean Meat plus ½ Other Carbohydrate
Low-sodium diets: Prepare Mustard Dressing without salt.

Pan-Grilled Scallops

Enjoy scallops often. They have almost no fat and are low in cholesterol too. These scallops can be enjoyed as an entree or on top of a pasta or green salad. If a grill is handy, quickly grill the marinated scallops. The grill marks, from an outdoor or stovetop grill, look nice on scallops.

2 teaspoons light (reduced-sodium) soy sauce
1 tablespoon Oriental dark-roasted sesame oil, divided
½ teaspoon Chinese five-spice powder
¼ teaspoon freshly ground pepper
1 pound large sea scallops

Combine soy sauce, 2 teaspoons of the sesame oil, five-spice powder, and pepper in bottom of a medium-sized bowl. Add scallops and toss to coat. Marinate scallops for 15 minutes.

Set nonstick skillet over high heat. Brush remaining 1 teaspoon sesame oil on bottom of skillet. Add scallops and sauté, turning constantly, about 3 minutes until scallops are lightly browned at the edges. Scallops, when cooked, should feel slightly springy to the touch.

4 servings
1 serving = ½ cup scallops

CAL.	CHO(g)	PRO.(g)	TOTAL FAT(g)	SAT. FAT(g)	CHOL.(mg)	FIBER(g)	SODIUM(mg)
135	3	19	4	0.5	35	0	285

Food exchanges per serving: 3½ Very Lean Meats
Low-sodium diets: This recipe is acceptable.

Spiced Grilled Scallops on Leeks

1 pound (about 2) leeks
1 tablespoon margarine
1 tablespoon + 1 teaspoon olive oil
¼ teaspoon salt

¼ teaspoon freshly ground pepper
1 pound large sea scallops
1 teaspoon blackening spice or
    Cajun seasoning

Wash leeks well and discard root ends. Cut leeks into ⅛- to ¼-inch slices, including most of green tops. Heat margarine and 1 tablespoon olive oil in a nonstick skillet. Sauté leeks over medium heat until tender, stirring often. Season with salt and pepper. Set aside.

Brush scallops with remaining 1 teaspoon olive oil and sprinkle with blackening spice. Arrange scallops on a broiler rack suitable for indoor cooking, on a sheet of aluminum foil, in an oiled rack for outdoor grilling, or on skewers. Broil scallops until they are just opaque, turning once.

Serve scallops on a bed of sautéed leeks.

4 servings
1 serving = 3 ounces cooked scallops plus ½ cup leeks

CAL.	CHO(g)	PRO.(g)	TOTAL FAT(g)	SAT. FAT(g)	CHOL.(mg)	FIBER(g)	SODIUM(mg)
210	12	21	9	1	35	1.5	580

Food exchanges per serving: 3 Lean Meats plus 2 Vegetables
Low-sodium diets: Omit salt. This recipe is acceptable for occasional use if sodium restriction is mild or moderate.

Dilled Shrimp

These shrimp are great for a shrimp cocktail. Try them with Dill Sauce, Caper Sauce, or Mustard Sauce (see Index), or use them to top a Caesar, Greek, or other green salad. Don't be concerned about the amount of salt used, as the poaching liquid is drained.

½ pound medium or large shrimp,
*   in shells*
1 tablespoon dill seeds
2 sprigs fresh dill

1 teaspoon salt
1 teaspoon peppercorns
1 tablespoon lemon juice

*F*ill a medium-sized saucepan half full of water. Add dill seeds, dill, salt, peppercorns, and lemon juice; bring to a rolling boil.

Add shrimp and boil until shrimp turn pink, about 2 minutes. Drain liquid; peel and devein shrimp, leaving tails on.

Serve shrimp hot or chilled.

3 servings
1 serving = 5–7 shrimp, depending on size

CAL.	CHO(g)	PRO.(g)	TOTAL FAT(g)	SAT. FAT(g)	CHOL.(mg)	FIBER(g)	SODIUM(mg)
65	1	13	1	0	90	0	180

Food exchanges per serving: 2 Very Lean Meats
Low-sodium diets: Omit salt.

Sesame Shrimp

1 tablespoon margarine

1 tablespoon sesame oil

½ cup diced green bell pepper

1 pound raw shrimp, peeled and
    deveined

⅓ cup diagonally sliced scallions

2 tablespoons minced fresh
    gingerroot

1½ tablespoons sesame seeds

1 tablespoon light (reduced-
    sodium) soy sauce

*H*eat margarine and sesame oil together in a large skillet or wok. Mix all other ingredients together in a bowl; stir to blend. Add shrimp mixture to hot oil; stir-fry about 4–5 minutes, until shrimp are opaque and vegetables are crisp but tender.

Taste and add more soy sauce if desired.

4 servings (makes 2⅔ cups)
1 serving = ⅔ cup

CAL.	CHO(g)	PRO.(g)	TOTAL FAT(g)	SAT. FAT(g)	CHOL.(mg)	FIBER(g)	SODIUM(mg)
185	4	20	10	1.5	140	0.5	320

Food exchanges per serving: 3 Lean Meats plus 1 Vegetable
Low-sodium diets: This recipe is suitable for occasional use if sodium restriction is mild or moderate.

Seafood Gumbo

One of my favorite one-dish meals, this gumbo can be made ahead and tastes even better when reheated. Gumbo blend is a convenient mixture of okra, corn, onions, and bell peppers found in the freezer case of many supermarkets. If the market doesn't have the blend, make it yourself. Choose a spicy sausage you like. It can be beef, pork, or turkey sausage, but it should be one labeled "lean" or "low-fat."

4 cups Chicken Stock (see Index) or chicken broth

2 10-ounce cans diced tomatoes with green chilies

8 ounces whiting or pollock fillets, cut into 1-inch cubes

½–1 pound crab clusters or crab legs in shells, broken in pieces

1 cup (6 ounces) cooked skinless chicken or 8 ounces skinless, boneless raw chicken breast, cut into small pieces

1 tablespoon gumbo filé

¼ teaspoon cayenne

2 cups (8 ounces total) frozen gumbo vegetable blend

1 lobster tail, cut into 1-inch sections, or 5–6 ounces imitation lobster

4 ounces lean smoked spicy sausage, sliced thin

⅓ cup uncooked rice

8 ounces medium-sized shrimp in shells

Put Chicken Stock, tomatoes, fish, crab, chicken, gumbo filé, and cayenne into a large pot; bring mixture to a boil. Simmer uncovered 15 minutes.

Add vegetable blend, lobster, sausage, and rice. Mix well and simmer 30 minutes more, stirring every few minutes.

Add shrimp and cook about 3 minutes more until shrimp turn pink.

6 servings
1 serving = 1½ cups

CAL.	CHO(g)	PRO.(g)	TOTAL FAT(g)	SAT. FAT(g)	CHOL.(mg)	FIBER(g)	SODIUM(mg)
295	19	36	9	1	140	3.5	810

Food exchanges per serving: 4 Lean Meats plus 1 Starch plus 1 Vegetable
Low-sodium diets: This recipe is not suitable.

Caper Sauce

Serve this as a dip or sauce for scallops or shrimp, or as a topping on seafood cocktails.

⅔ cup plain low-fat yogurt
1 tablespoon drained capers
1 tablespoon prepared mustard
1 tablespoon lemon juice

½ teaspoon Worcestershire sauce
3 drops hot-pepper sauce
¼ teaspoon salt

Combine all ingredients in a small bowl or jar. Chill mixture a few hours before serving for flavors to meld.

6 servings (makes ¾ cup)
1 serving = 2 tablespoons

CAL.	CHO(g)	PRO.(g)	TOTAL FAT(g)	SAT. FAT(g)	CHOL.(mg)	FIBER(g)	SODIUM(mg)
20	2	1	0.5	0.5	0	0	190

Food exchanges per serving: a Free Food (up to 2 tablespoons)
Low-sodium diets: Use only 1 tablespoon. Omit salt.

Dill Sauce

Try this sauce on simply cooked fish or vegetables.

1½ tablespoons margarine
2 tablespoons all-purpose flour
1 teaspoon seasoned salt
⅛ teaspoon ground white pepper
½ cup Chicken Stock or Vegetable
    Stock (see Index) or chicken
    broth

1 cup plain low-fat yogurt
1½ tablespoons minced fresh dill or
    1½ teaspoons dried dill

*M*elt margarine in a small saucepan. Stir in flour, salt and pepper; blend until smooth. Add stock, gradually stirring to blend. Cook over low heat, stirring constantly until thick and smooth. Remove from heat.

Stir in yogurt and dill; blend well. Stir over low heat, but do not allow to boil.

8 servings (makes 1½ cups)
1 serving = 3 tablespoons

CAL.	CHO(g)	PRO.(g)	TOTAL FAT(g)	SAT. FAT(g)	CHOL.(mg)	FIBER(g)	SODIUM(mg)
45	4	2	3	0.5	0	0	335

Food exchange per serving: ½ Low-Fat Milk
Low-sodium diets: Substitute light (reduced-sodium) seasoned salt and unsalted margarine.

Creole Gumbo Sauce

This versatile sauce can be served with fish, shellfish, veal, or poultry. If serving the sauce over very lean meat or seafood, do not count the Fat Exchange, and count the entree as Lean Meat Exchanges.

2 tablespoons margarine
¾ cup chopped onion
¾ cup chopped green bell pepper
½ cup thinly sliced okra
1 16-ounce can tomatoes with
    liquid

2 tablespoons tomato paste
1 cup tomato juice
1 tablespoon Creole or Cajun
    seasoning
1½ teaspoons sugar

Melt margarine in a heavy saucepan; add onion, green pepper, and okra. Cook gently, stirring frequently, until onions are tender. Cut up tomatoes and add with tomato liquid. Add all other ingredients; mix well. Bring to a boil; simmer gently 8–10 minutes.

7 servings (makes 3½ cups)
1 serving = ½ cup

CAL.	CHO(g)	PRO.(g)	TOTAL FAT(g)	SAT. FAT(g)	CHOL.(mg)	FIBER(g)	SODIUM(mg)
70	10	2	4	0.5	0	1.5	660

Food exchanges per serving: 1 Vegetable plus 1 Fat
Low-sodium diets: Omit Creole or Cajun seasoning; add ½ teaspoon chili powder, 2 cloves garlic, crushed, and ½ teaspoon unsalted herb blend.

Herb Seasoning for Fish

1 tablespoon finely chopped onion
1 tablespoon snipped fresh parsley
1 tablespoon Worcestershire sauce
¾ teaspoon seasoned salt

1 teaspoon snipped fresh rosemary
   or ¼ teaspoon crushed dried
   rosemary
¼ teaspoon freshly ground pepper
4 teaspoons melted margarine

*C*ombine all ingredients in a small bowl. Spread over fish fillets. Use regular method for baking or broiling fish.

4 servings (makes ¼ cup)
1 serving = 1 tablespoon

CAL.	CHO(g)	PRO.(g)	TOTAL FAT(g)	SAT. FAT(g)	CHOL.(mg)	FIBER(g)	SODIUM(mg)
40	1	0	4	0.5	0	0	325

Food exchange per serving: 1 Fat
Low-sodium diets: Substitute light (reduced-sodium) seasoned salt.

19

Eggs, Cheese, and Yogurt

Eggs

Egg Salad

4 hard-boiled eggs, peeled and
    chilled
2 tablespoons finely chopped
    scallions
2 tablespoons finely chopped celery
    with leaves

½ teaspoon salt
¼ teaspoon freshly ground pepper
⅓ cup light or reduced-fat
    mayonnaise
1 teaspoon spicy mustard

Mound on crisp lettuce, garnish with a dash of paprika, and serve as a salad
or enjoy as a spread or sandwich filling.
Finely dice eggs. Mix thoroughly with all other ingredients.

4 servings
1 serving = ⅓ cup

CAL.	CHO(g)	PRO.(g)	TOTAL FAT(g)	SAT. FAT(g)	CHOL.(mg)	FIBER(g)	SODIUM(mg)
135	2	7	11	3	220	0	460

Food exchanges per serving: 1 Medium-Fat Meat plus 1 Fat
Low-sodium diets: Omit salt.

Puffy Omelet

Use a 10-inch pan for a four-egg omelet to give it room to puff up and not overflow. Have eggs at room temperature before beating to maximize volume of the omelet.

4 large eggs, separated	⅛ teaspoon finely ground pepper
½ teaspoon salt	Dash paprika
3 tablespoons cold water	1 tablespoon margarine

Preheat oven to 325°F. Place egg whites in a 1-quart mixing bowl. Add salt and cold water. Beat until high peaks form but whites are still bright and shiny.

In another bowl, add pepper and paprika to egg yolks; beat until thick, lemon-colored, and well mixed. Fold yolks carefully but thoroughly into egg whites.

Heat margarine in a 10-inch ovenproof skillet over moderate heat until hot enough to sizzle a few drops of water. Pour in egg mixture; reduce heat to low. With flat side of spatula, gently even out top surface of egg mixture. Cook slowly about 5 minutes, until evenly puffed and lightly browned on bottom. To peek at bottom, carefully lift omelet at edge with tip of spatula.

Place skillet in oven and bake about 12–14 minutes or until a knife tip inserted in center comes out clean.

Serve immediately on warmed plates. To divide, use two forks and tear gently into pie-shaped pieces. Invert omelet on plates so browned bottom is on top. If desired, fold over before serving.

2 servings
1 serving = ½ omelet

CAL.	CHO(g)	PRO.(g)	TOTAL FAT(g)	SAT. FAT(g)	CHOL.(mg)	FIBER(g)	SODIUM(mg)
200	1	13	16	4	425	0	740

Food exchanges per serving: 2 High-Fat Meats
Low-sodium diets: Omit salt. Use unsalted margarine.

Classic French Omelet

This omelet is best made in a small nonstick skillet or an 8-inch omelet pan. It may be served plain or filled with cheese or a vegetable mixture. Especially tasty omelets include those stuffed with Ratatouille or Roasted Red Peppers (see Index).

2 large eggs or *½ cup egg substitute*
2 tablespoons water
¼ teaspoon salt

Dash freshly ground pepper
2 teaspoons margarine

*M*ix eggs, water, salt, and pepper with a fork. Heat margarine in a skillet over medium heat until hot enough to sizzle a drop of water. Pour in egg mixture. Allow edges to set, and lift mixture at edges with pancake turner to allow egg liquid to flow under the center. Slide pan back and forth over heat to keep omelet in motion so that it does not stick.

When bottom is set and top is still moist, fill if desired, or fold omelet in half and slide it onto a heated plate to serve.

1 serving
1 serving = 1 omelet

Made with whole eggs:

CAL.	CHO(g)	PRO.(g)	TOTAL FAT(g)	SAT. FAT(g)	CHOL.(mg)	FIBER(g)	SODIUM(mg)
215	1	13	18	4.5	425	0	755

Food exchanges per serving: 2 Medium-Fat Meats plus 2 Fats *or* 2 High-Fat Meats
Low-sodium diets: Omit salt. Use unsalted margarine.

Note: To make an omelet with half the cholesterol and less fat, substitute 1 egg and 1 egg white for the 2 whole eggs.

Made with egg substitute:

CAL.	CHO(g)	PRO.(g)	TOTAL FAT(g)	SAT. FAT(g)	CHOL.(mg)	FIBER(g)	SODIUM(mg)
130	2	12	8	1	0	0	830

Food exchanges per serving: 2 Lean Meats
Low-sodium diets: Omit salt. Use unsalted margarine.

Jeanette's Dutch Babies

This recipe is from Jeanette White, a dietitian who for many years counseled individuals with diabetes. Serve this as a dessert or as a main dish for a brunch or luncheon. If used as a main course, double the portion and the Exchange values.

2 eggs
1/3 cup all-purpose flour
1/3 cup skim milk
1/4 teaspoon salt
1/4 teaspoon grated lemon zest
1 1/2 teaspoons sugar

1 tablespoon margarine, at room
    temperature
1 tablespoon lemon juice
2 teaspoons powdered sugar
1 lemon, sliced thin

Preheat oven to 400°F. Prepare an 8- or 9-inch pie pan with nonstick cooking spray. Beat eggs until light yellow. Mix in flour, milk, salt, lemon zest, sugar, and margarine; beat until smooth. Pour into prepared pan.

Bake 20 minutes. Reduce heat to 350°F, and continue baking another 10 minutes.

To serve, cut into 4 wedges, sprinkle with lemon juice, dust with powdered sugar, and garnish with lemon slices.

4 servings (makes a 9-inch pancake)
1 serving = 1/4 pancake

CAL.	CHO(g)	PRO.(g)	TOTAL FAT(g)	SAT. FAT(g)	CHOL.(mg)	FIBER(g)	SODIUM(mg)
125	15	5	6	1.5	105	0.5	210

Food exchanges per serving: 1 Medium-Fat Meat plus 1 Fruit
Low-sodium diets: Omit salt. Use unsalted margarine.

Apple Pancake

A great brunch or luncheon entree. Both sugar and sugar substitute are used because real sugar caramelizes and adds texture and appearance as well as adding sweetness.

Cinnamon Topping

1 teaspoon ground cinnamon
Heat-stable sugar substitute
    equivalent to 2 tablespoons
    sugar
2 tablespoons sugar

Pancake

1 large tart apple
½ cup skim milk
½ cup all-purpose flour
3 eggs, beaten
1 teaspoon sugar
Dash salt
2 tablespoons margarine, divided
2 tablespoons fresh lemon juice

Preheat oven to 400°F. For cinnamon topping, combine cinnamon, sugar substitute, and sugar; mix well. Set aside.

Peel and cut apple into very thin slices, removing core. Combine skim milk, flour, eggs, 1 teaspoon sugar, and salt; mix until smooth; do not beat. Melt 1 tablespoon margarine in a 10-inch skillet, and "roll" it around so sides and bottom are covered. Add sliced apples and sauté slightly.

Pour batter evenly on top. Bake about 10 minutes or until pancake is puffy and nearly cooked. Sprinkle top with cinnamon mixture; dot with remaining 1 tablespoon margarine. Return to oven to brown pancake.

Before serving, sprinkle with lemon juice. Cut into quarters to serve.

4 servings
1 serving = ¼ pancake

CAL.	CHO(g)	PRO.(g)	TOTAL FAT(g)	SAT. FAT(g)	CHOL.(mg)	FIBER(g)	SODIUM(mg)
230	27	8	10	2	160	1	165

Food exchanges per serving: 1 Starch plus 1 Fruit plus 1 High-Fat Meat
Low-sodium diets: Omit salt.

Sourdough Orange French Toast

Serve this French toast warm with a Red Plum Spread or Pear Butter (see Index) or with fresh fruit. (Remember to add the nutritive values and exchanges.)

2 eggs, beaten very lightly
⅓ cup fresh-squeezed orange juice
½ teaspoon pure vanilla extract
1 teaspoon grated orange zest

4 slices sourdough bread (day-old bread is better than fresh)
2 teaspoons margarine

Mix together eggs, orange juice, vanilla, and orange zest in a pie plate. Dip each slice of bread into mixture until all liquid is absorbed into bread.

Melt margarine in a large nonstick skillet over medium heat. Lightly brown bread on both sides. Serve hot.

2 servings
1 serving = 2 slices French toast

CAL.	CHO(g)	PRO.(g)	TOTAL FAT(g)	SAT. FAT(g)	CHOL.(mg)	FIBER(g)	SODIUM(mg)
270	31	11	10	2.5	215	1.5	415

Food exchanges per serving: 2 Starches plus 1 High-Fat Meat
Low-sodium diets: Sourdough bread is higher in sodium than other white breads. Substitute white, French, or raisin bread.

Vegetable Frittata

What a wonderful way to clean out your vegetable bin! You can use almost any vegetable in this baked omelet. It can be made ahead and served warm or at room temperature. The calculated values use egg substitutes. If you use whole eggs, each slice will be 165 calories, contain 165 milligrams cholesterol, and provide 1 additional Fat Exchange.

1 teaspoon olive oil
1 medium yellow onion, sliced thin
1 medium (6-ounce) potato, boiled with skin on and sliced
1 medium zucchini, sliced
1 small red bell pepper, cored and sliced
6 Greek black olives, pitted and sliced

2 tablespoons minced fresh Italian parsley
4 ounces shredded light Jarlsberg or baby Swiss cheese
1½ cups egg substitute or 6 large eggs
¾ teaspoon salt
¼ teaspoon freshly ground black pepper

*P*reheat oven to 400°F. Put oil into bottom of an 8-inch ceramic quiche dish or pie plate. Arrange onion to cover bottom of pan. Bake 10 minutes while preparing other ingredients.

Remove baking dish from oven. Layer sliced potato, zucchini, red pepper, olives, and parsley on onions. Top vegetables with shredded cheese.

In a small bowl, beat egg substitute or eggs; add salt and black pepper. Gently pour egg mixture over casserole. Bake casserole 20–25 minutes until eggs are set.

8 servings
1 serving = ⅛ frittata

CAL.	CHO(g)	PRO.(g)	TOTAL FAT(g)	SAT. FAT(g)	CHOL.(mg)	FIBER(g)	SODIUM(mg)
115	8	10	4	1.5	5	1	395

Food exchanges per serving: 1 Lean Meat plus 1 Vegetable
Low-sodium diets: Omit salt. Add ½ teaspoon salt-free herb blend.

Cracker-Crusted Onion Quiche

A hearty, full-flavored treat for lunch or brunch!

Crust

1¼ cups soda cracker crumbs (20
    crackers crushed)
¼ cup melted margarine

Filling

2 tablespoons margarine
2½ cups thinly sliced onion
3 eggs, beaten
½ cup instant nonfat dry milk
    powder
⅔ cup water
6 ounces light Swiss cheese,
    shredded
¼ teaspoon salt
Dash freshly ground pepper
Dash ground nutmeg

Make the crust: Prepare a 9-inch pie plate with nonstick cooking spray. Combine crumbs and margarine thoroughly; press evenly with the back of a spoon into the bottom and sides of prepared pie plate. Set aside.

Prepare the filling: Preheat oven to 325°F. Melt margarine in a skillet. Add onion and sauté over low heat, stirring, until translucent. Turn onion into cracker crust and spread evenly. Combine all remaining filling ingredients in a medium saucepan; mix well. Heat over low heat, stirring only until cheese melts. Pour carefully on top of onion.

Bake about 40 minutes or until custard is set. Knife tip inserted in center should come out clean.

6 servings (makes a 9-inch pie)
1 serving = ⅙ pie

CAL.	CHO(g)	PRO.(g)	TOTAL FAT(g)	SAT. FAT(g)	CHOL.(mg)	FIBER(g)	SODIUM(mg)
310	17	15	19	7.5	120	1.5	520

Food exchanges per serving: 2 High-Fat Meats plus 1 Starch
Low-sodium diets: Omit salt. Substitute unsalted crackers.

Cheese

Spinach Ricotta Dumplings with Marinara Sauce

1 10-ounce package frozen chopped spinach, thawed and squeezed dry

1 15-ounce container part-skim ricotta cheese

1 cup seasoned bread crumbs

½ cup egg substitute or 2 eggs, beaten

¼ cup grated Parmesan cheese

2 cloves garlic, crushed

½ teaspoon ground nutmeg

¼ cup flour

1 28-ounce jar garden-style marinara sauce or 3 cups Chunky Tomato Sauce (see Index)

Combine spinach, ricotta, bread crumbs, egg substitute or eggs, Parmesan, garlic, and nutmeg. Form into balls about the size of golf balls. Roll lightly in flour. Chill at least 2 hours.

Heat marinara sauce. Cook half of dumplings in a large pot of boiling salted water. They will sink and then float to surface when cooked (about 6 minutes). Remove dumplings with a slotted spoon. Repeat with remaining dumplings.

Divide dumplings among six dishes. Top each with sauce.

6 servings
1 serving = 4 dumplings plus ½ cup sauce

CAL.	CHO(g)	PRO.(g)	TOTAL FAT(g)	SAT. FAT(g)	CHOL.(mg)	FIBER(g)	SODIUM(mg)
295	37	19	8	4.5	25	2.5	1,360

Food exchanges per serving: 2 Starches plus 2 Lean Meats plus 1 Vegetable
Low-sodium diets: Substitute plain bread crumbs and unsalted marinara sauce or Chunky Tomato Sauce prepared without salt. Cook dumplings in unsalted water.

Never-Fail Blintzes

Serve these blintzes topped with fresh berries, Red Plum Spread (see Index), or fat-free sour cream.

Filling

1 pound dry cottage cheese
    (or farmer's cheese)
1 egg, beaten
1 tablespoon margarine
1 tablespoon sugar
Dash salt

Batter

2 eggs, beaten until light and
    foamy
½ teaspoon salt
1 teaspoon sugar
1¼ cups water
½ teaspoon grated orange zest
2 tablespoons margarine, melted,
    divided
¼ teaspoon baking powder
1 cup sifted all-purpose flour

Make the filling: Press cheese through a ricer or finer strainer. Mix well with remaining filling ingredients; set aside.

Prepare the blintzes: Preheat oven to 400°F. Prepare a 7-inch nonstick skillet and a shallow baking pan with nonstick cooking spray. In a mixing bowl, combine eggs, salt, sugar, water, orange zest, 1 tablespoon of the melted margarine, baking powder, and flour; beat until smooth. Pour 2½ tablespoons batter at a time into a heated skillet. Tip skillet so batter spreads thinly over entire pan. Pour off excess. Cook over low to medium heat until top is dry and starts to blister.

Turn out onto a board. Put 1 tablespoon filling on the blintz, fold in the sides, and roll until filling is enclosed. Place blintzes in the prepared baking pan. When all blintzes are in the pan, brush tops with remaining 1 tablespoon melted margarine. Bake 20–25 minutes, until lightly browned.

5 servings (makes 15 blintzes)
1 serving = 3 small filled blintzes

CAL.	CHO(g)	PRO.(g)	TOTAL FAT(g)	SAT. FAT(g)	CHOL.(mg)	FIBER(g)	SODIUM(mg)
280	23	22	10	2.5	135	0.5	400

Food exchanges per serving: 3 Lean Meats plus 1½ Starches
Low-sodium diets: Omit salt. Use unsalted margarine.

Baked Macaroni and Cheese

It's difficult to make a good-tasting macaroni and cheese that's not very high in fat. Most reduced-fat cheeses either have poor flavor or seem to turn to the texture of rubber bands when heated. I used many cheeses in various combinations before I found a winner.

8 ounces elbow macaroni or pasta
    wheels
¾ cup skim milk
8 ounces light pasteurized cheese
    product (such as Velveeta
    Light)
2 tablespoons minced fresh parsley

¾ teaspoon dry mustard
¼ teaspoon crushed red pepper
    flakes
2 ounces (½ cup) grated sharp
    cheddar cheese

Preheat oven to 350°F. Prepare a 6- to 8-cup ovenproof casserole with nonstick cooking spray. Cook macaroni in a large pot of boiling salted water until tender, about 10 minutes; drain in a colander.

While pasta is cooking, heat skim milk in a small heavy saucepan or in top of a double boiler. Cut processed cheese into small chunks. Add to milk and stir over very low heat just until it melts. Be careful; this mixture burns easily.

Return pasta to large pot; stir in cheese sauce, parsley, mustard, and pepper. Transfer mixture to casserole and top with grated cheddar.

Bake 20 minutes until crusty and bubbly.

6 servings
1 serving = 1 cup

CAL.	CHO(g)	PRO.(g)	TOTAL FAT(g)	SAT. FAT(g)	CHOL.(mg)	FIBER(g)	SODIUM(mg)
270	34	16	8	5	25	1	640

Food exchanges per serving: 2 Lean Meats plus 2 Starches
Low-sodium diets: This recipe is not suitable.

Macaroni and Cheese with Salsa

When pasta is listed in ounces, you must weigh it, not measure it.

*8 ounces elbow macaroni or pasta
    wheels*
¾ cup skim milk
*8 ounces light pasteurized cheese
    product (such as Velveeta
    Light)*

2 tablespoons minced fresh parsley
¾ teaspoon dry mustard
*¼ teaspoon crushed red pepper
    flakes*
*½ cup chunky tomato salsa (hot or
    mild as you prefer)*

Cook macaroni in a large pot of boiling salted water until tender, about 10 minutes; drain in a colander.

While pasta is cooking, heat skim milk in a small heavy saucepan or in the top of a double boiler. Cut processed cheese into small chunks. Add to milk and stir over very low heat just until it melts. Be careful; this mixture burns easily.

Return pasta to large pot; stir in cheese sauce, parsley, mustard, pepper, and salsa. Serve hot.

6 servings
1 serving = 1 cup

CAL.	CHO(g)	PRO.(g)	TOTAL FAT(g)	SAT. FAT(g)	CHOL.(mg)	FIBER(g)	SODIUM(mg)
240	35	14	5	3	15	1	795

Food exchanges per serving: 2 Starches plus 1 Lean Meat plus 1 Vegetable
Low-sodium diets: This recipe is not suitable.

Mexican Bean and Cheese Rollups

Choose hot or mild salsa and regular or peppered Mexican cheese depending on your preference for spicy foods.

1 16-ounce can fat-free refried beans

2 tablespoons canned chopped green chilies

2 tablespoons chopped cilantro

1 cup chunky tomato salsa, divided

10 soft tortillas

8 ounces natural Mexican-style Chihuahua (also called queso blanco) cheese or Monterey Jack cheese

Preheat oven to 350°F. Mix refried beans, chilies, cilantro, and ¼ cup of the salsa. Shred or very thinly slice cheese.

Spread 3 tablespoons bean mixture and 2 tablespoons shredded cheese on each tortilla and roll up. Arrange rolls, seam side down, on an ovenproof platter. Sprinkle remaining cheese over the tops.

Bake until rolls are hot and cheese melts, about 8 minutes. Serve with remaining ¾ cup salsa.

5 servings
1 serving = 2 rolls plus 2 tablespoons salsa

CAL.	CHO(g)	PRO.(g)	TOTAL FAT(g)	SAT. FAT(g)	CHOL.(mg)	FIBER(g)	SODIUM(mg)
385	43	19	16	8.5	40	7	1,065

Food exchanges per serving: 3 Starches plus 2 High-Fat Meats
Low-sodium diets: This recipe is not suitable.

Whipped Cottage Cheese and Chives

Use this recipe as a base for dips, as a spread for bagels, and to top baked potatoes.

1 cup creamed (4% milk fat) cottage cheese	1 tablespoon snipped fresh chives
2 tablespoons water	⅛ teaspoon salt
1 tablespoon white vinegar	Dash white pepper

Place all ingredients in a food processor or blender. Cover tightly and whip at low speed for 30 seconds or until smooth. Chill at least 2 hours before serving for flavors to blend.

If using as a dip base, add other ingredients before chilling.

8 servings
1 serving = 2 tablespoons

CAL.	CHO(g)	PRO.(g)	TOTAL FAT(g)	SAT. FAT(g)	CHOL.(mg)	FIBER(g)	SODIUM(mg)
25	1	3	1	0.5	5	0	140

Food exchange per serving: ½ Lean Meat
Low-sodium diets: Omit salt.

Yogurt

Yogurt Cheese

The goal here is to concentrate the yogurt solids. Sometimes gelatin or stabilizers are added to yogurt to keep the liquid suspended within it. Look at the ingredients list, and choose a yogurt without gelatin or stabilizers.

> 1 quart plain nonfat or low-fat
>   yogurt

*P*lace yogurt into fine sieve or colander lined with cheesecloth or a large coffee filter. Place sieve over a bowl to catch liquid that will drain off. Cover and refrigerate 24 hours.

4 servings (makes 2 cups)
1 serving = ½ cup

Made with nonfat yogurt:

CAL.	CHO(g)	PRO.(g)	TOTAL FAT(g)	SAT. FAT(g)	CHOL.(mg)	FIBER(g)	SODIUM(mg)
80	8	9	0	0	0	0	80

Food exchanges per serving: 1 Skim Milk
Low-sodium diets: This recipe is acceptable.

Made with low-fat yogurt:

CAL.	CHO(g)	PRO.(g)	TOTAL FAT(g)	SAT. FAT(g)	CHOL.(mg)	FIBER(g)	SODIUM(mg)
100	5	11	3	0	5	0	70

Food exchanges per serving: ½ Low-fat Milk plus 1 Very Lean Meat
Low-sodium diets: This recipe is acceptable.

Lemon Yogurt Cups

Try these molded yogurt delights in the center of a fresh-fruit salad plate or as a dessert topped with a few berries.

2 tablespoons granulated gelatin
½ cup water
2 6-ounce cartons low-fat lemon
    yogurt

2 teaspoons grated lemon zest
4 sprigs fresh mint (optional)

*D*issolve gelatin in water in a small saucepan. Cook over medium heat, stirring often, until gelatin is dissolved. Stir in yogurt and lemon zest.

Spray 4 4-ounce molds with nonstick cooking spray. Pour yogurt mixture into the molds. Refrigerate until firm.

When ready to serve, unmold onto serving plates. Garnish with fresh mint sprigs.

4 servings (makes 2 cups)
1 serving = ½ cup

CAL.	CHO(g)	PRO.(g)	TOTAL FAT(g)	SAT. FAT(g)	CHOL.(mg)	FIBER(g)	SODIUM(mg)
100	16	7	1	0.5	5	0	55

Food exchange per serving: 1 Skim Milk
Low-sodium diets: This recipe is excellent.

20

Potatoes, Rice, Pasta, and Grains

Potatoes

Baked "French Fries"

2 large (about 1¼ pounds total)
    potatoes

1 tablespoon corn oil
½ teaspoon seasoned salt

Preheat oven to 450°F. Peel potatoes; cut into slices 4 inches long and ¼ inch wide. Place in a bowl of ice water to crisp.

Just before cooking, turn potatoes onto paper towels and pat dry. Spread pieces in one layer on a shallow baking pan. Brush with corn oil. Bake 30–40 minutes, turning frequently, until golden brown.

Empty potatoes onto paper towels. Sprinkle with seasoned salt.

5 servings (makes 50–60 pieces)
1 serving = 10–12 pieces

CAL.	CHO(g)	PRO.(g)	TOTAL FAT(g)	SAT. FAT(g)	CHOL.(mg)	FIBER(g)	SODIUM(mg)
90	15	2	3	0.5	0	1.5	130

Food exchange per serving: 1 Starch
Low-sodium diets: Substitute light (reduced-sodium) seasoned salt.

Cheddar Roasted Potato Fans

2 medium (about 1 pound total)
   baking potatoes
1 tablespoon margarine, melted
¼ teaspoon salt

⅛ teaspoon freshly ground pepper
¼ cup shredded sharp cheddar
   cheese

Preheat oven to 425°. Peel potatoes. Push skewer through 1 potato lengthwise ½ inch from bottom of potato. Put potato on cutting board with skewer close to bottom surface. Slice potato, with cuts ¼ inch apart, from top downward to skewer. This procedure will fan-slice the potato on top but keep the base intact. Remove skewer and repeat process with other potato. Cut each potato crosswise in half and fan slightly.

Prepare small ovenproof pan with nonstick cooking spray. Brush potatoes with margarine. Season with salt and pepper. Bake 45 minutes.

Remove potatoes from oven. Insert cheese between fanned slices across top of potatoes. Return to oven; bake 10 more minutes until cheese is melted and potatoes are soft inside.

4 servings
1 serving = 1 potato fan

CAL.	CHO*(g)*	PRO.*(g)*	TOTAL FAT*(g)*	SAT. FAT*(g)*	CHOL.*(mg)*	FIBER*(g)*	SODIUM*(mg)*
125	15	4	6	2	5	1.5	220

Food exchanges per serving: 1 Starch plus 1 Fat
Low-sodium diets: Omit salt.

Stuffed Baked Potatoes

2 large (about 1¼ pounds total)   ½ teaspoon salt
   baking potatoes   ¼ teaspoon freshly ground pepper
½ cup sour half-and-half   2 teaspoons minced fresh parsley
1 egg   ⅛ teaspoon paprika
3 tablespoons finely chopped
   scallions with tops

*P*reheat oven to 400°. Wash potatoes and prick with a fork. Bake 1 hour.

Cut each potato lengthwise to make 2 equal-sized potato shells. Scoop out hot potato from shells, leaving enough potato in skin for shells to remain firm. Mash hot potato in a mixer or in a bowl; add sour half-and-half, egg, scallions, salt, and pepper. Beat only until potatoes have no lumps. Divide filling to stuff potato shells. Top each with parsley and paprika.

Reduce heat to 350°F. Bake 15–20 minutes until potatoes are hot and edges browned.

4 servings
1 serving = 1 stuffed potato half

CAL.	CHO*(g)*	PRO.*(g)*	TOTAL FAT*(g)*	SAT. FAT*(g)*	CHOL.*(mg)*	FIBER*(g)*	SODIUM*(mg)*
165	26	5	5	2.5	65	2	310

Food exchanges per serving: 1½ Starches plus 1 Fat
Low-sodium diets: Omit salt.

Roasted Hash Browns

So good you won't miss the usual fried variety.

2 medium (about 1 pound total) onions	1 tablespoon virgin olive oil
2 medium (about 1 pound total) potatoes	1 teaspoon finely minced garlic
	¼ teaspoon paprika
¾ cup water	½ teaspoon salt
	¼ teaspoon freshly ground pepper

Preheat oven to 400°F. Peel and cut onions into bite-sized wedges. Wash potatoes and, with skins on, cut into bite-sized cubes. Put potatoes, onions, and water into a 13″ × 9″ baking pan. Cover tightly and roast 25 minutes; drain well.

In a large bowl, combine olive oil, garlic, and paprika. Add potato and onion mixture; toss to coat.

Return mixture to baking pan, distributing it into a single layer, if possible. Turn heat up to 425°F. Return baking pan to oven; roast uncovered another 20–30 minutes, turning every 5 minutes to brown. Add salt and pepper, and serve.

6 servings (makes 4 cups)
1 serving = ⅔ cup

CAL.	CHO(g)	PRO.(g)	TOTAL FAT(g)	SAT. FAT(g)	CHOL.(mg)	FIBER(g)	SODIUM(mg)
100	19	2	2	0.5	0	2.5	190

Food exchange per serving: 1 Starch
Low-sodium diets: Omit salt.

Roasted Potatoes

This dish is also delicious made with small red new potatoes. Use them unpeeled. The skins are tender and delicious.

2 medium (about 1 pound) baking
    potatoes
2 tablespoons margarine, melted
½ teaspoon salt

⅛ teaspoon freshly ground pepper
1 tablespoon finely minced fresh
    parsley or fresh dill

Prepare a pie plate with nonstick cooking spray. Wash potatoes; boil them in their skins in enough salted boiling water to cover for 20–25 minutes or until tender when pierced with a fork.

Preheat oven to 400°F. Drain potatoes and peel immediately. Cut each potato into 4 pieces; place on prepared pie plate. Baste each potato wedge with melted margarine; sprinkle with salt, pepper, and parsley.

Roast 15 minutes, until potatoes are nicely browned.

4 servings
1 serving = 2 potato wedges

CAL.	CHO(g)	PRO.(g)	TOTAL FAT(g)	SAT. FAT(g)	CHOL.(mg)	FIBER(g)	SODIUM(mg)
145	21	2	6	1	0	2	350

Food exchanges per serving: 1½ Starches plus 1 Fat
Low-sodium diets: Omit salt. Use unsalted margarine.

Giant Potato Pancake

Use Idaho potatoes in this recipe because they are more solid and grate better than most other varieties. The turning is tricky!

1½ pounds Idaho baking potatoes
½ cup finely chopped onion
1 teaspoon salt

¼ teaspoon freshly ground pepper
1 tablespoon margarine

*P*are potatoes with a vegetable peeler. Grate potatoes with food processor or with medium grater. Turn potatoes into a large bowl. Add onion, salt, and pepper; mix lightly but well with a blending fork.

Melt margarine in a 10-inch nonstick skillet, and rotate to coat bottom and sides of pan. Turn potatoes into pan; pat down and spread evenly. Cover pan tightly; turn heat low and let cook about 15 minutes or until underside is browned.

Take pan off heat temporarily. Put a 12-inch plate (or very large pie plate) upside down on top of potatoes and, with one hand on handle of skillet and the other hand guiding the plate, turn skillet upside down, then lift it off the pancake. This puts the pancake on the plate. Immediately slide pancake back into the skillet, browned side up.

Return to low heat. Do not cover. Let cook another 15 minutes or until bottom is browned.

To serve, cut evenly into 6 wedges.

6 servings
1 serving = ⅙ pancake

CAL.	CHO(g)	PRO.(g)	TOTAL FAT(g)	SAT. FAT(g)	CHOL.(mg)	FIBER(g)	SODIUM(mg)
90	17	2	2	0.5	0	1.5	395

Food exchange per serving: 1 Starch
Low-sodium diets: Omit salt. Use unsalted margarine.

Scalloped Potatoes

2–3 medium (about 1 pound total)
   potatoes
2 tablespoons all-purpose flour
½ teaspoon salt

⅛ teaspoon freshly ground pepper
2 tablespoons margarine
½ cup finely chopped onion

Preheat oven to 400°F. Prepare a 1½-quart casserole with nonstick cooking spray. Pare potatoes; slice crosswise in ⅛-inch slices; if potatoes are large, cut slices in half. Mix together flour, salt, and pepper.

Place half of potatoes in prepared casserole. Dot with half the margarine; sprinkle half the seasoned flour on top, then half the onion. Repeat with remaining potatoes, margarine, seasoned flour, and onion. Pour enough very hot water in, at one corner only, so that water barely comes to the top of potatoes.

Cover and bake 45 minutes. Uncover and bake another 20–25 minutes or until potatoes are browned and tender.

5 servings (makes 2½ cups)
1 serving = ½ cup

CAL.	CHO(g)	PRO.(g)	TOTAL FAT(g)	SAT. FAT(g)	CHOL.(mg)	FIBER(g)	SODIUM(mg)
115	16	2	5	1	0	1.5	275

Food exchanges per serving: 1 Starch plus 1 Fat
Low-sodium diets: Omit salt. Use unsalted margarine.

Pratie Cakes

Certain Irish folk refer to potato cakes as "praties." These cakes are great! Mix and shape them ahead, then chill before cooking.

2 cups cold mashed potatoes (fresh or prepared from flakes)	¼ teaspoon salt
½ cup unsifted all-purpose flour (reserve 1 tablespoon for flouring board)	¼ cup finely chopped onion
	2 tablespoons margarine, divided

*T*urn mashed potatoes into a large bowl. Add flour, salt, and onion. Mix thoroughly with hands and fingers until completely mixed and smooth. Turn onto a lightly floured board and pat down until ½ inch thick. Cut with a 3-inch floured cookie cutter or use the top of a water glass as a cutter. Place potato patties on a cookie sheet, cover lightly with waxed paper and refrigerate until just before cooking.

To cook, use 1 tablespoon margarine at a time. Melt margarine in a large skillet or stovetop griddle. Fry potato cakes over moderately high heat, turning to brown on both sides. Serve immediately.

7 servings (makes 7 cakes)
1 serving = 1 3-inch potato cake

CAL.	CHO(g)	PRO.(g)	TOTAL FAT(g)	SAT. FAT(g)	CHOL.(mg)	FIBER(g)	SODIUM(mg)
125	17	2	6	1	0	1.5	290

Food exchanges per serving: 1 Starch plus 1 Fat
Low-sodium diets: Omit salt from original mashed potato mixture and from recipe.

Colcannon

A delicious Irish comfort food—mashed potatoes with cabbage. Try it with baked or grilled ham or lean turkey sausage. If you don't have buttermilk, you can substitute 1 teaspoon lemon juice or vinegar mixed in ⅓ cup skim or low-fat milk.

1½ pounds potatoes, peeled and cut into pieces

⅓ cup cultured low-fat (1½% milk fat) buttermilk

4 cups finely chopped green cabbage

2 slices bacon, chopped

1 small onion, chopped fine

½ teaspoon salt

¼ teaspoon pepper

Bring salted water to boil in a large pot. Add potatoes; cook until tender. Remove potatoes from water, reserving water. Drain potatoes well; mash with buttermilk while still hot.

Add cabbage to boiling water; cook 5 minutes. Drain cabbage well; stir into potatoes.

In a large skillet, heat bacon over low heat until it starts to release fat. Add onions and cook until onions are translucent. Beat bacon-onion mixture, salt, and pepper into potato-cabbage mixture.

If mixture is not hot enough to serve, transfer to an ovenproof casserole and heat at 350°F for 10–15 minutes.

9 servings (makes 4½ cups)
1 serving = ½ cup

CAL.	CHO(g)	PRO.(g)	TOTAL FAT(g)	SAT. FAT(g)	CHOL.(mg)	FIBER(g)	SODIUM(mg)
90	13	2	3	1	5	1.5	255

Food exchanges per serving: 1 Starch plus ½ Fat
Low-sodium diets: Omit salt.

Mashed Sweet Potatoes

Because sweet potatoes are high in carbohydrates, the serving size is small. If you want more, eat a double portion and double the exchanges.

1½ pounds sweet potatoes
1½ tablespoons margarine, cut into
  pieces

½ teaspoon pumpkin pie spice
  mixture or ¼ teaspoon
  cinnamon plus a dash of
  nutmeg plus a dash of ginger

Scrub sweet potatoes thoroughly; cut off and discard small ends and inedible knobs. If large, cut into halves or thirds. Place in a deep cooking pot; add enough water to cover potatoes. Cover pot; bring to a boil. Cook over moderate heat until sweet potatoes are soft (about 25 minutes).

Drain at once. Hold each sweet potato with a fork, and peel quickly. Place potatoes in a bowl; mash. Beat in margarine and pumpkin pie spice.

6 servings (makes 2 cups)
1 serving = ⅓ cup

CAL.	CHO(g)	PRO.(g)	TOTAL FAT(g)	SAT. FAT(g)	CHOL.(mg)	FIBER(g)	SODIUM(mg)
110	20	1	3	0.5	0	2.5	45

Food exchanges per serving: 1 Starch plus ½ Fat
Low-sodium diets: This recipe is excellent.

Sweet Potato Coins

The liqueur is optional but adds a hint of almond flavor and a bit of glaze.

*2 small (about 1 pound total) sweet
  potatoes
4 teaspoons margarine or butter,
  melted*

*1 tablespoon amaretto (optional)
¼ teaspoon salt*

Preheat oven to 400°F. Peel sweet potatoes; cut crosswise into ¼-inch slices. Spray a cookie sheet with nonstick cooking spray. Spread sweet potato slices in a single layer on pan. Brush tops with 2 teaspoons margarine and 1½ teaspoons amaretto.

Bake sweet potato slices 10 minutes. Turn slices over; brush tops with remaining 2 teaspoons margarine and 1½ teaspoons amaretto. Bake another 10 minutes. Season with salt and serve hot.

4 servings (makes 2 cups)
1 serving = ½ cup coins

CAL.	CHO*(g)*	PRO.*(g)*	TOTAL FAT*(g)*	SAT. FAT*(g)*	CHOL.*(mg)*	FIBER*(g)*	SODIUM*(mg)*
130	20	1	4	0.5	0	2.5	330

Food exchanges per serving: 1 Starch plus 1 Fat
Low-sodium diets: Omit salt.

Rice

In all of the rice recipes, brown rice may be substituted for white rice. This will increase the fiber content of the recipes. Brown rice usually takes about 40 minutes to cook, so adjust cooking times.

Brown Rice Pilaf

3 tablespoons margarine
1 cup crumbled uncooked vermicelli
    or other thin noodles

1 cup uncooked brown rice
3 cups Chicken Stock (see Index) or
    chicken broth

Heat margarine in a large nonstick skillet. Sauté noodles until coated and slightly brown, stirring often. Add rice and stir to combine. Add Chicken Stock; cover, and continue cooking over low heat until stock is absorbed and rice is tender, about 40 minutes.

Turn off heat and let stand, covered, 5 minutes. Toss with a fork before serving.

8 servings (makes 4 cups)
1 serving = ½ cup

CAL.	CHO(g)	PRO.(g)	TOTAL FAT(g)	SAT. FAT(g)	CHOL.(mg)	FIBER(g)	SODIUM(mg)
185	30	5	6	1	0	1.5	95

Food exchanges per serving: 2 Starches plus 1 Fat
Low-sodium diets: Use unsalted chicken broth.

Golden Rice

Add color to any plate with this bright golden-orange rice. The cilantro makes it a good flavor combination with Mexican foods, Oriental flavors, and seafood.

2 teaspoons margarine	*½ cup uncooked white rice*
1 medium onion, chopped	*½ teaspoon salt*
1 clove garlic, minced	*2 tablespoons chopped cilantro*
½ teaspoon turmeric	
1 cup Chicken Stock or Vegetable	
Stock (see Index) or unsalted	
chicken or vegetable broth	

*H*eat margarine in a medium-sized nonstick saucepan. Add onion and garlic; sauté until onion is translucent. Stir in turmeric. Add Chicken Stock, rice, and salt. Mix well. Cover and simmer until liquid is absorbed, about 15 minutes.

Remove from heat and let rest for 5 minutes. Add cilantro, and fluff rice with a fork.

4 servings (makes 2 cups)
1 serving = ½ cup

CAL.	CHO*(g)*	PRO.*(g)*	TOTAL FAT*(g)*	SAT. FAT*(g)*	CHOL.*(mg)*	FIBER*(g)*	SODIUM*(mg)*
125	23	3	3	0.5	0	1	325

Food Exchanges per serving: 1½ Starches
Low-sodium diets: Omit salt.

Rizzi Bizzi

1½ cups Chicken Stock or Vegetable
    Stock (see Index)
½ teaspoon salt
1 tablespoon margarine

¾ cup uncooked white rice
1 10-ounce package frozen peas
¼ cup finely chopped scallions

Bring Chicken Stock, salt, and margarine to a boil in a medium-sized saucepan. Add rice slowly, stirring with a fork, and cook according to package directions.

In a separate saucepan, cook peas according to package directions until crisp-tender. When rice is cooked, add peas and scallions; mix well.

6 servings (makes 4 cups)
1 serving = ⅔ cup

CAL.	CHO(g)	PRO.(g)	TOTAL FAT(g)	SAT. FAT(g)	CHOL.(mg)	FIBER(g)	SODIUM(mg)
145	26	5	3	0.5	0	2	285

Food exchanges per serving: 2 Starches
Low-sodium diets: Omit salt. Used unsalted Chicken Stock or Vegetable Stock.

Rice with Mushrooms

2 cups Chicken Stock or Vegetable
  Stock (see Index) or unsalted
  chicken broth
½ teaspoon salt
1 cup uncooked rice
1 4-ounce can mushroom stems and
  pieces or 1 cup sliced fresh
  mushrooms

2 tablespoons margarine
⅛ teaspoon freshly ground pepper
Few sprigs parsley for garnish

*B*ring Chicken Stock and salt to a boil. Add rice slowly, stirring with a fork, and cook according to cooking time indicated on rice package. (Different types of rice vary in cooking times.)

Drain mushrooms, and pour liquid from can into water with the rice. All liquid should be absorbed when the rice is cooked.

Melt margarine in a small saucepan; sauté mushrooms until slightly browned. When rice is cooked, toss mushrooms and pepper into rice; stir with a fork to mix. Serve in a bowl topped with parsley sprigs.

5 servings (makes 3⅓ cups)
1 serving = ⅔ cup

CAL.	CHO(g)	PRO.(g)	TOTAL FAT(g)	SAT. FAT(g)	CHOL.(mg)	FIBER(g)	SODIUM(mg)
190	31	4	6	1	0	0.5	410

Food exchanges per serving: 2 Starches plus 1 Fat
Low-sodium diets: Omit salt; substitute unsalted margarine and fresh mushrooms.

Wild Rice with Fennel and Cherries

Delicious and festive, especially when served with poultry.

3 ounces (about ½ cup) uncooked
    wild rice
2 cups water
¼ teaspoon salt
½ cup reduced-sugar cranberry
    juice cocktail
2 tablespoons dried cherries

1 tablespoon margarine
1 small fennel bulb, diced (about
    1¼ cups)
1 large shallot, chopped
½ teaspoon salt
⅛ teaspoon freshly ground pepper

Rinse wild rice in a fine strainer under cold running water. Bring 2 cups water to a boil; add rice and salt. Return to a boil; cover, reduce heat, and simmer 35 minutes. Add cranberry juice cocktail and cherries; stir well. Cover and cook 15 minutes more.

While rice-cherry mixture is cooking, melt margarine in a nonstick saucepan. Add fennel and shallot; sauté over low heat, stirring often until fennel and shallots are tender, about 10 minutes. Season with salt and pepper. Stir vegetable mixture into rice.

5 servings (makes 2½ cups)
1 serving = ½ cup

CAL.	CHO(g)	PRO.(g)	TOTAL FAT(g)	SAT. FAT(g)	CHOL.(mg)	FIBER(g)	SODIUM(mg)
100	18	3	3	0.5	0	1	385

Food exchanges per serving: 1 Starch plus ½ Fat
Low-sodium diets: Omit salt.

Risotto Milanese

Double the ingredients and portions if you are serving the risotto as an entreé (and, of course, double the exchange values, too). Arborio rice is the traditional type of Italian rice used for risotto. It releases enough starch for the creamy texture of risotto.

1 tablespoon olive oil
1 onion, chopped
1 ounce prosciutto or smoked ham,
*   chopped fine*
½ cup Arborio rice

¼ teaspoon saffron threads
1½ cups Chicken Stock (see Index)
*   or unsalted chicken broth*
½ cup dry white wine
¼ cup grated Parmesan cheese

*H*eat olive oil in a medium-sized nonstick saucepan. Add onion and prosciutto; sauté until onion is soft. Add rice and saffron; cook 3 minutes over medium heat, stirring constantly.

In another saucepan, simmer Chicken Stock and white wine. Add ½ cup of stock-wine mixture to rice, stirring constantly. As stock is absorbed, add more stock, a few tablespoons at a time, continuing to stir between each addition. It should take about 25 minutes to incorporate all of the liquid.

When rice is creamy-looking and tender but grains are slightly firm in the center, stir in Parmesan cheese. Serve immediately in warmed bowls.

4 servings (makes 2 cups)
1 serving = ½ cup

CAL.	CHO(g)	PRO.(g)	TOTAL FAT(g)	SAT. FAT(g)	CHOL.(mg)	FIBER(g)	SODIUM(mg)
205	25	7	7	2	10	1	270

Food exchanges per serving: 1½ Starches plus 1 Vegetable plus 1 Fat
Low-sodium diets: This recipe is acceptable for occasional use.

Golden Asparagus Risotto

Carl Jerome, a wonderful chef with whom I have taught at the Cooking and Hospitality Institute of Chicago, included this recipe in his book *Cooking for a New Earth.* The microwave variation really works well and saves constant stirring.

1 tablespoon olive oil
2 shallots, peeled and chopped fine
1 small clove garlic, peeled and
*   chopped fine*
½-inch chunk fresh gingerroot,
*   peeled and grated*
1 cup medium-grain rice,
*   unwashed*
2¾ cups Chicken Stock (see Index)
*   or unsalted chicken or*
*   vegetable broth if*
*   microwaving, or 4 cups if*
*   preparing traditionally*

¼ teaspoon crushed saffron threads
6 ounces asparagus, trimmed of
*   woody bottom ends and cut on*
*   the bias into ½-inch pieces*
2 tablespoons grated Romano cheese
1 tablespoon finely chopped fresh
*   tarragon*

Traditional Procedure: Heat olive oil in a large saucepan set over medium heat. Add shallots, garlic, and gingerroot; sauté 5 minutes. Stir in rice; sauté until rice becomes white and opaque, about 2 minutes.

While shallots and rice are sautéing, bring Chicken Stock and saffron to a boil in a medium-sized pot. Reduce heat and keep at a simmer. Slowly ladle about a cup of the stock into the pot containing the rice; over medium-low heat, stir occasionally until the stock is absorbed. Continue adding stock, about ½ cup at a time, keeping the stock very hot and the risotto at a simmer the whole time, about 30–35 minutes, to incorporate all the stock. After 25 minutes, add asparagus. Just before serving, stir in Romano cheese and tarragon.

If stock is added too quickly, rice will be mushy on the outside and chalky inside; if it is added too slowly, risotto will become pasty. After about half the stock has been absorbed, risotto will need almost constant stirring.

Microwave Procedure: In a large, microwave-safe bowl, stir together the shallots, garlic, ginger, rice, and oil; stir until rice is evenly coated with oil. Cover tightly and microwave 4 minutes on High (100% power).

While rice is cooking, stir saffron into Chicken Stock. Uncover rice and add stock. Cover rice tightly and microwave 17 minutes on High.

Carefully uncover; using a fork, gently stir in asparagus. (The rice will be slightly undercooked and the risotto somewhat soupy at this point.) Cover again and microwave 6 minutes on High. The risotto should be creamy and moist, but not soupy; if still too liquid, return to the microwave for another 1–2 minutes.

When rice is ready, stir in the Romano cheese and tarragon with a fork. Serve immediately.

6 servings (makes 4 cups)
1 serving = ⅔ cup

CAL.	CHO*(g)*	PRO.*(g)*	TOTAL FAT*(g)*	SAT. FAT*(g)*	CHOL.*(mg)*	FIBER*(g)*	SODIUM*(mg)*
165	29	5	4	1	0	1	75

Food exchanges per serving: 2 Starches plus ½ Fat
Low-sodium diets: This recipe is excellent. Be sure to use unsalted Chicken Stock or chicken or vegetable broth.

Leek and Herb Risotto

A mixture of fresh herbs is essential to this dish. Use at least three different types. You can substitute a bulb of fennel for the leek if you wish.

½ cup mixed snipped fresh herbs
    (basil, dill, chives, oregano,
    rosemary, and/or tarragon),
    divided
1 medium (1½-inch-diameter)
    leek, well washed
1 tablespoon olive oil or chicken fat
    (removed from stock)

2 cloves garlic, minced
¾ cup Arborio rice
2 cups Chicken Stock or Vegetable
    Stock (see Index) or unsalted
    chicken or vegetable broth
½ teaspoon salt
¼ teaspoon freshly ground pepper

Mix herbs together in a small bowl or measuring cup. In a food processor, chop white part of leek and enough of the light green part to make 1 cup.

Heat oil in a medium-sized nonstick saucepan. Add leek and garlic; cook over low heat until soft but not browned. Add rice and cook, stirring constantly, 3–4 minutes until edges of rice are translucent.

In a small pot, heat Chicken Stock with ¼ cup mixed herbs, salt, and pepper.

Add ½ cup of the hot herbed stock to rice; cook over medium-high heat, stirring constantly until liquid is absorbed. Continue adding herbed stock, a few tablespoons at a time, stirring constantly until liquid is nearly absorbed after each addition. In about 25 minutes, all liquid should be added, the rice should be creamy-looking, and its grains tender but slightly firm in the center.

Stir in remaining ¼ cup fresh herbs. Serve immediately in warmed bowls.

5 servings (makes 2½ cups)
1 serving = ½ cup

CAL.	CHO(g)	PRO.(g)	TOTAL FAT(g)	SAT. FAT(g)	CHOL.(mg)	FIBER(g)	SODIUM(mg)
165	30	4	4	0.5	0	0.5	270

Food exchanges per serving: 2 Starches
Low-sodium diets: Omit salt.

Pasta

Pasta Primavera

This typical Italian pasta preparation has not a hint of tomato sauce. It is scrumptious hot but may also be served at room temperature as a pasta salad for a buffet or picnic.

½ pound thin spaghetti, cooked according to package directions
½ pound broccoli, asparagus, eggplant, or sweet bell peppers
2 tablespoons olive oil, divided
2 cloves garlic, crushed
½ pound young zucchini, sliced thin

½ pound mushrooms, sliced
1½ teaspoons dried basil or 1 tablespoon snipped fresh basil
½ teaspoon salt
½ teaspoon coarsely ground pepper
2 tablespoons water
2 tablespoons grated Parmesan cheese

*W*hile spaghetti is cooking, wash broccoli; cook in a small amount of boiling water until crisp-tender. Meanwhile heat 1 tablespoon of the olive oil in a large skillet; add garlic and sauté 3 minutes. Add zucchini and sauté until slightly browned. Add mushrooms; cook until mushrooms are tender.

Drain broccoli; slice into bite-sized pieces and add to zucchini and mushrooms. Stir in seasonings.

When spaghetti is al dente (cooked but not soft), stop cooking by pouring cold water into pot; drain spaghetti. Return it to the pot, stir in 2 tablespoons water, remaining 1 tablespoon olive oil, Parmesan cheese, and vegetable mixture. Cover and reheat over low heat.

6 servings (makes 6¼ cups)
1 serving = 1 cup

CAL.	CHO(g)	PRO.(g)	TOTAL FAT(g)	SAT. FAT(g)	CHOL.(mg)	FIBER(g)	SODIUM(mg)
215	34	8	6	1	0	2.5	230

Food exchanges per serving: 2 Starches plus 1 Vegetable plus 1 Fat
Low-sodium diets: Omit salt.

Fusilli with Puttanesca Sauce

Puttanesca sauce is named for "ladies of the night." It is a coarse, rather rough and spicy sauce. The sauce ingredients are just heated to a boil, so this dish is very quick to make.

12 ounces fusilli or rotini (spiral-shaped) pasta

1 tablespoon olive oil

2 cloves garlic, chopped

1 28-ounce can crushed tomatoes in tomato puree

12 Calamata (Greek) olives, pitted and chopped coarse

2 tablespoons chopped fresh basil leaves

¼ cup chopped fresh Italian parsley, divided

1 tablespoon drained capers

1 teaspoon crushed red pepper flakes

In a large pot of boiling salted water, cook fusilli about 14 minutes or until al dente (cooked but not soft).

Meanwhile, heat olive oil in a medium-sized pot. Add garlic; sauté 1 minute over low heat. Add tomatoes, olives, basil, 2 tablespoons of the parsley, capers, and red pepper flakes. Cook just until mixture comes to a boil.

Drain pasta well. Serve topped with sauce and garnished with remaining 2 tablespoons chopped parsley.

6 servings
1 serving = 1 cup pasta plus ⅔ cup sauce

CAL.	CHO(g)	PRO.(g)	TOTAL FAT(g)	SAT. FAT(g)	CHOL.(mg)	FIBER(g)	SODIUM(mg)
305	53	9	7	1	0	1.5	655

Food exchanges per serving: 3 Starches plus 1 Vegetable plus 1 Fat
Low-sodium diets: Substitute unsalted canned tomatoes in puree. Omit salt in water used to boil pasta. Use only 6 olives.

Pasta with Tomatoes and Chicken

This quick, easy, delicious pasta is very versatile. You can make it with your favorite type of pasta. Prepare it without the chicken if you prefer a vegetarian entree. For an appetizer or side dish, serve a smaller portion.

1 pound spaghetti, mostaccioli, or other pasta

8 ounces cooked chicken, chopped coarse

4 medium tomatoes, peeled, seeded, and chopped

¼ cup chopped fresh Italian parsley

6–8 leaves fresh basil, chopped

⅓ cup freshly grated Parmesan cheese, divided

¼ cup virgin olive oil

2 cloves garlic, minced

½ teaspoon salt

¼ teaspoon crushed red pepper flakes

Cook the pasta according to package directions.

While pasta is cooking, mix all remaining ingredients except 2 tablespoons Parmesan cheese. When pasta is al dente (cooked but not soft), drain well. In a large serving bowl, toss hot pasta with uncooked sauce. Top with 2 tablespoons reserved Parmesan cheese.

9 servings
1 serving = about 1 cup (depending on type of pasta used)

CAL.	CHO(g)	PRO.(g)	TOTAL FAT(g)	SAT. FAT(g)	CHOL.(mg)	FIBER(g)	SODIUM(mg)
315	40	16	10	2	25	2	215

Food exchanges per serving: 2 Starches plus 2 Vegetables plus 1 Lean Meat plus 1 Fat
Low-sodium diets: Omit salt.

Squash-Filled Ravioli with Ginger Cream Sauce

This easy and interesting technique uses packaged dough for wrapping wontons or egg rolls to make homemade ravioli. You can fill the ravioli with almost anything that cooks quickly. They are delicious filled with finely chopped scallops or shrimp mixed with equal amounts of fish. For the sauce, be sure to use unsalted Chicken Stock or broth. When you simmer the stock to concentrate its flavor, you don't want it to become too salty.

1 cup unsalted Chicken Stock (see Index) or unsalted chicken or vegetable broth
1 teaspoon finely minced gingerroot
¾ cup cooked winter squash, fresh or frozen
¾ cup part-skim ricotta cheese
1 tablespoon finely minced fresh chives, divided

½ teaspoon grated orange or tangerine zest
¼ teaspoon salt
¼ teaspoon freshly ground pepper
¼ teaspoon ground sage
10 6½-inch-square egg roll wrappers
1 egg white
2 tablespoons half-and-half

Simmer Chicken Stock and gingerroot in a small pot until volume is reduced by half. In a medium bowl, combine squash, ricotta cheese, 2 teaspoons of the chives, orange zest, salt, pepper, and sage.

Cut egg roll wrappers in half. Brush egg white around ½-inch edge of each wrapper. Put 1 tablespoon filling on one side of wrapper; fold over and seal edges with fingers to make ravioli packets. (They can be refrigerated at this point for later cooking if you wish.)

Fill a large pot with salted water; bring to a boil. Cook ravioli in small batches about 2–3 minutes, until they float to top. Drain ravioli.

Add half-and-half to gingered broth. Heat so that sauce is hot but not boiling.

To serve, put 5 ravioli on each plate. Divide sauce over ravioli; sprinkle with remaining 1 teaspoon chives.

4 servings
1 serving = 5 ravioli with sauce

CAL.	CHO(g)	PRO.(g)	TOTAL FAT(g)	SAT. FAT(g)	CHOL.(mg)	FIBER(g)	SODIUM(mg)
265	38	14	7	3	60	2.5	185

Food exchanges per serving: 2 Starches plus 1 Vegetable plus 1 Medium-Fat Meat
Low-sodium diets: Omit salt.

Fettuccine with Garlic, Tomatoes, and Basil

Make this pasta dish in the summer when tomatoes are at their reddest, ripest best. To seed and dice ripe tomatoes, just cut them in half crosswise and squeeze firmly over the sink to remove most of the seeds and interior liquid. Then dice the red pulp.

12 medium-sized fresh ripe tomatoes, seeded and diced
2 tablespoons olive oil
2 teaspoons minced fresh garlic
½ teaspoon cracked pepper
¼ teaspoon salt
6 ounces fettuccine
¼ cup chopped fresh basil
5 whole fresh basil leaves

*I*n a large saucepan combine tomatoes, olive oil, garlic, pepper, and salt; simmer 15 minutes.

While sauce is simmering, cook fettucine according to package directions. Drain pasta; toss with sauce and chopped basil.

Garnish each serving with a fresh basil leaf.

5 servings (makes 5 cups)
1 serving = 1 cup

CAL.	CHO(g)	PRO.(g)	TOTAL FAT(g)	SAT. FAT(g)	CHOL.(mg)	FIBER(g)	SODIUM(mg)
245	39	8	8	1	30	5	140

Food exchanges per serving: 2 Starches plus 2 Vegetables plus 1 Fat
Low-sodium diets: Omit salt.

Vegetarian Lasagna Roll-Ups

A nutrient-rich family favorite.

8 lasagna noodles
8 ounces fresh mushrooms, sliced
1 15-ounce container part-skim
   ricotta cheese
1 10-ounce package frozen chopped
   spinach, defrosted, well
   drained
2 cups shredded light or part-skim
   mozzarella cheese, divided

½ cup egg substitute or 2 eggs
3 tablespoons chopped fresh basil or
   1 tablespoon dried basil
½ teaspoon freshly ground pepper
1 27- to 30-ounce jar chunky
   garden-style pasta sauce
¼ cup shredded Parmesan cheese

*P*arboil lasagna noodles in boiling salted water 10 minutes; drain.

Heat a nonstick skillet over high heat. Add mushrooms and sauté (without fat) until mushrooms are browned around the edges.

Preheat oven to 375°F. In a large bowl, combine ricotta cheese, spinach, mushrooms, 1 cup of the mozzarella cheese, eggs, basil, and pepper; mix well. Spread cheese filling (about ½ cup per noodle) down length of each noodle; roll up to form lasagna rolls.

Put rolls in an ovenproof flat casserole, edge side up. Top with pasta sauce, the remaining 1 cup mozzarella, and Parmesan cheese. Bake 25–30 minutes.

8 servings
1 serving = 1 lasagna roll with sauce

CAL.	CHO(g)	PRO.(g)	TOTAL FAT(g)	SAT. FAT(g)	CHOL.(mg)	FIBER(g)	SODIUM(mg)
305	34	24	9	4.5	20	2	820

Food exchanges per serving: 2 Starches plus 2 Medium-Fat Meats plus 1 Vegetable
Low-sodium diets: Substitute unsalted pasta sauce or Chunky Tomato Sauce (see Index) prepared without salt. Reduce mozzarella to 1½ cups.

No-Fuss Beef Lasagna

This lasagna, provided by the Test Kitchens of the National Live Stock and Meat Board, is layered with uncooked lasagna noodles to save a step.

1 pound 85% lean ground beef
¼ teaspoon salt
1 26- to 30-ounce jar prepared
  pasta sauce
1 14½-ounce can Italian-style
  diced tomatoes, undrained
¼ teaspoon ground red pepper

1 15-ounce carton part-skim
  ricotta cheese
¼ cup grated Parmesan cheese
1 egg, beaten
10 uncooked lasagna noodles
1½ cups shredded part-skim
  mozzarella cheese

Heat oven to 375°F. In a large nonstick skillet, brown ground beef over medium heat 8–10 minutes or until it is no longer pink. Pour off drippings. Season beef with salt; stir in pasta sauce, tomatoes, and red pepper; set aside.

Meanwhile, in a medium bowl, combine ricotta cheese, Parmesan cheese, and egg.

Spread 2 cups beef sauce over bottom of a 13″ × 9″ nonstick baking dish. Arrange 4 lasagna noodles lengthwise in a single layer on top. Place a fifth noodle across end of baking dish, breaking noodle to fit dish; press noodles into sauce.

Spread ricotta cheese mixture over noodles; sprinkle with 1 cup mozzarella cheese, and top with 1½ cups beef sauce. Arrange remaining noodles in a single layer; press lightly into sauce. Top with remaining sauce.

Bake 45 minutes or until noodles are tender. Sprinkle top with remaining ½ cup mozzarella cheese; tent lightly with aluminum foil. Let stand 15 minutes; cut into 12 3-inch squares.

12 servings
1 serving = 1 3-inch square

CAL.	CHO(g)	PRO.(g)	TOTAL FAT(g)	SAT. FAT(g)	CHOL.(mg)	FIBER(g)	SODIUM(mg)
330	30	20	15	6	60	1	600

Food exchanges per serving: 2 Starches plus 3 Medium-Fat Meats
Low-sodium diets: Omit salt. Substitute unsalted pasta sauce and unsalted diced tomatoes.

Spaghetti and Meat Sauce

You can use this method to prepare your favorite type of pasta with this meat sauce.

> ½ pound spaghetti   ¼ cup grated Parmesan cheese
> 3 cups (½ recipe) Rich Meat Sauce
>   (recipe follows)

Bring a large pot of salted water to a boil. Add spaghetti and stir until water boils again. Cook pasta about 15 minutes or until al dente (cooked but not soft). Drain well in colander before adding sauce.

While pasta is cooking, heat sauce. Serve pasta topped with sauce and sprinkled with Parmesan cheese.

4 servings
1 serving = 1 cup spaghetti plus ¾ cup sauce plus 1 tablespoon cheese

CAL.	CHO(g)	PRO.(g)	TOTAL FAT(g)	SAT. FAT(g)	CHOL.(mg)	FIBER(g)	SODIUM(mg)
475	60	23	12	4.5	40	4	625

Food exchanges per serving: 3 Starches plus 3 Lean Meats plus 2 Vegetables
Low-sodium diets: Omit salt in water to boil pasta. Use unsalted pasta sauce in the Rich Meat Sauce.

Rich Meat Sauce

I usually make this multipurpose meat sauce with leftover red wine. If you don't want to use wine, substitute beef broth.

1 pound 90% lean ground beef
1 large onion, chopped coarse
1 26- to 27-ounce jar pasta sauce
   with mushrooms
¾ cup dry red wine
1 2¼-ounce can sliced ripe olives,
   drained

3 large cloves garlic, minced
2 tablespoons chopped fresh basil or
   1 teaspoon dried basil
¼ teaspoon crushed red pepper
   flakes

Sauté ground beef and onion in a deep nonstick skillet or pot until beef is no longer pink. Transfer mixture to a colander and rinse beef to remove the extra fat.

Return beef and onions to pot; add all other ingredients. Simmer 15–20 minutes over low heat, stirring occasionally.

8 servings (makes 6 cups)
1 serving = ¾ cup

CAL.	CHO(g)	PRO.(g)	TOTAL FAT(g)	SAT. FAT(g)	CHOL.(mg)	FIBER(g)	SODIUM(mg)
220	18	13	8	2.5	35	3	460

Food exchanges per serving: 2 Lean Meats plus 3 Vegetables *or* 2 Lean Meats plus 1 Fruit
Low-sodium diets: Substitute unsalted pasta sauce.

Chunky Tomato Sauce

This sauce can be prepared ahead of time and frozen. It is a good sauce to have on hand for topping pasta, seafood, or pizza.

¼ cup Chicken Stock or Vegetable Stock (see Index)
3 cloves garlic, minced
1½ cups minced onion
1 28-ounce can crushed tomatoes
1 6-ounce can tomato paste
1½ teaspoons dried basil

1½ teaspoons dried oregano
2 bay leaves
½ teaspoon fennel seeds
1 teaspoon honey
½ teaspoon salt
¼ teaspoon freshly ground pepper

*H*eat stock in a large saucepan over medium heat. Add garlic and onion; sauté a few minutes until onion is soft. Mix in tomatoes with juice, tomato paste, basil, oregano, bay leaves, fennel seeds, honey, salt, and pepper. Bring sauce to a boil.

Reduce heat to simmer, and continue cooking uncovered 35 minutes or until sauce thickens. Stir occasionally.

Discard bay leaves before serving.

6 servings (makes 3–3½ cups)
1 serving = ½ cup

CAL.	CHO*(g)*	PRO.*(g)*	TOTAL FAT*(g)*	SAT. FAT*(g)*	CHOL.*(mg)*	FIBER*(g)*	SODIUM*(mg)*
75	16	3	1	0	0	3	630

Food exchanges per serving: 3 Vegetables *or* 1 Other Carbohydrate
Low-sodium diets: Omit salt.

Pesto

In Genoa, pesto is traditionally made with a mortar and pestle. I take a shortcut and use a food processor. Pesto freezes well. Freeze it in 2-tablespoon portions in small freezer bags and use it to season pasta, rice, or vegetables. When used over pasta as an entree, the recipe is enough to season ½ pound of your favorite type of pasta.

1 cup fresh basil leaves
½ cup fresh Italian parsley leaves
½ cup grated Parmesan cheese
½ cup grated Romano cheese
¼ cup pine nuts
2 large garlic cloves

¾ teaspoon salt
¼ teaspoon crushed red pepper flakes
½ cup Chicken Stock (see Index) or chicken or vegetable broth
⅓ cup virgin olive oil

Put all ingredients except Chicken Stock and oil in a food processor or blender. Process 1 minute to grind ingredients. With motor running slowly add Chicken Stock, then very slowly, add olive oil.

10 servings (makes 1¼ cups)
1 serving = 2 tablespoons

CAL.	CHO(g)	PRO.(g)	TOTAL FAT(g)	SAT. FAT(g)	CHOL.(mg)	FIBER(g)	SODIUM(mg)
125	3	4	12	2	5	0.5	295

Food exchanges per serving: 2 Fats plus 1 Vegetable
Low-sodium diets: Omit salt.

Grains

Garlic Grits

Baked garlic gives the grits a mild and nutty flavor. Serve this dish with an entree that has gravy or sauce.

4 cloves garlic, unpeeled	*¼ teaspoon ground white pepper*
3 cups water	*¾ cup quick-cooking white hominy*
½ teaspoon salt	*grits*

Preheat oven to 375°F. Place garlic cloves on baking sheet; bake 10 minutes. Remove and discard outer skin. Chop garlic; reserve.

Bring water to a rolling boil; add salt and pepper. Stir grits into boiling water in a slow, steady stream. Cook, stirring constantly, 3 minutes. Turn off heat; let stand, covered, 5 minutes. Stir chopped garlic into grits.

6 servings (makes 3 cups)
1 serving = ½ cup

CAL.	CHO*(g)*	PRO.*(g)*	TOTAL FAT*(g)*	SAT. FAT*(g)*	CHOL.*(mg)*	FIBER*(g)*	SODIUM*(mg)*
70	15	2	0	0	0	1	185

Food exchange per serving: 1 Starch
Low-sodium diets: Omit salt.

Bulgur with Raisins and Cinnamon

Whole grains and dried fruits are excellent sources of fiber. This recipe has both.

1 tablespoon margarine
½ cup chopped onion
½ cup chopped celery
1 cup bulgur
2 cups Chicken Stock (see Index) or
    chicken or vegetable broth
½ teaspoon minced garlic

¼ teaspoon ground white pepper
½ teaspoon crumbled dried
    tarragon
½ cup raisins
½ teaspoon cinnamon
½ teaspoon salt

*I*n a nonstick pot, melt margarine. Add onion and celery; sauté until tender, stirring often. Stir in bulgur; continue cooking until bulgur is coated and turns a golden brown.

Blend in stock, garlic, pepper, and tarragon. Add raisins, cinnamon, and salt; mix well. Cover and continue cooking 15–17 minutes or until all liquid has been absorbed.

Serve hot as a cereal or as a grain side dish.

6 servings (makes 3 cups)
1 serving = ½ cup

CAL.	CHO(g)	PRO.(g)	TOTAL FAT(g)	SAT. FAT(g)	CHOL.(mg)	FIBER(g)	SODIUM(mg)
150	30	5	3	0.5	0	5.5	255

Food exchanges per serving: 1 Starch plus 1 Fruit
Low-sodium diets: Omit salt. Use unsalted Chicken Stock or broth.

Barley with Browned Onions

1 tablespoon olive oil
1 large sweet Spanish onion,
    chopped
1½ cups Chicken Stock (see Index)
    or chicken or vegetable broth

¾ cup quick-cooking pearled barley
2 tablespoons diced pimiento or
    roasted red pepper
2 tablespoons minced fresh parsley

*H*eat oil in nonstick skillet. Add onion; sauté until lightly browned.

In a medium saucepan, bring Chicken Stock to a boil. Add barley; stir and cover. Reduce heat and simmer 10 minutes. Add browned onions, pimiento, and parsley. Stir to blend.

8 servings (makes 4 cups)
1 serving = ½ cup

CAL.	CHO(g)	PRO.(g)	TOTAL FAT(g)	SAT. FAT(g)	CHOL.(mg)	FIBER(g)	SODIUM(mg)
85	15	3	2	0.5	0	2	25

Food exchange per serving: 1 Starch
Low-sodium diets: This recipe is excellent.

Wild Mushroom Couscous

The couscous picks up an earthy flavor from the dried mushrooms and mushroom liquid. Warm water is used to rehydrate dried mushrooms more quickly.

1 ounce dried shiitake or other dried mushrooms
2 cups warm water
1 cup couscous
1 tablespoon olive oil

1 cup chopped onion
2 tablespoons finely chopped fresh chives
½ teaspoon salt
¼ teaspoon freshly ground pepper

Soak dried mushrooms in warm water 30 minutes to allow mushrooms to soften. Remove from liquid; finely slice.

Pour soaking liquid and mushrooms into a medium-sized saucepan. Bring to a boil; add couscous and stir to mix. Cover, remove from heat, and allow to stand 5 minutes.

While couscous is resting, heat olive oil in a small nonstick skillet. Add onion; sauté until lightly browned. Stir sautéed onion, chives, salt, and pepper into couscous. Toss well to mix.

6 servings (makes 4½ cups)
1 serving = ⅔ cup

CAL.	CHO(g)	PRO.(g)	TOTAL FAT(g)	SAT. FAT(g)	CHOL.(mg)	FIBER(g)	SODIUM(mg)
160	30	5	3	0.5	0	1.5	185

Food exchanges per serving: 2 Starches
Low-sodium diets: Omit salt.

Gingered Apricot Carrot Couscous

For a special presentation, press scoops of warm couscous into a ½-cup metal measuring cup or mold. Unmold on a platter or individual plates. Top or surround the molded couscous with shrimp, steamed crab claws, or grilled scallops. The couscous can also be served at room temperature and is a lovely buffet item. While this is a rather sophisticated dish, I have found that kids (particularly toddlers) love it.

½ cup carrot juice, fresh or canned
½ cinnamon stick
1 teaspoon grated fresh gingerroot
½ teaspoon salt
1 cup couscous

¼ cup (2 ounces) dried apricots, sliced thin
3 scallions, minced
3 tablespoons lightly toasted pine nuts

*P*ut carrot juice, cinnamon stick, gingerroot, and salt in a medium-sized saucepan; bring to a boil. Stir in couscous; cover and remove from heat. Let stand 5 minutes.

Discard cinnamon stick. Toss couscous with apricots, scallions, and pine nuts.

9 servings (makes about 4½ cups)
1 serving = ½ cup

CAL.	CHO(g)	PRO.(g)	TOTAL FAT(g)	SAT. FAT(g)	CHOL.(mg)	FIBER(g)	SODIUM(mg)
140	27	5	2	0.5	0	2	155

Food exchanges per serving: 2 Starches
Low-sodium diets: Omit salt.

Classic Polenta

For a treat, serve Classic Polenta over grilled or broiled portobello mushrooms. A small amount of real butter and good-quality Parmesan from Reggiano make this simple dish both authentic and delicious.

2 cups water	2 teaspoons butter or margarine
¼ teaspoon salt	2 tablespoons freshly grated
½ cup instant polenta	Parmigiano-Reggiano cheese

In a medium-sized pot, bring water to a boil; add salt and polenta. Stir continuously 4–5 minutes over low heat.

Serve polenta in ½-cup portions. Top each portion with ½ teaspoon butter or margarine and 1½ teaspoons cheese.

4 servings (makes 2 cups)
1 serving = ½ cup

CAL.	CHO(g)	PRO.(g)	TOTAL FAT(g)	SAT. FAT(g)	CHOL.(mg)	FIBER(g)	SODIUM(mg)
150	27	4	3	1.5	5	3.5	170

Food exchanges per serving: 2 Starches
Low-sodium diets: Omit salt.

Grilled Polenta with Marinara Sauce

Try this polenta topped with Rainbow Pepper Sauté or Ratatouille, or serve it on a bed of Oven-Roasted Tomatoes (see Index). The triangles are easy, or you can use a cookie cutter to make moons, stars, or other shapes. If your meal includes other sauces, you can omit the marinara.

2 cups water
½ cup instant polenta
¼ teaspoon salt
1 tablespoon snipped fresh chives

1 cup prepared marinara or other
   pasta sauce with mushrooms
   or Chunky Tomato Sauce
   (see Index)
2 teaspoons butter, divided

Prepare an 8-inch baking pan with nonstick cooking spray. Bring water to a boil in a medium saucepan. Add polenta and salt; stir mixture continuously with a wooden spoon for 4–5 minutes over very low heat. Add chives and stir to mix.

Pour polenta into prepared pan; spread to level top of mixture. Allow to cool. In pan, cut polenta into quarters, each 4 inches square. Cut each quarter diagonally to make eight triangles.

Heat marinara sauce in a small pot.

Heat 1 teaspoon butter in a nonstick skillet over low heat. Add four polenta triangles and brown both sides; remove from pan. Wipe out browned butter from pan with paper towel. Add remaining 1 teaspoon butter; brown remaining polenta triangles.

To serve, top each triangle with heated sauce.

8 servings
1 serving = 1 triangle plus 2 tablespoons sauce

CAL.	CHO(g)	PRO.(g)	TOTAL FAT(g)	SAT. FAT(g)	CHOL.(mg)	FIBER(g)	SODIUM(mg)
110	18	2	2	1	5	2.5	200

Food exchange per serving: 1 Starch
Low-sodium diets: Omit salt.

21
Vegetables

Roasted Asparagus with Shredded Parmesan

Served hot, this is a wonderful spring and summer vegetable dish. I like it at room temperature as an appetizer or salad, and it is a beautiful addition to any buffet.

1 pound slender fresh asparagus
1 tablespoon virgin olive oil

1 tablespoon freshly shredded
Parmesan cheese

Preheat oven to 425°F. Snap off tough ends of asparagus. Cook in boiling salted water about 5 minutes. Drain.

Spread asparagus in a small roasting pan or on a cookie sheet in a single layer. Brush with olive oil; roast 10 minutes, turning once during roasting time. Put hot asparagus on a platter or individual plates. Sprinkle with cheese. Serve hot or at room temperature.

4 servings
1 serving = about 4 spears

CAL.	CHO(g)	PRO.(g)	TOTAL FAT(g)	SAT. FAT(g)	CHOL.(mg)	FIBER(g)	SODIUM(mg)
50	4	4	3	0.5	0	1	85

Food exchanges per serving: 1 Vegetable plus ½ Fat
Low-sodium diets: This recipe is suitable.

Tiny Bean Bundles

If you have a bottle of herb-infused oil—such as garlic, basil, or porcini mushroom oil—you can substitute 2 teaspoons of it for the lemon oil in this recipe.

½ pound fresh thin, tiny French green beans

2 or 3 scallions

2 teaspoons virgin olive oil

1 teaspoon fresh squeezed lemon juice

½ teaspoon finely grated lemon zest

Rinse beans and snap off stem ends. Cut off base of each scallion; slit scallions lengthwise several times to make long ribbonlike strips, including all of the green part.

Bring a large pot of salted water to a boil. Blanch scallion strips in boiling water 1 minute or until they wilt. Carefully remove strips from water.

Make 12 small bundles of beans; tie each bundle with a scallion ribbon, closing with a little knot or bow. Put bundles in a large colander or large steamer; immerse in boiling water 5 minutes until the beans are crisp tender.

In a small bowl, combine oil, lemon juice, and lemon zest.

Remove beans from pot; drain well. Brush each bundle with lemon oil.

Serve hot or at room temperature.

6 servings
1 serving = 2 bundles

CAL.	CHO*(g)*	PRO.*(g)*	TOTAL FAT*(g)*	SAT. FAT*(g)*	CHOL.*(mg)*	FIBER*(g)*	SODIUM*(mg)*
25	3	1	1	0	0	1	50

Food exchange per serving: 1 Vegetable
Low-sodium diets: This recipe is excellent.

Green Beans with Honey Ham

1 pound fresh green beans, washed
2 teaspoons margarine or butter
1 small sweet yellow onion, sliced
    thin
1 clove garlic, minced fine
2 ounces lean honey ham, diced
    fine, drained

¼ cup water
¼ teaspoon salt
¼ teaspoon freshly ground pepper
½ teaspoon chopped fresh thyme

Snap stem ends from beans. Boil 5 minutes in salted water; drain.

Melt margarine in a large skillet. Add onion and garlic; sauté over low heat until onion is translucent. Add ham, drained beans, and water. Simmer about 5 minutes until beans are tender.

Season with salt, pepper, and thyme. Serve hot.

6 servings (makes 4½ cups)
1 serving = ¾ cup

CAL.	CHO(g)	PRO.(g)	TOTAL FAT(g)	SAT. FAT(g)	CHOL.(mg)	FIBER(g)	SODIUM(mg)
55	8	3	2	0.5	5	1.5	255

Food exchanges per serving: 2 Vegetables
Low-sodium diets: Omit salt.

Green Beans Italiano

1 tablespoon margarine
1 medium yellow onion
2 cloves garlic, crushed
1 8-ounce can tomatoes
1 10-ounce package frozen green
    beans or 1 16-ounce can cut
    green beans, drained

¼ cup chopped green bell pepper
¼ teaspoon salt
½ teaspoon crushed dried oregano
1 tablespoon wine vinegar

Melt margarine in a heavy, deep saucepan. Peel onion and slice crosswise into thin rings; sauté onion and garlic in melted margarine. Stir over medium heat with a wooden spoon until onion is tender but not browned.

Cut tomatoes into bite-sized pieces. Add to onions with tomato liquid, green beans, and all remaining ingredients. Mix well. Bring to a boil and simmer gently about 5 minutes to blend flavors.

6 servings (makes 3 cups)
1 serving = ½ cup

CAL.	CHO(g)	PRO.(g)	TOTAL FAT(g)	SAT. FAT(g)	CHOL.(mg)	FIBER(g)	SODIUM(mg)
55	8	2	2	0.5	0	1.5	175

Food exchanges per serving: 2 Vegetables
Low-sodium diets: Omit salt. Use unsalted margarine, unsalted canned tomatoes, and unsalted green beans.

Bok Choy with Walnuts

If you don't have walnut oil, substitute another nut oil or a vegetable oil. Nut oils are a flavorful addition to vegetables and salad dressings. Because their flavors are intense, a little oil goes a long way.

1 tablespoon walnut oil
2 tablespoons chopped red bell pepper
2 cloves garlic, chopped fine
1 small head (1 pound) bok choy, sliced
½ cup Chicken Stock (see Index) or chicken broth

½ teaspoon salt
⅛ teaspoon crushed red pepper flakes
2 tablespoons coarsely chopped walnuts

*H*eat walnut oil in a large nonstick skillet. Add pepper and garlic; sauté until fragrant. Add bok choy and Chicken Stock; sauté about 4 minutes, just until greens start to wilt. Add salt, red pepper flakes, and walnuts; heat through.

6 servings (makes 4 cups)
1 serving = ⅔ cup

CAL.	CHO(g)	PRO.(g)	TOTAL FAT(g)	SAT. FAT(g)	CHOL.(mg)	FIBER(g)	SODIUM(mg)
50	3	1	4	0.5	0	1	235

Food exchanges per serving: 1 Vegetable plus 1 Fat
Low-sodium diets: Omit salt.

Jade Green Gingered Broccoli

Beautiful, tasty, nutritious—this broccoli recipe is a winner!

6 cups sliced trimmed broccoli pieces
⅓ cup Chicken Stock (see Index) or
    chicken or vegetable broth
2 cloves garlic, minced fine
1 teaspoon grated peeled fresh
    gingerroot

3 tablespoons light (reduced-
    sodium) soy sauce
1 tablespoon brown sugar
1 teaspoon sesame oil
1 tablespoon cornstarch
2 tablespoons cold water

Place broccoli in a large pan of boiling water. Return to boil and cook 2 minutes; drain and set aside.

Heat the Chicken Stock in a wok or large skillet over medium heat. Add garlic and ginger; stir for 1 minute. Add soy sauce, brown sugar, and sesame oil.

In a small bowl, dissolve cornstarch in cold water; add to skillet. Cook and stir until sauce thickens. Stir in broccoli.

6 servings (makes 4½ cups loosely packed)
1 serving = ¾ cup

CAL.	CHO(g)	PRO.(g)	TOTAL FAT(g)	SAT. FAT(g)	CHOL.(mg)	FIBER(g)	SODIUM(mg)
55	9	3	1	0	0	2.5	380

Food exchanges per serving: 2 Vegetables
Low-sodium diets: Use only 1 tablespoon light (reduced-sodium) soy sauce.

Broccoli with Lemon

Broccoli is rich in many nutrients—terrific in vitamin A, vitamin C, many minerals, and fiber. And, as a cruciferous vegetable, it may help to prevent cancer.

1½ pounds broccoli
2 tablespoons margarine
2 tablespoons fresh lemon juice

½ lemon, cut into thin wedges, for
garnish

On stovetop, bring to a boil a large pot of salted water.

Wash broccoli; trim off tough stems. Cut each stalk of broccoli from top to bottom into several pieces for more uniform cooking. Add broccoli to boiling water; reduce heat and simmer until broccoli is crisp-tender, about 6 minutes. Meanwhile, melt margarine in a small saucepan or bowl. Add lemon juice.

Arrange broccoli in a serving dish. Drizzle margarine-lemon mixture over broccoli, and garnish with lemon wedges.

8 servings (makes 6 cups loosely packed)
1 serving = ¾ cup

CAL.	CHO(g)	PRO.(g)	TOTAL FAT(g)	SAT. FAT(g)	CHOL.(mg)	FIBER(g)	SODIUM(mg)
40	4	2	3	0.5	0	1.5	220

Food exchanges per serving: 1 Vegetable plus ½ Fat
Low-sodium diets: Omit salt. Use unsalted margarine.

Herbed Broccoli-Cauliflower Puree

You can use fresh broccoli and cauliflower, but frozen works well and is so easy. Fresh herbs—whatever herbs you have in your refrigerator or on your windowsill—add great flavor.

1 cup Chicken Stock (see Index) or chicken or vegetable broth
1 pound frozen mixed broccoli and cauliflower
¼ cup fresh herbs (oregano, basil, chives, thyme, and/or tarragon)

1 tablespoon margarine or butter
1 teaspoon salt
¼ teaspoon freshly ground pepper
¼ teaspoon grated or ground nutmeg

*P*ut Chicken Stock in a medium-sized pot; add broccoli and cauliflower, and simmer 5 minutes. Vegetables will be partially cooked.

Transfer vegetables with liquid to bowl of a food processor fitted with a steel blade. Process until mixture is fairly smooth. Add herbs, margarine, and seasonings; process 30 seconds more.

Serve hot.

4 servings (makes 2 cups)
1 serving = ½ cup

CAL.	CHO*(g)*	PRO.*(g)*	TOTAL FAT*(g)*	SAT. FAT*(g)*	CHOL.*(mg)*	FIBER*(g)*	SODIUM*(mg)*
65	7	4	4	0.5	0	2.5	360

Food exchanges per serving: 1 Vegetable plus 1 Fat
Low-sodium diets: Omit salt. Use unsalted broth.

Low Country Cabbage

This recipe is inspired by a dish enjoyed by my colleague Karen Connit at Elizabeth's on 37th Street in Savannah, Georgia. Karen shared it with me; I modified it to reduce fat and share it with you.

1 strip bacon, diced
4 ounces leeks, mostly the white
    part, washed and sliced
1 pound shredded cabbage
1 cup Chicken Stock (see Index) or
    chicken or vegetable broth
1 small Granny Smith apple, diced
    with peel on

2 ounces diced lean smoked ham or
    Canadian bacon
1 teaspoon grated gingerroot
⅔ cup cultured low-fat (1½% milk
    fat) buttermilk
½ teaspoon salt
¼ teaspoon freshly ground pepper

Sauté bacon and leeks in a deep skillet over low heat. Add cabbage, Chicken Stock, apple, ham, and ginger. Simmer 15 minutes, covered; stir occasionally.

Add buttermilk; simmer uncovered to reduce liquid, about 5 more minutes. Season with salt and pepper.

8 servings (makes 4 cups)
1 serving = ½ cup

CAL.	CHO(g)	PRO.(g)	TOTAL FAT(g)	SAT. FAT(g)	CHOL.(mg)	FIBER(g)	SODIUM(mg)
70	8	4	3	1	5	2	305

Food exchanges per serving: 1 Vegetable plus ½ Fat
Low-sodium diets: Omit salt.

Sweet and Sour Red Cabbage

1 pound red cabbage, shredded
½ cup cider vinegar
½ cup water
2 tablespoons margarine

½ teaspoon salt
Sugar substitute equivalent to 3
    tablespoons sugar

Put cabbage, vinegar, water, margarine, and salt in a deep cooking pot. Cover, bring to a boil and simmer about 15 minutes or until crisp-tender, lifting and turning with a large kitchen fork two or three times.

Remove from heat. Add sweetener gradually, lifting and mixing well with a fork. Let cabbage rest in liquid 5–10 minutes, to absorb flavors. Drain off any liquid.

8 servings (makes 6 cups)
1 serving = ¾ cup

CAL.	CHO(g)	PRO.(g)	TOTAL FAT(g)	SAT. FAT(g)	CHOL.(mg)	FIBER(g)	SODIUM(mg)
30	4	1	1	0	0	1	90

Food exchange per serving: 1 Vegetable
Low-sodium diets: Omit salt. Use unsalted margarine.

Orange Spiced Baby Carrots

Enjoy carrots often. They are very rich in protective vitamins and minerals. You can use fresh or frozen baby carrots for this recipe. I've also made it with grated carrots sold in a bag in the produce department. Simmer grated carrots only 15 minutes.

½ cup water
½ cup orange juice
1 tablespoon margarine
1 pound peeled baby carrots

½ teaspoon pure vanilla extract
¼ teaspoon ground nutmeg
1½ teaspoons grated fresh orange
  zest

*P*ut water, orange juice, and margarine into a saucepan; add carrots. Cover tightly and simmer over low heat 25 minutes or until carrots are crisp-tender. Check occasionally to make sure that carrots don't burn, because most of the liquid will be absorbed; add a few tablespoons water if necessary.

Sprinkle carrots with vanilla, nutmeg, and orange zest; mix well.

4 servings (makes 2 cups)
1 serving = ½ cup

CAL.	CHO(g)	PRO.(g)	TOTAL FAT(g)	SAT. FAT(g)	CHOL.(mg)	FIBER(g)	SODIUM(mg)
90	15	1	3	0.5	0	3.5	75

Food exchanges per serving: 1 Vegetable plus ½ Fruit plus ½ Fat *or* 1 Starch
Low-sodium diets: This recipe is excellent.

Dill Roasted Carrots

If you have an outdoor grill going, you can roast these foil-packed carrots on the grill—about 30 minutes.

1 pound young tender carrots,
    without tops
1½ tablespoons margarine
¼ teaspoon dried dill or *1 teaspoon*
    snipped fresh dill

¼ teaspoon salt
Dash freshly ground pepper
1 tablespoon water

Preheat oven to 375°F. Pare carrots with a vegetable peeler, or scrub them very well with a vegetable brush. Cut into strips, like french fries.

Place carrots in the middle of a piece of heavy-duty foil. Dot with margarine; sprinkle with seasonings and water. Wrap carrots securely in foil, and crimp edges.

Bake 45 minutes or until carrots are tender.

5 servings (makes 2½ cups)
1 serving = ½ cup (about 7 strips)

CAL.	CHO(g)	PRO.(g)	TOTAL FAT(g)	SAT. FAT(g)	CHOL.(mg)	FIBER(g)	SODIUM(mg)
65	8	1	4	0.5	0	2.5	175

Food exchanges per serving: 1 Vegetable plus 1 Fat
Low-sodium diets: Omit salt. Use unsalted margarine.

Cauliflower Crown

1 small (1½-pound head) cauliflower	1 slice bread
1 teaspoon fresh lemon juice	¼ cup plain low-fat yogurt
1 teaspoon salt	1 tablespoon margarine
	¼ teaspoon paprika

Trim tough stem and soft or browned leaves off whole head of cauliflower, leaving tender leaves and stems. Even off the bottom.

In a deep pot, bring 1 quart water, lemon juice, and salt to a boil. Add cauliflower. Place bread slice on top to absorb odor. Let cauliflower cook briskly about 20 minutes or until cauliflower stem is fork-tender.

Preheat oven to 350°F.

Discard bread slice. Drain cauliflower carefully but thoroughly. Place cauliflower stem side down on a foil-lined baking sheet. Spoon yogurt over the center of the top of the cauliflower to form a "crown."

Divide margarine into small bits; dot margarine on top of yogurt. Sprinkle evenly with paprika. Bake cauliflower crown 10 minutes.

6 servings
1 serving = ⅙ head (about ¾ cup)

CAL.	CHO*(g)*	PRO.*(g)*	TOTAL FAT*(g)*	SAT. FAT*(g)*	CHOL.*(mg)*	FIBER*(g)*	SODIUM*(mg)*
35	4	2	2	0.5	0	1.5	125

Food exchange per serving: 1 Vegetable
Low-sodium diets: Omit salt. Use unsalted margarine.

Corn Cakes with Salsa

Try these as a brunch or lunch entree and serve a double portion.

1½ cups corn, cut from the cob or   1 tablespoon melted margarine
    frozen and thawed   ¼ teaspoon salt
2 tablespoons evaporated skim milk   ½ cup plus 2 tablespoons Chunky
1 egg, beaten   Salsa (see Index), at room
1 tablespoon finely chopped fresh   temperature
    parsley

Combine all ingredients except salsa in a bowl; mix well.

Heat a large nonstick skillet or griddle over medium heat. Spray skillet or griddle with butter-flavored nonstick cooking spray.

Drop batter, in 2-tablespoon scoops per corn cake, onto skillet. Cook until lightly browned; turn to brown other side. Spray pan between each batch.

Serve hot corn cakes topped with Chunky Salsa.

5 servings
1 serving = 2 corn cakes plus 2 tablespoons salsa

CAL.	CHO(g)	PRO.(g)	TOTAL FAT(g)	SAT. FAT(g)	CHOL.(mg)	FIBER(g)	SODIUM(mg)
95	12	3	4	1	45	1.5	480

Food exchanges per serving: 1 Starch plus 1 Fat
Low-sodium diets: Omit salt. Use unsalted salsa.

Smothered Corn

One of my favorite casual restaurants in Chicago is called Heaven on Seven. There they call this dish Macque Choix and often serve it with added shrimp or crayfish. It's delicious with or without the seafood.

4 ears corn	*1 clove garlic, minced*
1 tablespoon corn oil	*½ cup water*
1 small onion, chopped	*6 ripe cherry tomatoes, chopped*
½ green bell pepper, chopped	*1 teaspoon Cajun seasoning*

Cut kernels from corn cobs. Heat a large nonstick skillet; add oil, onion, pepper, and garlic. Sauté 2–3 minutes until onion is translucent.

Add corn and ½ cup water; simmer 5 minutes, stirring often. Stir in tomatoes and Cajun seasonings; simmer about 10 minutes, stirring often.

6 servings (makes 3 cups)
1 serving = ½ cup

CAL.	CHO*(g)*	PRO.*(g)*	TOTAL FAT*(g)*	SAT. FAT*(g)*	CHOL.*(mg)*	FIBER*(g)*	SODIUM*(mg)*
85	14	2	3	0.5	0	2.5	150

Food exchanges per serving: 1 Starch plus ½ Fat
Low-sodium diets: This recipe is acceptable.

Corn and Red Bean Medley

1 cup canned whole-kernel corn,
   with liquid
¼ cup chopped onion
¾ cup canned red kidney beans,
   drained

¾ teaspoon chili powder
¼ teaspoon crushed red pepper
   flakes (or to taste)

*D*rain liquid from canned corn and heat it in a nonstick saucepan. Add onion; sauté until tender, about 2 minutes. Add corn, beans, and seasonings; heat, stirring often. Taste and adjust seasonings. Serve hot.

4 servings (makes 2 cups)
1 serving = ½ cup

CAL.	CHO(g)	PRO.(g)	TOTAL FAT(g)	SAT. FAT(g)	CHOL.(mg)	FIBER(g)	SODIUM(mg)
80	17	4	1	0	0	3	230

Food exchange per serving: 1 Starch
Low-sodium diets: Substitute unsalted canned vegetables if available.

Kale Timbales

You can make this with other leafy greens—collard or mustard greens, Swiss chard, or spinach. Kale is a thick, tough green and requires about 8 minutes to parboil. Use the same method for the other greens but reduce the boiling time to 4–5 minutes. Parboiling is a technique used to tenderize and partially cook vegetables that need a longer cooking time than other ingredients that will be added to a recipe. Or you can save several steps by using ¾ cup frozen chopped greens, thawed and drained.

4 cups (4–5 ounces) kale, thick stems removed

1 medium onion, cut into chunks

1 cup evaporated skim milk

¾ cup egg substitute or *3 eggs*

¼ teaspoon ground nutmeg

*P*reheat oven to 350°F. Cook kale 8 minutes in boiling salted water; kale should wilt but remain bright green. Drain.

Put kale and onions in bowl of a food processor; process until kale is chopped. Add evaporated milk, egg, and nutmeg; process another 30 seconds.

Prepare 10 cups of a 12-cup muffin tin with nonstick cooking spray. Divide kale mixture among the cups. Bake about 25 minutes until timbales are firm.

Unmold immediately. Serve hot, or chill to serve later.

10 servings
1 serving = 1 timbale

CAL.	CHO*(g)*	PRO.*(g)*	TOTAL FAT*(g)*	SAT. FAT*(g)*	CHOL.*(mg)*	FIBER*(g)*	SODIUM*(mg)*
45	6	4	0	0	0	1	80

Food exchange per serving: 1 Vegetable
Low-sodium diets: This recipe is acceptable.

Thai Grilled Leeks

Leeks are a tasty and unusual accompaniment to grilled fish, poultry, or meat. Think of leeks when you barbecue; they are delicious grilled. Marinate them for a few minutes with a marinade, or simply brush them with a little olive oil.

2 (about 1 pound total) medium leeks

2 tablespoons Thai-Style Vinaigrette (see Index)

Bring a medium-sized pot of water to a boil. Remove base from leeks and most of the greens from their tops, leaving about 2 inches of the green part. Split leeks lengthwise. Holding leeks firmly together, rinse dirt from between layers.

Push four toothpicks through each leek half, about 2 inches apart, to hold layers together. Cut each leek into 5- to 6-inch lengths. Parboil leeks 4–5 minutes; drain. (If you prefer, you can cook the leeks in a microwave oven 2–3 minutes.)

Brush hot leeks with vinaigrette; marinate for 15 minutes. Grill over white-ashed coals for about 10 minutes, turning several times until leeks are tender and browned.

Remove toothpicks and serve.

4 servings
1 serving = 2 pieces

CAL.	CHO(g)	PRO.(g)	TOTAL FAT(g)	SAT. FAT(g)	CHOL.(mg)	FIBER(g)	SODIUM(mg)
40	7	1	1	0	0	0.5	85

Food exchange per serving: 1 Vegetable
Low-sodium diets: This recipe is acceptable.

Mushrooms au Jus

These mushrooms with their natural juices are great with steak, roast beef, or burgers.

1 pound fresh mushrooms
1 tablespoon margarine, broken into bits

¼ teaspoon salt
Dash freshly ground pepper

Preheat oven to 350°F or prepare grill. Wash mushrooms thoroughly and remove tough tips from bottom of stems. Cut a large piece of aluminum foil; place mushrooms in the middle of the foil, dot with margarine, and sprinkle with salt and pepper. Fold foil around mushrooms; seal package tightly by crimping edges.

Bake 20–30 minutes in oven or on grill. Remove package; open very carefully to avoid spilling the delicious juices from the mushrooms.

7 servings (makes 3½ cups)
1 serving = ½ cup

CAL.	CHO(g)	PRO.(g)	TOTAL FAT(g)	SAT. FAT(g)	CHOL.(mg)	FIBER(g)	SODIUM(mg)
30	3	1	2	0.5	0	1	100

Food exchange per serving: 1 Vegetable
Low-sodium diets: Omit salt. Use unsalted margarine.

Balsamic Red Onions

Red onions are usually milder than white onions, and they contain a phytochemical that some experts believe lowers blood cholesterol.

 2 (about 1 pound total) red onions   2 tablespoons water
 2 tablespoons balsamic vinegar

Clean, peel, and remove stem ends from onions; cut each onion into six wedges. Put balsamic vinegar and water in a small bowl or zip-top bag. Add onions; mix well with marinade. Refrigerate at least 1 hour, turning onions in marinade once or twice.

   Preheat oven to 400°F. Spread onions and liquid in a nonstick baking pan. Roast 20–25 minutes until onions are tender and edges are browned. Turn onions once during cooking.

4 servings
1 serving = 3 wedges

CAL.	CHO(g)	PRO.(g)	TOTAL FAT(g)	SAT. FAT(g)	CHOL.(mg)	FIBER(g)	SODIUM(mg)
40	10	2	0	0	0	1.5	10

Food exchange per serving: 1 Vegetable
Low-sodium diets: This recipe is excellent.

Sesame Sugar Snaps

This quick and easy recipe adds color and pizzazz to any plate. It can be served hot or chilled as a salad or buffet item. The technique of adding sesame oil and black sesame seeds to crisp-tender vegetables is also good for green beans, asparagus, and broccoli.

1 pound sugar snap peas, fresh or frozen
1 tablespoon Oriental dark-roasted sesame oil

1 teaspoon black sesame seeds or toasted sesame seeds

*I*f sugar snap peas are fresh, snap off stem ends. (Frozen ones are already trimmed.) Bring a pot of salted water to a boil; add peas and cook just until crisp and tender, about 3–5 minutes. Drain in colander.

Return to pot and toss with oil and seeds.

6 servings (makes 4½ cups)
1 serving = ¾ cup

CAL.	CHO(g)	PRO.(g)	TOTAL FAT(g)	SAT. FAT(g)	CHOL.(mg)	FIBER(g)	SODIUM(mg)
65	8	3	3	0.5	0	2.5	80

Food exchanges per serving: 1 Vegetable plus ½ Fat
Low-sodium diets: This recipe is acceptable.

Rainbow Pepper Sauté

Serve this colorful, tasty vegetable as a side dish or over simple grilled steak, pork chops, fish, or chicken breasts. For slightly different flavors, you can substitute other herbs—thyme, oregano, herbes de Provence, or cilantro.

1 large sweet Spanish onion
1 medium red bell pepper
1 medium green bell pepper
1 medium yellow bell pepper
1 tablespoon olive oil

2 large cloves garlic, minced
2 tablespoons chopped fresh basil or
    ¾ teaspoon dried basil
¼ teaspoon salt
⅛ teaspoon freshly ground pepper

Peel onion and cut into wedges. Wash peppers; remove stems, seeds, and cores. Cut peppers into ¼-inch strips.

Heat oil in a large, nonstick skillet over medium heat. Add onion; sauté, stirring often, 5 minutes. Add peppers; sauté, stirring, 3 minutes more. Add garlic; continue sautéing until vegetables are crisp but tender. Stir in basil, salt, and pepper.

7 servings (makes 3½ cups)
1 serving = ½ cup

CAL.	CHO(g)	PRO.(g)	TOTAL FAT(g)	SAT. FAT(g)	CHOL.(mg)	FIBER(g)	SODIUM(mg)
40	5	1	2	0.5	0	1	80

Food exchange per serving: 1 Vegetable
Low-sodium diets: Omit salt.

Roasted Red Peppers

Roasted red, yellow, or orange bell peppers are great to have on hand. Freeze extras in plastic freezer bags. They add color, flavor, and a hint of sweetness to recipes. While all kinds of peppers can be roasted, green bell peppers lose their bright color, and they aren't really sweet enough. Use them in stir-fried dishes instead. Red and yellow peppers are a nutritional marvel. One 3½-ounce serving provides a whole day's vitamin A plus many other vitamins and minerals. Red bell peppers have twice the vitamin C of green peppers (which themselves are an excellent source).

3 red, yellow, or orange bell peppers

Method 1: Using tongs or a long fork, hold peppers over the flame of a gas stove or lay peppers on top of the hot burner of an electric stove. Rotate with the tongs until all sides are blackened.

Place peppers in a paper bag. Seal the top and allow them to steam for 7–10 minutes. Remove peppers; cut out seeds, cores, and stems. Peel off blackened skin. To set color, plunge into ice water for 1 minute.

Method 2: Preheat oven to 500°F. Place peppers on a cookie sheet; roast until the skins wrinkle and turn brown. Turn peppers every few minutes so they are cooked uniformly.

Remove from oven and place in a brown paper bag. Seal the top and allow peppers to steam 7–10 minutes. Remove peppers; cut out seeds, cores, and stems. Peel off blackened skin. To set color, plunge into ice water for 1 minute.

3 servings
1 serving = 1 pepper

CAL.	CHO(g)	PRO.(g)	TOTAL FAT(g)	SAT. FAT(g)	CHOL.(mg)	FIBER(g)	SODIUM(mg)
20	5	1	0	0	0	1	0

Food exchange per serving: 1 Vegetable (A serving of less than 1 whole pepper is a Free Food.)
Low-sodium diets: An excellent choice.

Mashed Rutabaga and Apple

Wonderful with pork and an excellent source of potassium.

1 medium rutabaga	2 tablespoons margarine or butter
1 large potato	½ teaspoon salt
1 large tart apple	¼ teaspoon freshly ground pepper

*B*ring a large pot of salted water to a boil. Peel rutabaga, potato, and apple; cut each into 1-inch cubes. Cook rutabaga 15 minutes; add potato and cook another 10 minutes; add apple and cook 5 minutes more.

Drain rutabaga, potato, and apple; put hot cubes in a mixer or food processor. Add margarine; process until almost smooth. Season with salt and pepper.

6 servings (makes 4 cups)
1 serving = ⅔ cup

CAL.	CHO(g)	PRO.(g)	TOTAL FAT(g)	SAT. FAT(g)	CHOL.(mg)	FIBER(g)	SODIUM(mg)
100	15	1	4	0.5	0	2.5	290

Food exchanges per serving: 1 Starch plus 1 Fat
Low-sodium diets: Omit salt. Use unsalted margarine.

Oven-Roasted Shallots

You can use these shallots as a side dish with meat, atop couscous or barley, or as an ingredient in other dishes. Chopped roasted shallots add great flavor to salad dressings and savory sauces.

1 pound shallots	*½ teaspoon salt*
2 teaspoons olive oil	*¼ teaspoon coarsely ground pepper*

*P*reheat oven to 375°F. Peel shallots; cut large ones in half. Wrap tightly in a packet of foil. Roast 30 minutes.

Open top of foil to expose shallots. Brush with olive oil; roast another 20 minutes. Season with salt and pepper.

8 servings (makes 2⅔ cups)
1 serving = ⅓ cup shallots

CAL.	CHO(g)	PRO.(g)	TOTAL FAT(g)	SAT. FAT(g)	CHOL.(mg)	FIBER(g)	SODIUM(mg)
50	10	1	1	0	0	0.5	145

Food exchange per serving: 1 Vegetable
Low-sodium diets: Omit salt.

Gently Steamed Spinach

You can use other seasonings to alter the flavor of this tasty, nutrient-rich, and simple vegetable. Try it with ⅛ teaspoon crushed red peppers flakes, ½ teaspoon orange zest, or a clove of crushed garlic instead of the nutmeg.

> 1 10-ounce bag washed, trimmed spinach
> 2 teaspoons margarine or butter
>
> ⅛ teaspoon grated or ground nutmeg

*R*inse spinach in cold water. Trim any thick stems. Put wet spinach in large nonstick skillet. Cut margarine into small pieces. Put margarine pieces on top of spinach and sprinkle nutmeg over it. Cover skillet tightly with lid.

Cook over medium heat only until spinach begins to wilt, about 2–3 minutes. Be careful not to overcook. Turn spinach to mix seasonings throughout. Serve immediately.

4 servings (makes 2 cups)
1 serving = ½ cup

CAL.	CHO(g)	PRO.(g)	TOTAL FAT(g)	SAT. FAT(g)	CHOL.(mg)	FIBER(g)	SODIUM(mg)
35	3	2	2	0.5	0	2	80

Food exchange per serving: 1 Vegetable
Low-sodium diets: Use unsalted margarine.

Pineapple Squash

Winter squash is a great source of antioxidants that help prevent heart disease, cancer, and even the aging of cells.

2 4½-inch-diameter acorn squash (1½–2 pounds total)	2 teaspoons margarine
1 8-ounce can unsweetened crushed pineapple with juice	½ teaspoon cinnamon

Preheat oven to 375°F. Cut each squash in half; scoop out and discard seeds and pulp. Trim tip off bottom if necessary so that each squash cup stands up straight. Fill each squash cup with ¼ cup crushed pineapple, ½ teaspoon margarine, and a sprinkle of cinnamon.

Put squash into a flat baking dish, and pour hot water around the bottoms to a depth of ½ inch. Cover pan tightly with foil. Bake 1 hour or until squash is tender and can be easily pierced with a fork.

4 servings
1 serving = ½ stuffed squash

CAL.	CHO(g)	PRO.(g)	TOTAL FAT(g)	SAT. FAT(g)	CHOL.(mg)	FIBER(g)	SODIUM(mg)
105	23	1	2	0.5	0	0	25

Food exchanges per serving: 1 Starch plus ½ Fruit
Low-sodium diets: This recipe is excellent.

Baked Tomatoes

4 small ripe tomatoes (about 1
   pound)
1 slice bread, crumbled fine (¾ cup
   soft crumbs), divided
½ teaspoon herb or Italian
   seasoning

½ teaspoon salt
⅛ teaspoon coarsely ground pepper
1 tablespoon finely chopped scallion
1 teaspoon margarine, melted

Preheat oven to 350°F. Wash tomatoes and cut a thin slice off the top of
each. Scoop out pulp into a bowl, leaving shells. Mix pulp, ½ cup of the
bread crumbs, seasonings, and scallion.

Place tomato shells in an 8-inch square pan or a pie pan. Divide pulp
mixture evenly among the tomatoes, placing in hollows carefully. Mix melted
margarine with remaining ¼ cup bread crumbs; sprinkle on top of tomatoes.

Bake about 25 minutes, until tomatoes are tender.

4 servings
1 serving = 1 tomato

CAL.	CHO(g)	PRO.(g)	TOTAL FAT(g)	SAT. FAT(g)	CHOL.(mg)	FIBER(g)	SODIUM(mg)
50	8	1	2	0	0	1.5	330

Food exchange per serving: 1 Vegetable or ½ Starch
Low-sodium diets: Omit salt.

Oven-Roasted Tomatoes

Roasting concentrates the tomatoes' rich flavor. Use very ripe red tomatoes for maximum sweetness and flavor.

1 pint ripe cherry or small plum
tomatoes
¼ teaspoon salt

¼ teaspoon freshly ground pepper
2 tablespoons chopped fresh basil
2 teaspoons virgin olive oil

Preheat oven to 400°F. Put a wire cooling rack on top of a cookie sheet. Cut tomatoes in half, gently squeezing out most of soft center and seeds. Arrange tomatoes on rack, cut side down. Season with salt and pepper; roast 20–25 minutes.

Transfer tomatoes to a bowl; toss with basil and oil. Taste and add more seasonings if desired.

4 servings (makes 2 cups)
1 serving = ½ cup

CAL.	CHO(g)	PRO.(g)	TOTAL FAT(g)	SAT. FAT(g)	CHOL.(mg)	FIBER(g)	SODIUM(mg)
30	3	1	2	0.5	0	0.5	140

Food exchange per serving: 1 Vegetable
Low-sodium diets: Omit salt.

Mashed Turnips

1 pound turnips, without tops
1½ tablespoons margarine
½ teaspoon salt

⅛ teaspoon freshly ground pepper
Paprika or chopped fresh parsley for
    garnish (optional)

Bring a medium-sized pot of water to a boil.

Remove tops and root ends of turnips; pare and cut into small cubes. Put turnips in boiling water; cover pan, reduce heat to low, and cook about 20 minutes or until tender.

Drain any remaining water (most of it should be cooked away). Mash turnips thoroughly with a potato masher or an electric mixer; add margarine, salt, and pepper. Beat until blended and fluffy.

If garnish is desired, sprinkle with paprika or finely cut parsley.

4 servings (makes 2 cups)
1 serving = ½ cup

CAL.	CHO(g)	PRO.(g)	TOTAL FAT(g)	SAT. FAT(g)	CHOL.(mg)	FIBER(g)	SODIUM(mg)
65	6	1	4	0.5	0	1.5	385

Food exchanges per serving: 1 Vegetable plus 1 Fat
Low-sodium diets: Omit salt.

Ratatouille

This versatile vegetable mixture is great served either hot or cold. Try it warm in Herbed Phyllo Cups (see Index) as an appetizer or chilled on Boston lettuce with additional capers on top. I always make enough so that I can serve it hot once and cold once. It travels well in lunch bags and is a fine lunch with bread and cheese or cold roast chicken.

3 tablespoons virgin olive oil
4 tablespoons margarine
3 cloves garlic, crushed
3 medium onions, chopped
1 1-pound eggplant, peeled and cubed
2 medium (8–9 ounces total) green bell peppers, cored and sliced
2 medium (about 12 ounces) zucchini, sliced

3 tablespoons all-purpose flour
1 16-ounce can tomatoes, cut up, with liquid
¾ cup water
1 6-ounce can tomato paste
1 teaspoon salt
½ teaspoon coarsely ground pepper
¼ cup chopped fresh parsley
2 teaspoons drained capers

*H*eat oil and margarine in a large pot. Add garlic and onions; sauté until onions are translucent. Add eggplant, green pepper, and zucchini; sauté, stirring often, until vegetables wilt.

Sprinkle flour over vegetable mixture; stir in tomatoes with liquid, water, and tomato paste. Cover and cook over low heat 20 minutes, stirring often to prevent vegetables and sauce from sticking to bottom of pot. Add salt and pepper and cook, uncovered, 10 more minutes; stir often.

Serve topped with chopped parsley and capers.

16 servings (makes 8 cups)
1 serving = ½ cup

CAL.	CHO*(g)*	PRO.*(g)*	TOTAL FAT*(g)*	SAT. FAT*(g)*	CHOL.*(mg)*	FIBER*(g)*	SODIUM*(mg)*
90	9	2	6	1	0	1.5	315

Food exchanges per serving: 2 Vegetables plus 1 Fat
Low-sodium diets: Omit salt. Substitute unsalted tomato paste and unsalted canned tomatoes.

Roasted Root Vegetables

Use three root vegetables for this recipe. You can substitute turnips, carrots, potato, or other varieties of squash for the butternut squash.

1 1-pound rutabaga	2 teaspoons olive oil
1 small (1½ pounds) butternut squash	½ teaspoon salt
2 medium (1 pound total) onions	¼ teaspoon freshly ground pepper

*P*reheat oven to 400°F. Prepare a 10″ × 14″ baking pan with nonstick cooking spray. Cut rutabaga and squash into 1-inch cubes or wedges. Spread them in pan; add ¼ cup water. Cover tightly with foil and roast 15 minutes.

Peel onion; cut into small wedges. Remove foil from pan, add onions, and mix. Brush tops of vegetables with oil. Roast uncovered 30 40 minutes, turning every 10 minutes, until vegetables are tender and edges are browned. Season with salt and pepper.

8 servings (makes 4 cups)
1 serving = ½ cup

CAL.	CHO*(g)*	PRO.*(g)*	TOTAL FAT*(g)*	SAT. FAT*(g)*	CHOL.*(mg)*	FIBER*(g)*	SODIUM*(mg)*
75	15	2	1	0	0	3	150

Food exchange per serving: 1 Starch
Low-sodium diets: Omit salt.

Escarole, Beans, and Pepperoni

This wonderful bean-based entree uses a little pepperoni for flavor. The serving given is an entree-sized portion.

1 1-pound head escarole
1 tablespoon virgin olive oil
1 medium onion, sliced thin
1 shallot, sliced thin (optional)
2 cloves garlic, minced
2 ounces thinly sliced pepperoni
1 15-ounce can cannellini beans
    (white kidney beans)

1 cup Chicken Stock (see Index) or
    chicken broth
1 teaspoon dried oregano or
    1 tablespoon snipped fresh
    oregano
¼ teaspoon crushed red pepper
    flakes

Bring a large pot of salted water to a boil. Wash escarole. Cut off base; cut head crosswise into 1-inch slices so escarole will be in pieces. Blanch escarole in boiling water 2–3 minutes. Drain in colander.

Put olive oil in a large pot; add onion, shallot, and garlic. Sauté vegetables over low heat until onions are translucent. Cut pepperoni slices in half. Add pepperoni, beans with liquid, Chicken Stock, escarole, oregano, and red pepper flakes. Simmer 20 minutes, stirring occasionally.

4 servings (makes 5 cups)
1 serving = 1¼ cup

CAL.	CHO*(g)*	PRO.*(g)*	TOTAL FAT*(g)*	SAT. FAT*(g)*	CHOL.*(mg)*	FIBER*(g)*	SODIUM*(mg)*
235	25	11	11	3	10	10	780

Food exchanges per serving: 1½ Starches plus 1 Medium-Fat Meat plus 1 Fat
Low-sodium diets: This recipe is not suitable.

Zucchini Sauté

You can use any type of summer squash for this recipe—try it with crookneck, pattypan, or baby squash.

4 medium (about 1 pound) zucchini
1 tablespoon virgin olive oil
½ cup thinly sliced red onion

1 teaspoon minced fresh basil or ¼ teaspoon dried basil
¼ teaspoon salt
Dash freshly ground black pepper

Trim off stems and slice zucchini into thin strips or bite-sized pieces.

Heat oil in a large nonstick skillet. Add onion and stir-fry quickly until onion is soft but not browned. Add zucchini, cover skillet, and sauté 3–4 minutes, until zucchini is wilted.

Sprinkle with basil, salt, and pepper and mix well.

6 servings (makes 3 cups)
1 serving = ½ cup

CAL.	CHO(g)	PRO.(g)	TOTAL FAT(g)	SAT. FAT(g)	CHOL.(mg)	FIBER(g)	SODIUM(mg)
35	3	1	2	0.5	0	0.5	95

Food exchange per serving: 1 Vegetable
Low-sodium diets: Omit salt. Add ¼ teaspoon light (sodium-reduced) seasoned salt.

22

Relishes, Chutneys, and Salsas

Relishes

Dilled Vegetable Pickles

Use this pickling solution and method to pickle broccoli flowerets, sliced zucchini, or green beans. This process is not home canning with a water bath, so these vegetable pickles must be eaten within a week to ensure safety and good texture.

¾ cup white vinegar
¾ cup cold water
1 teaspoon salt
1½ teaspoons dill seed
1 small (3-ounce) pickling
   cucumber

4–5 small white pickling onions,
   peeled
1 cup small cauliflowerets
Sugar substitute equivalent to 2
   tablespoons sugar

Combine vinegar, cold water, salt, and dill seeds; bring to a boil. Simmer 5 minutes.

Slice cucumber crosswise into coins. Slice onions crosswise into thin slices and separate into rings. Add cauliflowerets, cucumbers, and onions to hot vinegar; bring to a boil and cook gently for 1 minute.

Remove from heat. Add sweetener and stir until dissolved. Spoon vegetables carefully into a hot, clean pint jar. Pour vinegar mixture on top;

441

cover and cool. Seal jar and store in refrigerator. Use after at least 24 hours but within 1 week.

8 servings (makes 1 pint)
1 serving = ¼ cup

CAL.	CHO*(g)*	PRO.*(g)*	TOTAL FAT*(g)*	SAT. FAT*(g)*	CHOL.*(mg)*	FIBER*(g)*	SODIUM*(mg)*
10	2	1	0	0	0	0.5	140

Food exchange per serving: a Free Food (up to ½ cup)
Low-sodium diets: May be used occasionally if sodium restriction is mild or moderate. These contain far less sodium than traditional pickles.

Sweet Pickled Cherries

A delightful treat for everyone and so easy to make! Serve with a salad, as an unusual garnish, or as finger food on relish trays.

3 cups (1 pound) Bing cherries
  with stems
1 cup cold water

1 cup white vinegar
1 teaspoon brown sugar
1 tablespoon salt

*P*ick over cherries to select firm, ripe ones. Leave on as many stems as possible. Carefully wash and drain cherries. Pack lightly into a 1-quart jar, shaking, but not pressing down.

Combine remaining ingredients and stir until salt dissolves; pour over cherries. Seal jar tightly and turn upside down. Leave for 2 hours in a cool place.

Turn upright. Store in refrigerator. Use after at least 24 hours, but within 1 month. Drain liquid before serving.

8–10 servings (makes 1 quart, or 50–60 cherries)
1 serving = 6–8 cherries

CAL.	CHO(g)	PRO.(g)	TOTAL FAT(g)	SAT. FAT(g)	CHOL.(mg)	FIBER(g)	SODIUM(mg)
35	8	1	0.5	0	0	0.5	185

Food exchange per serving: ½ Fruit (A serving of 2–3 cherries would be a Free Food.)
Low-sodium diets: For occasional use only. Limit to a maximum of 1 serving.

Pickled Ginger

This ginger relish is used in the Gingered Chicken Breasts recipe (see Index). It can also be used as a spicy accompaniment to roast pork or lamb chops.

½ cup sliced, peeled fresh gingerroot   *Sugar substitute equivalent to 2*
   (paper thin)   *tablespoons sugar*
1 cup boiling water   *1 tablespoon water*
½ cup rice vinegar   *¼ teaspoon salt*

*P*lace ginger slices in a bowl; cover with boiling water. Allow ginger to stand 1 minute; drain. Add remaining ingredients; stir well until sugar substitute dissolves.

Refrigerate until ready to serve. Drain pickled ginger before serving.

4 servings (makes ¼ cup)
1 serving = 1 tablespoon

CAL.	CHO(g)	PRO.(g)	TOTAL FAT(g)	SAT. FAT(g)	CHOL.(mg)	FIBER(g)	SODIUM(mg)
10	2	0	0	0	0	0	35

Food exchange per serving: a Free Food
Low-sodium diets: This recipe is acceptable.

Cranberry and Orange Relish

Serve with hot or cold sliced baked poultry or ham. If you freeze this relish, omit sweetener and add it at time of serving.

*2 cups (½ pound) fresh or frozen
   cranberries*
1 medium orange

*Sugar substitute equivalent to
   ¼ cup sugar*

*W*ash and pick over cranberries; discard overripe berries. Wash orange, and cut into small chunks with peel on; remove and discard seeds and center core. Put both fruits through a food grinder using a coarse blade, or chop in a food processor. Add sweetener; mix well.

Chill in a covered container for at least 1 hour. Taste and add more sweetener if desired.

8 servings (makes 1½ cups)
1 serving = 3 tablespoons

CAL.	CHO(g)	PRO.(g)	TOTAL FAT(g)	SAT. FAT(g)	CHOL.(mg)	FIBER(g)	SODIUM(mg)
25	7	1	0	0	0	1	0

Food exchange per serving: ½ Fruit
Low-sodium diets: This recipe is excellent.

Chutneys

Mango Chutney

Pumpkin pie spice as an ingredient is a shortcut. It's a blend of cinnamon, ginger, nutmeg, and allspice that saves measuring several spices. The ingredient list for this recipe is long, but the dish is simple to make because everything is simmered together in one step. If mangoes are unavailable (or if you live in peach territory), substitute ripe fresh peaches.

2 (about 1¼ pounds total) ripe mangoes	*3 scallions, chopped*
1 medium-sized sweet yellow onion, chopped	*2 tablespoons fresh lemon juice*
	1 tablespoon grated gingerroot
½ cup apple juice	*2 cloves garlic, minced*
⅓ cup packed dark brown sugar	*2 teaspoons mustard seeds*
¼ cup apple cider vinegar	*1 teaspoon pumpkin pie spice*
¼ cup golden raisins	*⅛ teaspoon crushed red pepper flakes*

*P*eel and seed mangoes; dice into ½-inch pieces. Put mangoes and all other ingredients in a nonstick saucepan. Bring to a boil; reduce heat and simmer 30 minutes, stirring every few minutes.

Serve warm or refrigerate. Use within 2 weeks.

12 servings (makes 3 cups)
1 serving= ¼ cup

CAL.	CHO(g)	PRO.(g)	TOTAL FAT(g)	SAT. FAT(g)	CHOL.(mg)	FIBER(g)	SODIUM(mg)
70	17	1	0	0	0	1	5

Food exchange per serving: 1 Fruit
Low-sodium diets: This recipe is excellent.

Raisins Indienne

Keep this raisin chutney in the refrigerator to serve with roast duckling, chicken, lamb, or pork or on top of hot cooked rice (plain or curried). One tablespoon over cottage cheese or roast chicken or pork adds a wonderful flavor contrast.

1 cup seedless raisins	*2 tablespoons chopped prepared*
½ cup finely chopped green bell	*chutney or Mango Chutney*
pepper	*(see preceding recipe)*
½ cup finely chopped celery	*¼ cup slivered blanched almonds*
½ cup finely chopped scallion	*3 tablespoons diced pimiento*
1½ tablespoons margarine	*1½ tablespoons apple cider vinegar*
¼ cup boiling water	*1½ tablespoons brown sugar*

Combine raisins, green pepper, celery, scallion, margarine, and water in a heavy pan. Bring to a boil. Reduce heat to low; cover and simmer gently until crisp-tender. Add all remaining ingredients. Stir over moderate heat to blend and heat together.

Store in the refrigerator up to 1 month.

12 servings (makes 1½ cups)
1 serving = 2 tablespoons

CAL.	CHO(g)	PRO.(g)	TOTAL FAT(g)	SAT. FAT(g)	CHOL.(mg)	FIBER(g)	SODIUM(mg)
85	15	1	3	0.5	0	1	30

Food exchanges per serving: 1 Fruit plus ½ Fat
Low-sodium diets: This recipe is excellent.

Apple Pear Chutney

This recipe makes a good side dish or sauce for chicken, turkey, or pork. It's also tasty over a scoop of cottage cheese or frozen vanilla yogurt.

1 orange
1 large Rome or other tart apple
1 large Anjou pear
1 medium-sized sweet yellow
    onion
½ cup apple cider or juice
¼ cup dried cherries or cranberries

1 tablespoon grated fresh
    gingerroot
1 teaspoon mustard seeds
¼ teaspoon cumin
¼ teaspoon ground allspice
¼ teaspoon ground nutmeg

Grate 1 tablespoon zest from orange. Squeeze juice from orange into a small bowl.

Slice and core, but do not peel, apple and pear. Chop apple, then pear, then onion by hand or in a food processor. (Don't chop them together, or you will puree the fruit.)

Combine all ingredients in a nonstick pot. Bring to a boil. Reduce heat and simmer 8–10 minutes until apple is tender but not mushy.

Chill at least 1 hour to blend flavors.

18 servings (makes 4½ cups)
1 serving = ¼ cup

CAL.	CHO(g)	PRO.(g)	TOTAL FAT(g)	SAT. FAT(g)	CHOL.(mg)	FIBER(g)	SODIUM(mg)
30	7	0	0	0	0	0.5	0

Food exchange per serving: ½ Fruit
Low-sodium diets: This recipe is excellent.

Salsas

Chunky Salsa

1 pound red, ripe tomatoes
½ cup chopped onion
½ cup finely chopped green bell
    pepper
⅓ cup chopped cilantro

3 cloves garlic, minced
1 small or ½ large jalapeño pepper,
    seeded and chopped fine
1½ tablespoons lemon juice
½ teaspoon salt

Cut tomatoes in half; squeeze out seeds and liquid. Chop coarsely with a knife or in a food processor using pulsing motion. Be careful not to puree.

Transfer tomatoes to a large bowl. Add remaining ingredients and mix well.

Use within 1 week.

12 servings (makes 3 cups)
1 serving = ¼ cup

CAL.	CHO(g)	PRO.(g)	TOTAL FAT(g)	SAT. FAT(g)	CHOL.(mg)	FIBER(g)	SODIUM(mg)
15	3	0	0	0	0	0.5	95

Food exchange per serving: a Free Food (Count ½ cup as 1 Vegetable.)
Low-sodium diets: Omit salt.

Pineapple Jalapeño Salsa

Terrific with simply grilled fish, chicken, or roasted pork. This recipe calls for a ripe, juicy pineapple. If the pineapple isn't very sweet, you may want to add more sugar substitute or use a small can of crushed pineapple instead. Taste it after the flavors blend, and add more sweetener if desired.

1 large ripe tomato
6 ounces ripe fresh pineapple, finely chopped
½ cup finely chopped onion
1 tablespoon finely chopped jalapeño pepper

Sugar substitute equivalent to 1 tablespoon sugar
½ teaspoon salt
¼ teaspoon freshly ground black pepper

Cut tomato in half; squeeze out seeds and liquid. Finely chop; combine with all other ingredients.

Chill at least 2 hours for flavors to blend. Serve at room temperature.

8 servings (makes 2 cups)
1 serving = ¼ cup

CAL.	CHO(g)	PRO.(g)	TOTAL FAT(g)	SAT. FAT(g)	CHOL.(mg)	FIBER(g)	SODIUM(mg)
20	5	0	0	0	0	0.5	140

Food exchange per serving: 1 Vegetable (A serving of less than ¼ cup is a Free Food.)
Low-sodium diets: Omit salt.

Cilantro Salsa

This recipe was shared by my colleague Karen Connit, who serves it on fish and chicken and as a dip with tortillas. It's also great with Easy Quesadillas (see Index).

2 large ripe tomatoes, diced
1 small white onion, chopped fine
1 cup minced cilantro
1 large or 2 small jalapeño peppers,
    peeled and diced fine

2 tablespoons fresh lime juice
½ teaspoon salt

Combine all ingredients. Taste and adjust seasonings.

Refrigerate for 2–3 hours for flavors to blend. Bring to room temperature before serving.

8 servings (makes 2 cups)
1 serving = ¼ cup

CAL.	CHO(g)	PRO.(g)	TOTAL FAT(g)	SAT. FAT(g)	CHOL.(mg)	FIBER(g)	SODIUM(mg)
15	4	1	0	0	0	0.5	140

Food exchange per serving: a Free Food (If more than ¼ cup is eaten, count each serving as 1 Vegetable.)
Low-sodium diets: Omit salt.

23
Desserts

Fruit

Grand Marnier Fruit Cup

1 small peach or nectarine, peeled
2 small purple plums
1 small red apple
24 green seedless grapes, cut in half

2 teaspoons fresh lemon juice
Sugar substitute equivalent to 2
  tablespoons sugar
1½ tablespoons Grand Marnier

Cut fruit into small bite-sized pieces, removing stones from peach and plums and core from apple. Mix all fruits well with remaining ingredients.

Spoon into a jar; cover and chill for at least one hour to blend flavors.

4 servings (makes 2 cups)
1 serving = ½ cup

CAL.	CHO(g)	PRO.(g)	TOTAL FAT(g)	SAT. FAT(g)	CHOL.(mg)	FIBER(g)	SODIUM(mg)
80	18	1	0	0	0	2	0

Food exchange per serving: 1 Fruit
Low-sodium diets: This recipe is excellent.

453

Citrus Ambrosia

1 cup fresh orange sections   Sugar substitute equivalent to 2
1 cup fresh grapefruit sections   teaspoons sugar
2 medium red apples   ⅓ cup sliced banana
2 tablespoons dry sherry (optional) 2 tablespoons shredded coconut
1 teaspoon fresh lemon juice   3 maraschino cherries, drained

Cut orange sections in half, grapefruit sections into quarters, and apples into small bite-sized cubes. Core but do not pare apples. Mix these fruits with sherry, lemon juice, and sugar substitute.

Cover and chill 1 hour or longer. Just before serving, add banana; mix well. Spoon into six individual desert dishes. Scatter coconut on top of fruits. Slice maraschino cherries; place a few slices on top of coconut.

6 servings (makes 3 cups)
1 serving = ½ cup

CAL.	CHO(g)	PRO.(g)	TOTAL FAT(g)	SAT. FAT(g)	CHOL.(mg)	FIBER(g)	SODIUM(mg)
750	17	1	1	0.5	0	2	5

Food exchange per serving: 1 Fruit
Low-sodium diets: This recipe is excellent.

Pears Poached in Red Wine

You can use any pears in this recipe, but I like the shape of Bosc pears. Half of the sauce is used with the pears. Save the other half (4 tablespoons) to use over other fruit, pudding, or frozen yogurt.

¾ cup freshly squeezed orange juice
¾ cup red wine
1 cinnamon stick
4 (about 1¼ pounds total) firm but ripe pears

Sugar substitute equivalent to
2 tablespoons sugar

*P*ut orange juice, wine, and cinnamon stick in a medium-sized pot. Bring to a boil.

Peel pears, leaving stems on. Remove core from bottom of pear with a melon baller, and slice off thin layer of bottom so pears will stand up straight when served. (They will weigh about 1 pound total when cored and trimmed.)

Put pears in boiling liquid; cover and gently simmer for 20 minutes, turning every 5 minutes. Gently remove pears to a refrigerator container.

Remove sauce from heat; let cool 5 minutes. Discard cinnamon stick, add sweetener, and stir to mix. Pour sauce over pears and chill. Turn pears occasionally.

Serve pears standing up, each drizzled with 1 tablespoon sauce.

4 servings
1 serving = 1 pear plus 1 tablespoon sauce

CAL.	CHO*(g)*	PRO.*(g)*	TOTAL FAT*(g)*	SAT. FAT*(g)*	CHOL.*(mg)*	FIBER*(g)*	SODIUM*(mg)*
105	23	1	1	0	0	3.5	0

Food exchanges per serving: 1½ Fruits
Low-sodium diets: This recipe is excellent.

Peter's Favorite Strawberries

My husband, Peter, particularly likes this simple but elegant dessert. I serve it in champagne or brandy glasses. Never have vitamins and fiber looked and tasted so good!

1 pint ripe, very red strawberries   *2 tablespoons sweet vermouth*
1 medium orange   *Sugar substitute equivalent to 1*
2 tablespoons orange juice   *   tablespoon sugar (optional)*

Wash and hull strawberries; cut each in half. Slice ends off orange; quarter orange lengthwise and slice orange wedges crosswise with rinds left on, as thin as possible. Put strawberries and oranges in a bowl; mix well.

Mix together orange juice and sweet vermouth; drizzle over fruit mixture, and stir to mix. Check to see if berries have enough natural sweetness for your taste; if not, add sweetener.

Cover bowl and refrigerate 2 hours before serving. Stir gently several times to blend flavors.

3 servings (makes 3 cups)
1 serving = 1 cup

CAL.	CHO(g)	PRO.(g)	TOTAL FAT(g)	SAT. FAT(g)	CHOL.(mg)	FIBER(g)	SODIUM(mg)
70	17	1	0.5	0	0	3	0

Food exchange per serving: 1 Fruit
Low-sodium diets: This recipe is excellent.

Grapes with Orange Zest

This recipe is my favorite fruit standby because an orange and some grapes are usually in my refrigerator. It makes a pretty and simple dessert when served in small glass dishes and is equally nice as a fruit with breakfast or on a buffet.

1 navel orange
½ pound seedless red grapes
½ pound seedless green grapes

1 tablespoon chopped fresh mint
leaves (optional)

Remove 2 teaspoons zest from orange, using a zester or fine grater. Squeeze juice from orange into a 1-quart refrigerator container. Stir in zest.

Wash grapes and remove stems. If grapes are large, cut them in half. Put grapes into container with orange juice. Cover and shake to marinate grapes. Add mint if desired.

If time permits, refrigerate at least 1 hour for flavors to blend.

4 servings (makes 4 cups)
1 serving = 1 cup

CAL.	CHO(g)	PRO.(g)	TOTAL FAT(g)	SAT. FAT(g)	CHOL.(mg)	FIBER(g)	SODIUM(mg)
90	22	1	1	0	0	2	0

Food exchanges per serving: 1½ Fruits
Low-sodium diets: An excellent choice.

Granny Smith Applesauce

So many people love this recipe! Be sure to try it.

2 pounds firm Granny Smith apples	¼ teaspoon ground cinnamon
2 tablespoons fresh lemon juice	Sugar substitute equivalent to 3 tablespoons sugar
1 cup water	

*P*are apples. Remove cores, and cut apples into bite-sized pieces.

Put apples in a large heavy pot. Add lemon juice and water; mix well. Bring to a boil; cover and simmer gently until apples are very soft and tender.

Remove from heat. Add cinnamon and sweetener; mix thoroughly with a wooden spoon (a metal spoon may darken the sauce). Taste and add more sweetener if desired. Serve warm or chilled.

6 servings (makes 3 cups)
1 serving = ½ cup

CAL.	CHO(g)	PRO.(g)	TOTAL FAT(g)	SAT. FAT(g)	CHOL.(mg)	FIBER(g)	SODIUM(mg)
80	19	1	0	0	0	2.5	0

Food exchange per serving: 1 Fruit
Low-sodium diets: This recipe is excellent.

Honey Baked Grapefruit

1 large (12–14 ounces) white
    grapefruit
1 large (12–14 ounces) ruby red
    grapefruit
1½ tablespoons honey

2 teaspoons finely grated orange
    zest
2 teaspoons finely chopped walnuts
    or pecans

*P*reheat oven to 350°F. Peel and section grapefruits, removing all white pith and seeds. There should be about 2 cups white and red segments.

Mix segments in a small ovenproof casserole. Drizzle honey over top; sprinkle with orange zest and nuts. Bake about 10–12 minutes until grapefruit is hot.

4 servings (makes 2 cups)
1 serving = ½ cup

CAL.	CHO(g)	PRO.(g)	TOTAL FAT(g)	SAT. FAT(g)	CHOL.(mg)	FIBER(g)	SODIUM(mg)
60	15	1	1	0	0	0.5	0

Food exchange per serving: 1 Fruit
Low-sodium diets: This recipe is excellent.

Stewed Fruit Compote

Serve this old-fashioned stewed fruit in small individual dessert bowls, or serve a half portion over a slice of angel food cake or sponge cake dessert shells.

¾ cup prunes   1 cinnamon stick
¾ cup dried apricots   2½ cups water
½ cup raisins or dried cranberries
1 tablespoon + 1 teaspoon slivered
    orange zest

Put all ingredients into a medium saucepan. Bring to a boil; cover, reduce heat, and simmer about 20–25 minutes until fruits are tender.

    Remove cinnamon stick. Serve warm or chilled.

7 servings (makes 3½ cups)
1 serving = ½ cup

CAL.	CHO(g)	PRO.(g)	TOTAL FAT(g)	SAT. FAT(g)	CHOL.(mg)	FIBER(g)	SODIUM(mg)
105	28	1	0	0	0	3	5

Food exchanges per serving: 2 Fruits
Low-sodium diets: This recipe is excellent.

Stewed Rhubarb

Frozen unsweetened rhubarb is sold in 1-pound packages. The amount of fresh rhubarb to pick or buy, in order to end up with the same quantity—4 cups uncooked—depends upon how much top and bottom is left on before cleaning and cutting. Be sure all leaves are removed, because they are poisonous.

1 pound (4 cups) diced fresh or frozen rhubarb	*Sugar substitute equivalent to 6 tablespoons sugar*
¼ cup water	

*P*lace diced rhubarb and water in a deep saucepan. Cover and bring to a boil. Reduce heat; simmer gently until rhubarb is very tender, about 10–15 minutes, stirring occasionally.

Remove from heat, add sweetener, and mix well. The amount of artificial sweetener required depends largely upon the acidity or "sour" taste of the rhubarb you use. Taste and adjust amount of sweetener accordingly.

Serve warm or chilled.

4 servings (makes 2 cups)
1 serving = ½ cup

CAL.	CHO*(g)*	PRO.*(g)*	TOTAL FAT*(g)*	SAT. FAT*(g)*	CHOL.*(mg)*	FIBER*(g)*	SODIUM*(mg)*
35	6	2	0	0	0	2	5

Food exchange per serving: ½ Fruit
Low-sodium diets: This recipe is excellent.

Broiled Bananas

This recipe, adapted from one developed by Barbara Stone, was developed for my earlier book, *A Healthy Head Start: A Worry-Free Guide to Feeding Young Children*. It's easy and fun, and adults like it, too.

> 2 small ripe bananas, unpeeled
> 2 tablespoons vanilla low-fat
>   yogurt

Preheat broiler.

Make three small crosswise slits in the banana skin. Place banana, in peel, slit side up on a piece of aluminum foil or small broiler pan.

Broil 5–10 minutes or until banana is browned and softened. Slit skin lengthwise to expose banana and create a banana boat. Serve topped with a dollop of yogurt.

2 servings
1 serving = 1 banana

CAL.	CHO(g)	PRO.(g)	TOTAL FAT(g)	SAT. FAT(g)	CHOL.(mg)	FIBER(g)	SODIUM(mg)
95	23	2	1	0	0	1.5	10

Food exchanges per serving: 1½ Fruits
Low-sodium diets: This recipe is excellent.

Strawberry Shortcake

You can lighten this by using light whipped topping, but the Vanilla Crème Fraîche is truly delicious and well worth the extra fat exchange.

3 cups fresh ripe strawberries,
  hulled and sliced
Sugar substitute equal to
  1 tablespoon sugar (optional)
6 Baking Powder Biscuits
  (see Index) or small biscuits
  prepared from refrigerated
  dough

¾ cup Vanilla Crème Fraîche
  (recipe follows)

*P*ut strawberries in a bowl; taste and add sweetener if desired. Split each biscuit, and arrange two halves on each plate.

Spread ½ cup sliced strawberries over each half. Top each serving with 2 tablespoons Vanilla Crème Fraîche.

6 servings
1 serving = 1 strawberry shortcake

CAL.	CHO(g)	PRO.(g)	TOTAL FAT(g)	SAT. FAT(g)	CHOL.(mg)	FIBER(g)	SODIUM(mg)
185	23	4	9	3	15	2.5	330

Food exchanges per serving: 1 Starch plus ½ Fruit plus 2 Fats
Low-sodium diets: Modify biscuit recipe as directed.

Vanilla Crème Fraîche

Use this topping on berries, other fruits, and desserts.

¼ cup whipping cream   1 teaspoon pure vanilla extract
¼ cup plain low-fat yogurt

In a small chilled bowl, whip cream until almost stiff. Gently fold in yogurt and vanilla

Chill in a covered container at least 2 hours to allow flavors to blend. Store in refrigerator no longer than 2 days.

6 servings (makes ¾ cups)
1 serving = 2 tablespoons

CAL.	CHO(g)	PRO.(g)	TOTAL FAT(g)	SAT. FAT(g)	CHOL.(mg)	FIBER(g)	SODIUM(mg)
45	1	1	4	2.5	15	0	10

Food exchange per serving: 1 Fat
Low-sodium diets: This recipe is excellent.

Fresh Vanilla Custard Sauce

Enjoy this sauce over fresh berries or poached fruit. In strawberry season, arrange ripe strawberries around a bowl of this sauce—a feast!

¾ cup skim milk
½ vanilla bean, split lengthwise
⅓ cup part-skim ricotta cheese
1 egg
2 tablespoons sugar

1 teaspoon cornstarch
½ teaspoon pure vanilla extract
Sugar substitute equivalent to 2
    tablespoons sugar

*P*our milk into a small nonstick saucepan. Scrape seeds from vanilla bean; add seeds and pod to milk. Heat milk over low heat just until it is scalded and bubbles form around edge of pan. Remove from heat and cool 10 minutes, allowing vanilla to flavor milk.

In a food processor or blender, combine ricotta cheese, egg, sugar, and cornstarch. Process about 30 seconds until smooth. Remove beans from milk, leaving seeds; add to cheese mixture. Process again for a few seconds to combine.

Wash the small saucepan to remove any milk residue. Pour mixture back into saucepan; cook over very low heat, stirring constantly until mixture is the consistency of heavy cream. Do not overheat, or mixture will curdle.

While hot, pour through a fine strainer into a 1-pint refrigerator container. Stir in vanilla extract and sweetener. Cover and chill before serving.

8 servings (makes 1 cup)
1 serving = 2 tablespoons

CAL.	CHO*(g)*	PRO.*(g)*	TOTAL FAT*(g)*	SAT. FAT*(g)*	CHOL.*(mg)*	FIBER*(g)*	SODIUM*(mg)*
50	5	3	1	0.5	30	0	35

Food exchange per serving: ½ Skim Milk
Low-sodium diets: This recipe is excellent.

Sorbets and Ices

Mango Sorbet

The same technique can be used with peaches, berries, or other soft fruits. Use amounts equal to 1¼ cups pureed fruit.

2 large (about 1½ pounds total) mangoes
¼ cup fresh orange juice

Sugar substitute equivalent to 1 tablespoon sugar

Peel and slice mangoes; puree in a food processor fitted with a steel blade. Add orange juice and sweetener; mix well.

Pour into a shallow pan; freeze mixture until solid. Remove sorbet from freezer; break into pieces with a fork. Return to food processor and process 10 seconds until smooth and frosty. Serve immediately.

3 servings (makes 1½ cups)
1 serving = ½ cup

CAL.	CHO(g)	PRO.(g)	TOTAL FAT(g)	SAT. FAT(g)	CHOL.(mg)	FIBER(g)	SODIUM(mg)
125	32	1	0	0	0	2	5

Food exchanges per serving: 2 Fruits
Low-sodium diets: This recipe is excellent.

Blackberry Sherbet

This fruit ice is refreshing and handy to have in the freezer if guests drop by. Use individually quick-frozen blackberries, or if berries are in season, freeze them before beginning the recipe.

*1½ cups (8 ounces total) frozen
    blackberries*
*⅓ cup apple juice concentrate,
    thawed*
*6 ounces cherry-vanilla custard-
    style nonfat yogurt, sweetened
    with aspartame (or other
    fruit-flavored nonfat light
    yogurt)*

*Sugar substitute equivalent to 1
    tablespoon sugar*

*R*eserve 6 blackberries. In bowl of a food processor, combine remaining blackberries and apple juice concentrate; process 30–45 seconds. Add yogurt and sweetener; process 15 seconds. The mixture should be the consistency of soft-serve frozen yogurt. Taste and add more sweetener if desired.

Put paper liners in a six-cup muffin pan. Divide blackberry ice to fill cups. Top each cup with a reserved blackberry. Cover lightly with plastic film or foil; freeze at least 1 hour.

Allow sherbet to thaw about 10 minutes before serving.

6 servings
1 serving = 1 individual cup

CAL.	CHO*(g)*	PRO.*(g)*	TOTAL FAT*(g)*	SAT. FAT*(g)*	CHOL.*(mg)*	FIBER*(g)*	SODIUM*(mg)*
60	14	2	0	0	0	1.5	20

Food exchange per serving: 1 Fruit
Low-sodium diets: An excellent choice.

Custards, Puddings, and Mousses

Crème Caramel

½ cup sugar, divided
1 tablespoon hot water, divided
1¾ cups low-fat (2% milk fat)
    milk or whole milk

½ cup egg substitute or 2 eggs
¾ teaspoon pure vanilla extract
Dash ground cinnamon
Dash salt

Preheat oven to 350°F. Heat ¼ cup of the sugar in a small heavy saucepan over low heat, stirring constantly until it is a straw-colored syrup. Add water and continue stirring about 5 minutes until melted sugar is a dark caramel color. Divide sugar mixture among six custard cups or ½-cup soufflé dishes.

In a medium bowl, gently stir remaining ¼ cup sugar with milk, eggs, vanilla, cinnamon, and salt. Don't whip mixture, or you will create bubbles and ruin the smooth texture of the custard. Divide mixture among the six cups.

Place cups in a roasting pan. Pour hot water into the roasting pan to surround cups. Water should be about 1 inch deep, with tops of cups at least ½ inch over the water level so water doesn't flow into cups as it simmers. Gently set pan in oven; bake 1 hour until custard is set.

Remove cups from water; cool on a wire rack. Refrigerate at least 3 hours.

Before serving, run edge of sharp knife around each custard. Put individual serving plate on top of each cup, and invert custard onto plate.

6 servings
1 serving = 1 individual crème caramel

CAL.	CHO(g)	PRO.(g)	TOTAL FAT(g)	SAT. FAT(g)	CHOL.(mg)	FIBER(g)	SODIUM(mg)
110	21	4	1	0.5	5	0	90

Food exchanges per serving: 1 Other Carbohydrate plus ½ Skim Milk
Low-sodium diets: This recipe is acceptable.

Baked Custard

If you want to unmold this custard, leave cups in the refrigerator 2–3 extra hours.

1½ cups skim milk　　　　　*1 teaspoon pure vanilla extract*
2 large eggs, beaten slightly　*⅛ teaspoon ground nutmeg*
2 tablespoons sugar　　　　　*(optional)*
⅛ teaspoon salt

Preheat oven to 325°F. Heat milk in the top of a double boiler over simmering water until the surface of the milk begins to wrinkle.

In a medium bowl, blend together eggs, sugar, salt, and vanilla. Add hot milk gradually, stirring to mix well. Pour into 4 6-ounce individual custard cups. Sprinkle lightly with nutmeg.

Set cups in a deep baking pan; pour hot water around custard cups to come to within ½ inch of tops. Bake 50–60 minutes or until a knife tip inserted in center of custard comes out clean.

Remove from heat and water pan. Refrigerate custard to chill before serving.

4 servings (makes 2 cups)
1 serving = ½ cup

CAL.	CHO*(g)*	PRO.*(g)*	TOTAL FAT*(g)*	SAT. FAT*(g)*	CHOL.*(mg)*	FIBER*(g)*	SODIUM*(mg)*
95	11	6	3	1	110	0	150

Food exchange per serving: 1 Skim Milk
Low-sodium diets: Omit salt.

Strawberry Trifle

I use custard mix because it is a shortcut. The mix itself has no cholesterol but needs the single egg yolk for a truer custard taste and texture. It is beautiful in a pretty crystal bowl, and because it is made ahead, it's great for entertaining.

1 2.9-ounce package custard dessert mix
2 cups skim milk
1 egg yolk, well beaten
½ teaspoon pure orange extract or 2 tablespoons Grand Marnier

1 pint ripe, fresh strawberries
Sugar substitute equivalent to 1 tablespoon sugar
1 cup nondairy light whipped topping, thawed, divided
24 vanilla wafers

Stir custard mix into 2 cups skim milk in a small heavy saucepan. Add beaten egg yolk. Stirring constantly, cook over medium heat just until mixture comes to a boil. The mixture will be thin.

Remove from heat. Stir in orange extract or Grand Marnier. Pour custard into a bowl; refrigerate uncovered for 20 minutes or until it is cool but only softly set.

While custard is cooling, slice strawberries, reserving 6 with hulls for garnish. Mix sliced strawberries with the sweetener.

Gently fold ½ cup whipped topping into the custard with a rubber spatula.

Arrange 16 vanilla wafers, round side toward glass, on bottom and around sides of a medium-sized glass dessert bowl. Spread half of the strawberries over the cookies. Gently spoon on half of the custard. Arrange the remaining 8 cookies in a layer on top of custard; add layers of sliced strawberries with liquid and custard. Cover trifle with plastic wrap; chill at least 2 hours.

At serving time, top trifle with remaining ½ cup whipped topping. Garnish with reserved strawberries.

6 servings (makes 4½ cups)
1 serving = ¾ cup

CAL.	CHO(g)	PRO.(g)	TOTAL FAT(g)	SAT. FAT(g)	CHOL.(mg)	FIBER(g)	SODIUM(mg)
190	32	5	4	2	35	1.5	170

Food exchanges per serving: 1 Fruit plus ½ Low-Fat Milk plus ½ Starch *or* 1 Fruit plus 1 Starch
Low-sodium diets: This recipe is acceptable.

Cranberry Tapioca Pudding

2 tablespoons quick-cooking tapioca
1½ cups water
2 cups fresh cranberries

½ teaspoon pure orange extract
Sugar substitute equivalent to ½
    cup sugar

Combine tapioca and water in a medium saucepan; let stand 5 minutes. Bring to a boil and simmer 3 minutes, stirring frequently. Add cranberries and cook until all berries have popped.

Remove from heat; cool 5–10 minutes. Add orange extract and sweetener; mix well. Chill thoroughly.

4 servings (makes 2 cups)
1 serving = ½ cup

CAL.	CHO(g)	PRO.(g)	TOTAL FAT(g)	SAT. FAT(g)	CHOL.(mg)	FIBER(g)	SODIUM(mg)
60	13	2	0	0	0	2	25

Food exchange per serving: 1 Fruit *or* 1 Starch
Low-sodium diets: This recipe is excellent.

Rice Pudding

This is a favorite way of using leftover steamed rice after Chinese meals. Most people think of rice pudding as a dessert or snack, but it's also great for breakfast.

2 cups skim milk	¼–½ teaspoon ground cinnamon
2 eggs, beaten	1 teaspoon pure vanilla extract
2 tablespoons sugar	1 cup cold cooked rice
¼ teaspoon salt	2 tablespoons golden seedless raisins

Preheat oven to 350°F. Prepare a 1-quart casserole with nonstick cooking spray. Scald (heat) milk in the top of a double boiler over simmering water.

In a medium bowl, combine eggs, sugar, salt, cinnamon, and vanilla. Pour hot milk on top slowly, stirring to mix well.

Spread rice in the bottom of the casserole. Scatter raisins evenly over rice; pour milk mixture carefully on top. Place casserole in a pan of hot water with the hot water ½ inch from the top of the casserole. Bake about 45 minutes or until a knife tip inserted in center of the casserole comes out clean.

This pudding may be served warm or chilled, as you prefer.

6 servings (makes 3 cups)
1 serving = ½ cup

CAL.	CHO(g)	PRO.(g)	TOTAL FAT(g)	SAT. FAT(g)	CHOL.(mg)	FIBER(g)	SODIUM(mg)
115	18	6	2	0.5	70	0	155

Food exchanges per serving: 1 Starch plus ½ Skim Milk
Low-sodium diets: Omit salt.

Bread Pudding

Try serving this old-fashioned favorite topped with Berry Coulis or Strawberry Sauce (the following two recipes).

3 slices bread	*2 tablespoons sugar*
2 teaspoons margarine, softened	*1 teaspoon pure vanilla extract*
2 tablespoons seedless raisins	*¼ teaspoon ground cinnamon*
2 cups skim milk	*¼ teaspoon salt*
2 large eggs	

*P*reheat oven to 350°F. Prepare a 1½-quart casserole with butter-flavored cooking spray. Spread bread with margarine; cut each slice into small cubes. Place bread cubes in bottom of prepared casserole. Scatter raisins evenly over the top.

Scald (heat) milk in the top of a double boiler over simmering water. Remove from heat.

In a large bowl, beat eggs until light. Beat in remaining ingredients. Pour hot milk on top, stirring to blend well. Pour carefully on top of bread cubes. Place casserole in a pan of hot water (enough to come up to half the depth of the casserole).

Bake 50 minutes or until knife inserted halfway between center and outside edge comes out clean. Remove dish from water. Chill pudding in refrigerator at least 3 hours, or serve warm.

4 servings (makes 3 cups)
1 serving = ¾ cup

CAL.	CHO(g)	PRO.(g)	TOTAL FAT(g)	SAT. FAT(g)	CHOL.(mg)	FIBER(g)	SODIUM(mg)
195	26	9	6	1.5	110	0.5	355

Food exchanges per serving: 1 Starch plus 1 Low-Fat Milk
Low-sodium diets: Omit salt.

Berry Coulis

Put this colorful coulis in a plastic squeeze bottle and use as "paint" to decorate or drizzle over desserts. Individually quick-frozen blackberries, blueberries, and raspberries are often better quality and less expensive than fresh berries.

1½ cups frozen blackberries, blueberries, or raspberries, thawed, or fresh berries

1 tablespoon Crème de Cassis, Liqueur de Framboise, or other fruit liqueur
Sugar substitute to taste

*P*uree berries in a food processor. Place a fine strainer over bowl, and pour berry puree into strainer. With a spoon, press mixture through strainer to remove seeds.

Add fruit liqueur; stir to mix. Taste and add sugar substitute if desired.

12 servings (makes ¾ cup)
1 serving = 1 tablespoon

CAL.	CHO(g)	PRO.(g)	TOTAL FAT(g)	SAT. FAT(g)	CHOL.(mg)	FIBER(g)	SODIUM(mg)
15	3	0	0	0	0	0	0

Food exchange per serving: a Free Food (If ¼ cup is used, count as ½ Fruit.)
Low-sodium diets: An excellent choice.

Strawberry Sauce

Try this versatile sauce over one of our puddings, frozen yogurt, ladyfingers, or angel food cake.

> 1½ cups whole fresh strawberries
> Sugar substitute equivalent to 1
>   tablespoon sugar

*W*ash berries; remove hulls and soft spots. Cut berries into bite-sized pieces. Place in a bowl, crushing berries slightly with a fork. Add sweetener, if desired, by mixing it thoroughly with 1 tablespoon water and adding to berries. Mix well.

   Chill until ready to serve.

4 servings (makes 1⅓ cups)
1 serving = ⅓ cup

CAL.	CHO(g)	PRO.(g)	TOTAL FAT(g)	SAT. FAT(g)	CHOL.(mg)	FIBER(g)	SODIUM(mg)
15	4	0	0	0	0	1.5	0

Food exchange per serving: a Free Food (If ⅔ cup is used, count as ½ Fruit.)
Low-sodium diets: This recipe is excellent.

Tapioca Nectar Fluff

¼ cup quick-cooking tapioca

6 ounces apricot nectar

6 ounces unsweetened pineapple
    juice

1 tablespoon fresh lemon juice

¾ cup water

1 egg, separated

Sugar substitute equivalent to ½
    cup sugar

½ teaspoon pure vanilla extract

¼ teaspoon pure orange extract

1 additional egg white

3 maraschino cherries, sliced thin
    (optional)

Mix tapioca, apricot nectar, pineapple juice, lemon juice, water, and beaten egg yolk in a heavy pan; let stand 5 minutes. Bring to a full boil over medium heat; cook and stir constantly 6–8 minutes. Remove from heat.

Add sweetener and flavorings; mix well. Beat egg whites to soft peaks. Gradually add tapioca mixture, stirring quickly only until blended.

Serve warm or chilled. Garnish with sliced maraschino cherries if desired.

5 servings (makes 2½ cups)
1 serving = ½ cup

CAL.	CHO(g)	PRO.(g)	TOTAL FAT(g)	SAT. FAT(g)	CHOL.(mg)	FIBER(g)	SODIUM(mg)
100	20	3	1	0.5	45	0	60

Food exchanges per serving: 1 Fruit plus ½ Starch or 1 Starch plus ½ Fruit
Low-sodium diets: This recipe is suitable.

Frozen Nectarine Banana Mousse

Truly yummy. You can substitute ripe peaches or mangoes for the nectarine, but be sure all fruit used is very ripe and sweet.

2 large ripe nectarines
1 ripe banana
¼ cup part-skim ricotta cheese

⅓ cup skim milk
1 teaspoon pure vanilla extract

Peel nectarines and banana; cut each into 6 pieces. Place fruit in a heavy plastic bag; seal tightly. Freeze at least 6 hours or until solidly frozen.

Break pieces apart; put them into the bowl of a food processor with a steel blade. Add remaining ingredients. Process, occasionally scraping frozen parts into softened mixture with a spatula, until mousse is smooth and creamy. Serve immediately.

4 servings (makes 2 cups)
1 serving = ½ cup

CAL.	CHO(g)	PRO.(g)	TOTAL FAT(g)	SAT. FAT(g)	CHOL.(mg)	FIBER(g)	SODIUM(mg)
100	19	4	2	1	5	2	30

Food exchanges per serving: 1 Fruit plus ½ Skim Milk
Low-sodium diets: This recipe is excellent.

Raspberry Mousse

2½ cups frozen raspberries, divided   1 teaspoon pure vanilla extract
⅔ cup part-skim ricotta cheese   1 teaspoon grated orange zest
⅓ cup fresh orange juice

Reserve 2 tablespoons berries for garnish. Put remaining frozen raspberries in the bowl of a food processor fitted with a steel blade. Process 1 minute.

Add ricotta, orange juice, and vanilla. Continue processing, scraping sides often, until bits of berries are incorporated. Add orange zest; process until smooth and well blended—the consistency of soft frozen yogurt. Serve immediately.

6 servings (makes 3 cups)
1 serving = ½ cup

CAL.	CHO(g)	PRO.(g)	TOTAL FAT(g)	SAT. FAT(g)	CHOL.(mg)	FIBER(g)	SODIUM(mg)
90	12	5	3	1.5	10	2	40

Food exchanges per serving: ½ Fruit plus ½ Low-Fat Milk
Low-sodium diets: This recipe is excellent.

Pumpkin Soufflé with Praline Crumbs

Soufflé

2 egg whites
1 cup solid-pack canned pumpkin
¾ cup evaporated skim milk
⅓ cup packed dark brown sugar
½ cup egg substitute or *2 whole eggs*
1 teaspoon pumpkin pie spice
1 teaspoon pure vanilla extract

Praline Crumbs

1 tablespoon granulated sugar
2 tablespoons (1 ounce) broken pecans

Preheat oven to 350°F. Prepare a 6- to 8-cup soufflé dish with butter-flavored cooking spray.

In bowl of a mixer, whip egg whites to soft peaks. Transfer beaten whites to another bowl. In mixer bowl, combine pumpkin, milk, brown sugar, egg substitute, pumpkin pie spice, and vanilla. Whip until well blended. Gently fold in beaten egg whites with a rubber spatula.

Pour mixture into soufflé dish. Bake 1 hour on center rack of oven or until soufflé is set and puffed.

While soufflé is cooking, melt granulated sugar over low heat in a small nonstick skillet. (Be careful, as sugar will burn easily.) Add pecans; stir quickly about 15 seconds until nuts are coated. Turn candied pecans onto waxed paper to cool.

Fold waxed paper around and over cooled pecans. Using a heavy glass or the side of a meat mallet, crush pecans to coarse crumbs, or chop them in a food processor. This step will yield 3 tablespoons praline crumbs.

When soufflé is ready, serve immediately. Sprinkle praline crumbs over each serving.

6 servings
1 serving = 1 ¾- to 1-cup soufflé plus 1½ teaspoons praline crumbs

CAL.	CHO(g)	PRO.(g)	TOTAL FAT(g)	SAT. FAT(g)	CHOL.(mg)	FIBER(g)	SODIUM(mg)
145	23	6	4	0.5	1.5	1	95

Food exchanges per serving: 1 Other Carbohydrate plus ½ Whole Milk
Low-sodium diets: This recipe is acceptable.

Classic Strawberry-Banana Gelatin

If molding gelatin or adding fruit, create a firmer gel by using 1¾ cups of water instead of the 2 cups as directed on the package. Almost any cut fruit, except pineapple, can be added to fruit gelatin.

1 3-ounce package sugar-free strawberry-banana gelatin dessert mix	¾ cup cold water
	¾ cup sliced strawberries
	½ small banana, thinly sliced
1 cup boiling water	

*E*mpty gelatin mixture into a medium bowl. Add boiling water, stirring until gelatin is completely dissolved. Add ¾ cup ice water. Refrigerate at least 1 hour or until liquid is consistency of raw egg whites.

Fold strawberries and banana into gelatin. Chill mixture in bowl or a small mold until firm.

5 servings (makes 2½ cups)
1 serving = ½ cup

CAL.	CHO(g)	PRO.(g)	TOTAL FAT(g)	SAT. FAT(g)	CHOL.(mg)	FIBER(g)	SODIUM(mg)
22	4	1	0	0	0	0.5	35

Food exchange per serving: a Free Food (If 1 cup is used, count as ½ Fruit.)
Low-sodium diets: This recipe is excellent.

Pies and Cobblers

Graham Cracker Pie Shell

Packaged graham cracker crumbs are higher in carbohydrate than plain graham crackers. Fill this crust with your favorite flavor of sugar-free fat-free pudding. Or use the crumb mixture as a crust for a fruit tart.

8 2½″ × 5″ plain graham crackers   3 tablespoons margarine, melted

Break graham crackers into small pieces. Place in a plastic bag; close opening, and press with a rolling pin or a large jar to make crumbs. Continue until all crumbs are fine (total of 1¼ cups). Empty into bowl.

Melt margarine; add to crumbs, and mix well with a fork. Set aside 2 tablespoons to use later as a garnish on the pie.

Prepare a 9-inch pie plate with butter-flavored nonstick cooking spray. Using the back of a spoon, press crumb mixture evenly on bottom and sides of pie plate.

Chill in refrigerator 3 hours or longer before filling.

8 servings (makes a 9-inch pie shell)
1 serving = ⅛ pie shell

CAL.	CHO(g)	PRO.(g)	TOTAL FAT(g)	SAT. FAT(g)	CHOL.(mg)	FIBER(g)	SODIUM(mg)
95	11	1	6	1	0	0.5	135

Food exchanges per serving: 1 Starch plus 1 Fat
Low-sodium diets: Use unsalted margarine.

Vanilla Wafer Crumb Crust

2 teaspoons margarine, melted,   ¼ teaspoon pure vanilla extract
    divided
30 1¾-inch-diameter vanilla
    wafers

Prepare a 9-inch pie plate by rubbing inside, bottom, and sides with 1 teaspoon of the margarine. Place vanilla wafers in a plastic bag; seal tightly. Crush with a rolling pin or large jar to make very fine crumbs (1¼ cups).

Transfer crumbs to a large bowl. Combine vanilla and remaining 1 teaspoon melted margarine; drizzle all over crumbs. Mix thoroughly with a fork to make sure all is well blended. Remove about 2 tablespoons of crumb mixture and set aside to use if desired as a garnish on top of pie.

With back of a large spoon, press remaining crumbs evenly all over bottom and sides of prepared pie pan. Chill in refrigerator 2 hours or longer before filling.

8 servings (makes a 9-inch pie shell)
1 serving = ⅛ pie shell

CAL.	CHO(g)	PRO.(g)	TOTAL FAT(g)	SAT. FAT(g)	CHOL.(mg)	FIBER(g)	SODIUM(mg)
75	8	1	5	1	0	0	70

Food exchanges per serving: ½ Starch plus 1 Fat
Low-sodium diets: Use unsalted margarine.

Jo's Cranberry Pie

This is a special pie that is unique and quite low in calories. Josephine Anderson's original recipe is a Thanksgiving favorite at my home and is not for people with diabetes. This modified version is sure to please.

1 Vanilla Wafer Crumb Crust (see preceding recipe)
1 tablespoon granulated gelatin
2 cups cold water, divided
3 cups fresh or frozen raw cranberries

½ teaspoon grated orange zest
½ teaspoon pure orange extract
Sugar substitute equivalent to 12 tablespoons (¾ cup)
1½ cups frozen light whipped topping, thawed

Make crumb crust according to recipe. Chill in refrigerator at least 2 hours before filling.

Soak gelatin in ½ cup of the cold water; set aside. Pick over fresh or frozen cranberries; wash and measure. Put in a deep, heavy saucepan with 1½ cups water and orange zest. Cook over moderate heat until all cranberries pop, stirring occasionally. Remove from heat.

Stir in gelatin, orange extract, and sweetener; mix until gelatin is dissolved. Let cool about 30 minutes, stirring occasionally. Taste to see if enough sweetener has been added, because cranberries vary greatly in tartness. Spoon carefully and slowly into pie crust; smooth evenly with the back of a spoon.

Chill in refrigerator. When cool, spread whipped topping on pie, smoothing and swirling evenly. Chill in refrigerator 3–4 hours before serving.

8 servings (makes a 9-inch pie)
1 serving = ⅛ pie

CAL.	CHO(g)	PRO.(g)	TOTAL FAT(g)	SAT. FAT(g)	CHOL.(mg)	FIBER(g)	SODIUM(mg)
140	18	3	6	2.5	0	1.5	70

Food exchanges per serving: 1 Starch plus 1 Fat
Low-sodium diets: This recipe is excellent.

Banana Cream Pie

1 Vanilla Wafer Crumb Crust (see
    Index)
1 0.9-ounce package sugar-free
    banana cream pudding and
    pie filling mix

2 cups skim milk
1 pound ripe bananas
1½ cups nondairy light whipped
    topping, thawed

Prepare pie crust; chill 2 hours or longer before filling.
Prepare pudding with skim milk according to package directions. Refrigerate 5 minutes.

Peel bananas and slice thin. Arrange 1 cup of sliced bananas in bottom of pie shell; very carefully spoon or pour filling evenly over bananas. Gently spread whipped topping to cover the pudding. Arrange remaining sliced bananas on top.

Cover whole pie carefully with plastic wrap. Chill 2–3 hours, until set and firm. To serve, cut into 8 equal wedges.

8 servings (makes a 9-inch pie)
1 serving = ⅛ pie

CAL.	CHO(g)	PRO.(g)	TOTAL FAT(g)	SAT. FAT(g)	CHOL.(mg)	FIBER(g)	SODIUM(mg)
170	25	3	6	2.5	0	0.5	235

Food exchanges per serving: 1 Starch plus 1 Fruit plus 1 Fat
Low-sodium diets: This recipe is acceptable.

Chocolate Dream Pie

1 1.4-ounce package sugar-free,
   fat-free chocolate instant
   pudding mix
2 cups skim milk
1 8-ounce container nondairy light
   whipped topping, thawed,
   divided

1 Vanilla Wafer Crumb Crust (see
   Index), chilled
1 tablespoon semisweet chocolate
   chips

*P*repare pudding with skim milk according to package directions. Refrigerate 30 minutes.

Fold 1 cup of the whipped topping into pudding. Spoon chocolate mixture carefully into pie shell; chill until pudding is firm.

Gently spread remainder of whipped topping across top of pie with a small spatula. Sprinkle chips over top of pie. Cover pie carefully with plastic wrap. Chill 2–3 hours until set and firm.

To serve, cut into eight equal wedges.

8 servings (makes a 9-inch pie)
1 serving = ⅛ pie

CAL.	CHO(g)	PRO.(g)	TOTAL FAT(g)	SAT. FAT(g)	CHOL.(mg)	FIBER(g)	SODIUM(mg)
190	23	3	8	4.5	0	0.5	250

Food exchanges per serving: 1 Starch plus 1 Fat plus ½ Other Carbohydrate
Low-sodium diets: This recipe is acceptable.

Holiday Pumpkin Chiffon Pie

1 tablespoon granulated gelatin
½ cup cold water
3 eggs, separated
½ cup whole milk
1¼ cups solid-pack canned
    pumpkin
½ teaspoon salt
¼ teaspoon ground nutmeg
¾ teaspoon ground cinnamon

½ teaspoon ground ginger
½ teaspoon ground allspice
Sugar substitute equivalent to
    ½ cup sugar
2 tablespoons sugar
1 tablespoon brandy
1 Graham Cracker Pie Shell
    (see Index)

Dissolve gelatin in cold water; set aside.

Beat egg yolks lightly; stir in milk, pumpkin, salt, and spices; blend well. Cook in the top of a double boiler, stirring constantly until thick and smooth, about 8 minutes. Remove from heat.

Add gelatin and sweetener; stir until completely dissolved. Cool, then chill in refrigerator until mixture thickens to consistency of unbeaten egg white.

Remove from refrigerator. Beat egg whites until soft peaks form. Add sugar and brandy gradually to egg whites, beating constantly until stiff and shiny. Fold carefully but thoroughly into pumpkin mixture.

Turn carefully into the prepared pie shell; sprinkle top with reserved 2 tablespoons graham cracker crumbs. Chill several hours.

8 servings (makes a 9-inch pie)
1 serving = ⅛ pie

CAL.	CHO(g)	PRO.(g)	TOTAL FAT(g)	SAT. FAT(g)	CHOL.(mg)	FIBER(g)	SODIUM(mg)
175	19	6	8	2	80	1	305

Food exchanges per serving: 1 Starch plus 1 Fat plus ½ Low-Fat Milk
Low-sodium diets: Omit salt.

Strawberry Tart

In the summer top this pretty tart with any type of berries or a mixture of berries. In the winter top it with sliced kiwifruit or seedless green and red grapes.

*1 Graham Cracker Pie Shell
    (see Index)
2 cups low-fat (2% milk fat) milk
1 0.9- to 1-ounce package sugar-
    free, fat-free vanilla instant
    pudding mix*

*1 teaspoon freshly grated orange
    zest
2 cups cleaned and hulled
    strawberries or other berries*

*U*se a 9-inch tart pan with a removable bottom. Spray bottom and sides of pan with butter-flavored nonstick cooking spray. Firmly pat Graham Cracker Pie Shell mixture into tart pan. Set aside.

Blend milk with instant pudding mix in a deep bowl using a whisk or an electric mixer. Continue mixing 2 minutes or until pudding thickens. Add grated orange zest. Let stand 5 minutes; pour into pie shell. Chill 15 minutes or until set.

Shortly before serving, arrange strawberries or other fruit decoratively over pudding. Chill 1 hour before slicing.

8 servings (makes a 9-inch tart)
1 serving = ⅛ tart

CAL.	CHO(g)	PRO.(g)	TOTAL FAT(g)	SAT. FAT(g)	CHOL.(mg)	FIBER(g)	SODIUM(mg)
150	19	3	7	2	5	1.5	310

Food exchanges per serving: 1 Starch plus 1 Fat
Low-sodium diets: This recipe is suitable for occasional use. Use unsalted margarine in pie shell.

French Apple Clafouti

Also try this recipe with firm but ripe pears, peaches, or plums.

4 cups (4 medium to large) sliced   ½ cup all-purpose flour, sifted
    peeled Granny Smith or Rome   ¼ cup sugar
    apples   1½ teaspoons pure vanilla extract
1½ cups whole milk   ½ teaspoon ground cinnamon
4 eggs

Preheat oven to 350°F. Prepare a deep 10-inch pie plate with butter-flavored nonstick cooking spray, or use a nonstick pie plate. Arrange apple slices evenly in pie plate.

Use a blender or food processor to combine milk and eggs. Add remaining ingredients; blend 5 seconds. Scrape down sides of blender with a spatula; blend until ingredients are mixed together, about 30 seconds. A bowl and whisk can be used to prepare batter by hand.

Spread batter over apples. Bake 1 hour or until custard forms and cake tests done by inserting a toothpick that comes out clean. Serve warm or at room temperature.

8 servings (makes a 10-inch clafouti)
1 serving = 1 2½-inch wedge

CAL.	CHO(g)	PRO.(g)	TOTAL FAT(g)	SAT. FAT(g)	CHOL.(mg)	FIBER(g)	SODIUM(mg)
155	23	6	4	2	115	1	55

Food exchanges per serving: 1½ Fruits plus 1 Medium-Fat Meat
Low-sodium diets: This recipe is excellent.

Pear Crumble

¼ cup margarine, cut into ½-inch
   pieces
⅓ cup uncooked quick-cooking oats
¼ cup all-purpose flour
Sugar substitute equivalent to 2
   tablespoons sugar

2 cups chopped, cored firm ripe
   pears (½-inch pieces)
2 teaspoons fresh lemon juice
½ teaspoon ground cinnamon
¼ teaspoon ground nutmeg
½ teaspoon grated lemon zest

*P*reheat oven to 400°F. Prepare an 8-inch pie plate with butter-flavored nonstick cooking spray. In a medium mixing bowl, toss together margarine, oats, flour, and sweetener. Place pears in a separate mixing bowl; toss with lemon juice, cinnamon, nutmeg, and lemon zest.

Arrange pears in the prepared pan. Sprinkle oat mixture over fruit. Bake 15 minutes. Serve warm or cool.

6 servings (makes an 8-inch pie)
1 serving = ⅙ pie

CAL.	CHO*(g)*	PRO.*(g)*	TOTAL FAT*(g)*	SAT. FAT*(g)*	CHOL.*(mg)*	FIBER*(g)*	SODIUM*(mg)*
140	16	2	8	1.5	0	2	90

Food exchanges per serving: 1 Fruit plus 1½ Fats
Low-sodium diets: This recipe is excellent.

Apple Cobbler

1¾ pounds (about 4) medium-
    sized cooking apples (such as
    Jonathan or Granny Smith)
1½ tablespoons fresh lemon juice
1 teaspoon grated lemon zest
1 tablespoon cornstarch

1 teaspoon apple pie spice
¼ teaspoon salt, divided
Sugar substitute equivalent to
    ¼ cup sugar
½ cup flour
3 tablespoons margarine

Preheat oven to 425°F. Prepare a 9-inch pie plate with butter-flavored nonstick cooking spray. Pare apples, remove cores, and cut apples into ⅛-inch slices. Measure 4 cups.

In a medium bowl, combine apple slices, lemon juice, and zest. In a small bowl, combine cornstarch, spice, ⅛ teaspoon of the salt, and sweetener; mix thoroughly. Add to apples; stir lightly with a fork to coat all slices. Spread apples evenly in prepared pie plate; set aside.

Mix together flour and remaining ⅛ teaspoon salt. Cut in margarine with pastry blender or fork until crumbly; scatter all over top of apples. Bake about 35 minutes or until top is golden brown. Serve warm.

8 servings (makes a 9-inch cobbler)
1 serving = ⅛ recipe

CAL.	CHO(g)	PRO.(g)	TOTAL FAT(g)	SAT. FAT(g)	CHOL.(mg)	FIBER(g)	SODIUM(mg)
125	20	1	5	1	0	2	120

Food exchanges per serving: 1 Fruit plus 1 Fat plus ½ Starch
Low-sodium diets: Omit salt. Use unsalted margarine.

Grape Cobbler

This dessert can cook while you are eating dinner.

2 cups (about 10 ounces) seedless red grapes
1 tablespoon all-purpose flour
1 tablespoon granulated sugar
½-inch cube crystallized ginger, minced fine

½ cup ready-to-eat oat flake cereal
1½ tablespoons melted margarine
1½ tablespoons dark brown sugar
½ cup low-fat vanilla frozen yogurt

Preheat oven to 375°F. Prepare a 1-quart casserole or glass pie plate with butter-flavored nonstick cooking spray.

Remove grapes from stem; cut grapes in half. Put grapes in a mixing bowl with granulated sugar and ginger; toss to mix. Pour grape mixture into casserole.

In the same mixing bowl, combine oat cereal, melted margarine, and brown sugar. Spread oat mixture over grapes.

Bake 35 minutes. Serve warm, topped with a dollop of vanilla frozen yogurt.

4 servings
1 serving = ¼ cobbler plus 2 tablespoons frozen yogurt

CAL.	CHO(g)	PRO.(g)	TOTAL FAT(g)	SAT. FAT(g)	CHOL.(mg)	FIBER(g)	SODIUM(mg)
175	33	2	5	1	0	1.5	100

Food exchanges per serving: 1 Fruit plus 1 Other Carbohydrate plus 1 Fat
Low-sodium diets: This recipe is acceptable.

Cakes

Chocolate Mint Cake

½ cup firmly packed Dutch-process
    cocoa powder
½ cup very hot, strong coffee
1 teaspoon pure vanilla extract
2 eggs, separated
½ cup granulated sugar, divided

2 egg whites
¾ teaspoon mint extract
½ cup cake flour, sifted
Pinch salt
2 teaspoons powdered sugar
8 sprigs mint (optional)

Preheat oven to 350°F. Line the bottom of an 8-inch round cake pan with parchment paper or nonstick oven liner film. Spray liner and sides of pan with butter-flavored nonstick cooking spray.

Place cocoa powder, hot coffee, and vanilla in a medium-sized bowl. Whisk to dissolve cocoa. Set aside to cool.

Combine 2 egg yolks and ¼ cup of the granulated sugar in the top of a double boiler or in a small saucepan placed in a skillet half-filled with water. Heat bottom pan of water to a simmer, and whisk the egg-sugar mixture just until the mixture thickens and the sugar crystals are dissolved. (Do not overheat, or you will make sweet scrambled eggs.)

Transfer the yolk mixture to the bowl of a mixer. Beat mixture until it is the consistency of a light frosting and has doubled in volume. Gently fold this into the chocolate mixture with a spatula.

Place 4 egg whites in a dry, grease-free mixing bowl. Beat whites until soft peaks form. Very gradually add the remaining ¼ cup granulated sugar and mint extract, beating the meringue until stiff peaks form.

Sift cake flour and salt onto chocolate mixture. Fold flour into chocolate with a rubber spatula until no flour shows. Transfer half of chocolate mixture to the bowl of meringue. Fold it in very gently. Repeat process with remainder of chocolate. Turn the mixture into the prepared pan; use a spatula to level the top.

Put pan on middle rack of oven; bake about 20 minutes until cake is puffed but springs back to the touch or an inserted toothpick comes out clean. Remove from oven; cool 5–10 minutes on a wire rack. Put rack on top of cake; invert to remove cake from pan. Cool cake completely.

When ready to serve, sift powdered sugar over cake. Cut into eight wedges. If desired, garnish each piece with a sprig of mint.

8 servings (makes an 8-inch cake)
1 serving = ⅛ cake

CAL.	CHO(g)	PRO.(g)	TOTAL FAT(g)	SAT. FAT(g)	CHOL.(mg)	FIBER(g)	SODIUM(mg)
115	22	4	3	1	55	0	85

Food exchanges per serving: 1 Starch plus ½ Other Carbohydrate
Low-sodium diets: Omit salt.

Louis's Boston Cream Cake

This cake is a favorite of Dr. Louis Kraus, who used to live in Boston. Louis is the son of Barbara Grunes, who developed the recipe for this book.

5 eggs
½ cup sugar
3 packets heat-stable sugar
     substitute equivalent to
     2 tablespoons sugar
1 teaspoon pure vanilla extract
¾ cup flour
2 tablespoons cornstarch

1 teaspoon baking powder
2 cups skim milk
1 0.9- to 1-ounce package sugar-
     free, fat-free vanilla instant
     pudding mix
½ teaspoon ground cinnamon
1 teaspoon cocoa powder

Preheat oven to 400°F. Spray with nonstick cooking spray and line two 8-inch round cake pans with parchment paper or waxed paper. Beat eggs with an electric mixer until light and fluffy. Sprinkle sugar, sugar substitute, and vanilla over eggs; continue beating 2 minutes.

In a small bowl, sift together flour, cornstarch, and baking powder. Sprinkle half the mixture over batter. Fold in with a rubber spatula. Repeat with remaining flour mixture.

Use a rubber spatula to spread batter evenly in pans. Bake on center rack of oven 15–20 minutes or until cake is golden and springs back when lightly touched. Invert cake onto a wire rack; cool 5 minutes. Remove pan; set aside to cool.

Using an electric mixer, blend milk with instant pudding mix in a mixing bowl. Continue mixing at low speed 1 minute or until pudding mix is dissolved. Set pudding aside 10 minutes or until it thickens.

To assemble, arrange a single cake layer on a serving dish. Spread two-thirds of firm pudding evenly over bottom cake layer. Place remaining cake layer evenly on top. Stir cinnamon and cocoa into remaining pudding. Spread over top of cake as chocolate frosting.

Refrigerate until ready to serve. Cut with a serrated knife.

8 servings (makes an 8-inch cake)
1 serving = ⅛ cake

CAL.	CHO(g)	PRO.(g)	TOTAL FAT(g)	SAT. FAT(g)	CHOL.(mg)	FIBER(g)	SODIUM(mg)
190	30	7	4	1	135	0.5	290

Food exchanges per serving: 1 Starch plus 1 Medium-Fat Meat plus 1 Other Carbohydrate
Low-sodium diets: This recipe is suitable for occasional use.

Pumpkin Gingercakes with Orange Cream

A nutrient-rich, festive, and interesting dessert. The number of individual servings depends on the size of the cupcake tins or molds you use. You can also make the cake in a small bundt pan. Adjust cooking time based on size and type of pan.

Orange Cream

1 cup nondairy light whipped
    topping
½ teaspoon pure orange oil or ¾
    teaspoon orange extract

Cakes

¾ cup solid-pack canned pumpkin
½ cup cultured low-fat (1½% milk
    fat) buttermilk
¼ cup blackstrap molasses
¼ cup honey
2 tablespoons corn oil
2 eggs
½ teaspoon pure orange oil or
    ¾ teaspoon orange extract
1⅓ cups flour
2 teaspoons ground ginger
1 teaspoon crystallized ginger,
    finely chopped
1 teaspoon baking soda
1 teaspoon ground cinnamon
½ teaspoon ground nutmeg
1 tablespoon powdered sugar

Gently mix together whipped topping and orange oil. Refrigerate orange cream for flavors to blend.

Preheat oven to 350°F. Prepare a 12-cup muffin tin or 12 small molds with nonstick cooking spray. In a medium bowl, whisk together pumpkin, buttermilk, molasses, honey, corn oil, eggs, and orange oil.

In a large bowl, combine flour, ginger, crystallized ginger, baking soda, cinnamon, and nutmeg. Add pumpkin mixture; whisk until well blended. Fill muffin cups or molds ⅔ full. Bake about 20 minutes or until an inserted toothpick comes out clean.

Let cool in the pan on wire rack about 5 minutes. Invert onto wire rack to complete cooling.

At serving time, sprinkle powdered sugar over gingercakes and top each gingercake with a dollop of Orange Cream.

12 servings
1 serving = 1 gingercake plus 1 rounded tablespoon Orange Cream

CAL.	CHO(g)	PRO.(g)	TOTAL FAT(g)	SAT. FAT(g)	CHOL.(mg)	FIBER(g)	SODIUM(mg)
155	25	3	5	115	35	0.5	130

Food exchanges per serving: 1 Starch plus 1 Fat plus ½ Other Carbohydrate
Low-sodium diets: This recipe is suitable.

Plum Jelly Roll

If you don't have Red Plum Spread, use a prepared fruitspread with no added sugar.

5 eggs
½ cup sugar
3 packets heat-stable sugar
    substitute equivalent to
    2 tablespoons sugar
1 teaspoon pure vanilla extract

¾ cup all-purpose flour
2 tablespoons cornstarch
1 teaspoon baking powder
1¼ cups Red Plum Spread (recipe
    follows)

Preheat oven to 400°F. Spray bottom of a 10″ × 15″ jelly roll pan with nonstick cooking spray and line with waxed paper or baking pan liner.

With an electric mixer, beat eggs in a large bowl until fluffy. Sprinkle sugar, sugar substitute, and vanilla over eggs; continue beating 2 minutes.

In a small bowl, sift together flour, cornstarch, and baking powder. Sprinkle half the flour mixture over batter; fold in with a spatula. Repeat with remaining flour mixture. Spread batter evenly in pan.

Bake on center rack in oven for 10–12 minutes or until cake is golden and springs back when lightly touched.

Arrange a towel on work surface; cover with aluminum foil. Loosen edges of cake; unmold on foil. Roll cake jelly roll style. Leave cake rolled until it cools into jelly roll shape. Unroll; spread with the sweet spread and reroll. Cut into 1-inch slices and serve.

15 servings
1 serving = 1 1-inch-thick slice

CAL.	CHO(g)	PRO.(g)	TOTAL FAT(g)	SAT. FAT(g)	CHOL.(mg)	FIBER(g)	SODIUM(mg)
100	17	3	2	0.5	70	1	60

Food exchange per serving: 1 Starch
Low-sodium diets: This recipe is excellent.

Red Plum Spread

1¼ cups (about 1 pound) chopped
  pitted fresh red plums (small
  bite-sized pieces)
¾ cup cold water, divided

1 teaspoon fresh lemon juice
1½ teaspoons granulated gelatin
Sugar substitute equivalent to
  ¼ cup sugar

*I*n a heavy saucepan, combine plums with ½ cup of the water and the lemon juice. Bring to a boil; reduce heat and simmer gently about 8 minutes, stirring frequently.

Meanwhile, soak gelatin in remaining ¼ cup cold water. Remove cooked plums from heat. Stir in gelatin and sweetener, and mix well.

Store in the refrigerator no longer than 2 weeks.

20 servings (makes 1¼ cups)
1 serving = 1 tablespoon

CAL.	CHO(g)	PRO.(g)	TOTAL FAT(g)	SAT. FAT(g)	CHOL.(mg)	FIBER(g)	SODIUM(mg)
15	3	0	0	0	0	0.5	0

Food exchange per serving: a Free Food (up to 2 tablespoons)
Low-sodium diets: This recipe is excellent.

Chocolate-Filled Cake Roll

Cake

5 eggs
½ cup sugar
Heat-stable sugar substitute
    equivalent to 2 tablespoons
    sugar
1 teaspoon pure vanilla extract
¾ cup all-purpose flour
2 tablespoons cornstarch
1 teaspoon baking powder

Filling

2 cups skim milk
1 1.4-ounce package sugar-free
    chocolate instant pudding mix

Topping

2 teaspoons sugar-free cocoa mix

Preheat oven to 400°F. Spray the bottom of a 10″ × 15″ jelly roll pan with nonstick cooking spray and line with waxed paper. With an electric mixer, beat eggs in a large bowl until fluffy. Sprinkle sugar, sugar substitute, and vanilla over eggs; continue beating for 2 minutes. In a small bowl, sift together flour, cornstarch, and baking powder. Sprinkle half the mixture over batter; fold in with a spatula. Repeat with remaining flour mixture.

Spread batter evenly in pan. Bake on center rack in oven 10–12 minutes or until cake is golden and springs back when lightly touched.

Arrange a towel on work surface, cover with aluminum foil. Loosen edges of cake; unmold on foil. Roll cake jelly roll style. Leave cake rolled until it cools into jelly roll shape.

Meanwhile, to make filling, blend milk with pudding mix according to package directions. Refrigerate pudding until it thickens.

Unroll cake, spread evenly with pudding and reroll. Sprinkle cocoa mix over the top to decorate. Cut into 1-inch slices and serve.

15 servings
1 serving = 1 1-inch-thick slice

CAL.	CHO(g)	PRO.(g)	TOTAL FAT(g)	SAT. FAT(g)	CHOL.(mg)	FIBER(g)	SODIUM(mg)
100	17	4	2	0.5	70	0.5	155

Food exchange per serving: 1 Starch
Low-sodium diets: This recipe is acceptable.

Raspberry Dream

For this recipe, I used a fruit spread that has a nice flavor but only half the calories and sugar of regular preserves.

1½ cups nondairy light whipped topping, divided

¼ cup reduced-calorie raspberry fruit spread

6 ounces prepared angel food cake

½ pint fresh raspberries

*I*n a small bowl, very gently fold together 1 cup of the whipped topping and the raspberry spread.

Tear angel food cake into 1-inch pieces; put pieces into a large bowl. Add topping mixture to cake; toss gently to coat most of cake cubes.

Divide mixture among six individual dessert dishes. Top each dish with berries and a dollop of the remaining whipped topping.

6 servings
1 serving = 1 individual dessert

CAL.	CHO*(g)*	PRO.*(g)*	TOTAL FAT*(g)*	SAT. FAT*(g)*	CHOL.*(mg)*	FIBER*(g)*	SODIUM*(mg)*
150	30	2	2	2	0	1.5	210

Food exchanges per serving: 1 Starch plus 1 Fruit
Low-sodium diets: This recipe is acceptable.

Cookies

Brownie Squares

⅓ cup margarine

1 1-ounce square unsweetened
    chocolate

½ cup sugar

1 large egg

1 teaspoon pure vanilla extract

½ cup oat bran cereal

⅓ cup all-purpose flour

½ cup chopped walnuts, divided

Heat oven to 350°F. Prepare an 8-inch square pan with nonstick cooking spray. In a medium saucepan, melt margarine and chocolate over medium heat; cool. Add sugar, egg, and vanilla; mix well. Add oat bran cereal, flour, and ¼ cup of the nuts; mix just until well blended.

    Spread into prepared pan; sprinkle with remaining nuts. Bake about 18 minutes or until firm to the touch. Cool and cut into 2-inch squares.

8 servings (makes 16 brownies)
1 serving = 2 2-inch-square brownies

CAL.	CHO(g)	PRO.(g)	TOTAL FAT(g)	SAT. FAT(g)	CHOL.(mg)	FIBER(g)	SODIUM(mg)
230	22	4	15	3	25	2	100

Food exchanges per serving: 2 Fats plus 1½ Starches
Low-sodium diets: This recipe is suitable.

Almond Slices

3 large eggs
⅓ cup sugar
3 tablespoons vegetable shortening
    at room temperature
¾ teaspoon pure almond extract

¾ teaspoon pure vanilla extract
1½ cups all-purpose flour
1 teaspoon baking powder
½ cup golden raisins

*P*reheat oven to 350°F. Prepare bottom of a 9″ × 13″ pan with nonstick cooking spray. With an electric mixer, beat eggs and sugar until light. Add shortening, almond extract, vanilla, flour, and baking powder; mix well. Blend in raisins.

Divide batter and arrange into two 2-inch tube-shaped loaves in the prepared pan. Bake 25 minutes.

Remove pan from oven; cut cookies into ⅓-inch-thick slices. Turn cookies on their sides and bake 5 minutes more or until cookies are firm to the touch. Cool cookies and store in a tightly covered container.

22 servings (makes 44 almond slices)
1 serving = 2 cookies

CAL.	CHO*(g)*	PRO.*(g)*	TOTAL FAT*(g)*	SAT. FAT*(g)*	CHOL.*(mg)*	FIBER*(g)*	SODIUM*(mg)*
80	12	2	3	0.5	30	0.5	30

Food exchange per serving: 1 Starch
Low-sodium diets: This recipe is excellent.

Cranberry Pistachio Biscotti

Use natural pistachios for this recipe, not the ones colored red.

2 eggs
⅓ cup sugar
2 tablespoons margarine, at room
    temperature
1½ teaspoons pure vanilla extract

1 cup all-purpose flour
1 teaspoon baking powder
⅓ cup shelled pistachios
⅓ cup dried cranberries

Preheat oven to 350°F. Prepare a cookie sheet with nonstick cooking spray.

With an electric mixer, beat eggs and sugar until light and frothy. Add margarine and vanilla extract; mix about 30 seconds. Add flour and baking powder; mix well. Mix in pistachios and dried cranberries.

In the center of the cookie sheet, shape batter into a tube-shaped loaf about 2 inches wide and about 15 inches long. Bake 25 minutes.

Using a serrated knife, cut loaf into ⅓-inch-thick slices. Return slices to cookie sheet; bake 5 minutes more. Turn off oven, and let biscotti dry in the oven about 30 minutes.

Cool cookies. Store in a tightly covered tin.

12 servings (makes 3 dozen cookies)
1 serving = 3 cookies

CAL.	CHO(g)	PRO.(g)	TOTAL FAT(g)	SAT. FAT(g)	CHOL.(mg)	FIBER(g)	SODIUM(mg)
120	17	3	5	1	35	1	75

Food exchanges per serving: 1 Starch plus 1 Fat
Low-sodium diets: This recipe is acceptable.

Hazelnut Chocolate Biscotti

¼–⅓ cup raw shelled hazelnuts
2 tablespoons margarine
¼ cup sugar
2 egg whites
1½ teaspoons pure vanilla extract
2 teaspoons finely grated orange
     zest

1½ cups sifted all-purpose flour
½ teaspoon baking powder
¼ teaspoon salt
¼ cup semisweet chocolate chips

Preheat oven to 375°F. Place hazelnuts on an ungreased cookie sheet; toast in oven 8 minutes. Remove pan; rub hazelnuts between palms to remove most of their brown papery skin. Finely chop nuts. Reduce oven temperature to 325°F.

Combine margarine and sugar in a medium bowl; mix well. Add egg whites, vanilla, and orange zest; mix. Add flour, baking powder, salt, and ½ of the nuts. Mix until dough forms a ball.

Spray cookie sheet with nonstick cooking spray. Roll dough into a log about 12 inches long. Flatten log to about 2½ inches wide by ½ inch high. Bake log 25 minutes. Remove from oven; cool 5 minutes on a wire rack.

Spray cookie sheet again with nonstick cooking spray. With a serrated knife, slice log into ½-inch-thick slices. Place slices on cookie sheet and bake 10 minutes. Turn slices; bake 10 minutes more. Cool biscotti on wire rack.

Melt chocolate chips in a microwave oven, or pour chips into a glass measuring cup and melt by putting the cup in a small pan of boiling water. While biscotti are still warm, brush or drizzle melted chocolate over tops. Sprinkle with remaining chopped hazelnuts. Allow biscotti to cool and chocolate to harden.

Store in a tightly covered tin with waxed paper between layers.

12 servings (makes 2 dozen biscotti)
1 serving = 2 biscotti

CAL.	CHO(g)	PRO.(g)	TOTAL FAT(g)	SAT. FAT(g)	CHOL.(mg)	FIBER(g)	SODIUM(mg)
130	19	2	5	1	0	1	95

Food exchanges per serving: 1 Starch plus 1 Fat
Low-sodium diets: Omit salt.

Apple Spice Bar Cookies

1¾ cups sifted cake flour
½ teaspoon baking soda
1 teaspoon ground cinnamon
½ teaspoon ground allspice
⅛ teaspoon ground cloves
½ teaspoon salt

¼ cup margarine
¾ cup sugar
1 large egg
½ cup unsweetened applesauce
½ cup seedless raisins

*P*reheat oven to 375°F. Prepare bottom of an 11″ × 7″ pan with nonstick cooking spray.

In a medium bowl, sift together flour, baking soda, spices, and salt. In a separate bowl, cream margarine until soft and fluffy; beat in sugar gradually. Add egg; beat until light and fluffy. Add sifted dry ingredients and applesauce, alternately, stirring just enough to blend well. Add raisins; stir until all ingredients are thoroughly mixed. Turn into the prepared pan.

Bake about 30 minutes. Let cool on a baking rack 10 minutes, then cut into 24 1¾-inch squares.

24 servings
1 serving = 1 1¾-inch square

CAL.	CHO(g)	PRO.(g)	TOTAL FAT(g)	SAT. FAT(g)	CHOL.(mg)	FIBER(g)	SODIUM(mg)
80	15	1	2	0.5	10	0	95

Food exchange per serving: 1 Starch
Low-sodium diets: Omit salt.

Lemon Rings

1½ cups all-purpose flour
¼ cup sugar
Grated zest of 1 lemon
6 tablespoons margarine, cut into
    small pieces

1 large egg
1 egg white, beaten lightly

Preheat oven to 375°F. Prepare a cookie sheet with nonstick cooking spray. Using a food processor fitted with a steel blade, combine all ingredients except egg white. Flatten dough slightly; cover in plastic wrap. Chill 30 minutes.

Break off a tablespoonful of dough; roll out to form a 3-inch pencil-shaped rope. Attach edges to shape a ring. Place on prepared cookie sheet. Continue with remaining dough. Brush tops of cookies with lightly beaten egg white. Bake 10–12 minutes or until lightly golden.

Remove cookies from baking sheet and cool on a wire rack. Store in a tightly covered tin.

12 servings (makes 2 dozen cookies)
1 serving = 2 cookies

CAL.	CHO(g)	PRO.(g)	TOTAL FAT(g)	SAT. FAT(g)	CHOL.(mg)	FIBER(g)	SODIUM(mg)
135	16	2	6	1	15	0.5	75

Food exchanges per serving: 1 Starch plus 1 Fat
Low-sodium diets: This recipe is suitable.

Raisin Cookies

½ cup margarine
¼ cup sugar
Heat-stable sugar substitute
    equivalent to 2 tablespoons
    sugar
1 teaspoon pure vanilla extract
1 large egg

1½ cups all-purpose flour
½ cup uncooked quick-cooking oats
2 teaspoons baking powder
½ cup raisins
1 teaspoon all-purpose flour
    (to flour glass)

In large bowl of an electric mixer, cream together margarine, sugar, sugar substitute, vanilla, and egg until batter is light. Add flour, oats, baking powder, and raisins; blend well. Gather dough together, roll into a ball, and cover with plastic wrap. Chill 2 hours or overnight.

Preheat oven to 375°F. Roll dough into ¾-inch balls; place 1½ inches apart on a nonstick cookie sheet. Flatten cookies with bottom of a lightly floured glass. Bake cookies about 8–10 minutes or until they are firm and golden brown. Cool cookies before serving.

20 servings (makes about 3½ dozen cookies)
1 serving = 2 cookies

CAL.	CHO(g)	PRO.(g)	TOTAL FAT(g)	SAT. FAT(g)	CHOL.(mg)	FIBER(g)	SODIUM(mg)
110	14	2	5	1	10	0.5	105

Food exchanges per serving: 1 Starch plus 1 Fat
Low-sodium diets: This recipe is suitable.

Chocolate Meringue Clouds

Top clouds with fresh berries or sliced ripe peaches. The nutrient values are for the clouds only—add exchange values for the filling you use. You can use the same recipe to make about 2 dozen meringue kisses. Just put 1-tablespoon blobs on the lined pans. Use a spoon to pull the soft meringue blobs into a kiss shape. Four kisses—with 60 calories and 15 grams of carbohydrate—count as 1 Other Carbohydrate Exchange.

2 egg whites
½ teaspoon fresh lemon juice
¼ cup extra-fine sugar
½ teaspoon pure vanilla extract

¼ cup powdered sugar
2 tablespoons cocoa powder
1 cup fresh raspberries

Preheat oven to 225°F. Line a cookie sheet with parchment paper or nonstick oven liner film. Using an electric mixer, beat egg whites with lemon juice until soft peaks form. With mixer on, very gradually add the extra-fine sugar; beat until mixture forms stiff peaks. Add vanilla.

In a medium bowl, sift together powdered sugar and cocoa powder. Gently fold this mixture into the meringue.

Divide meringue into four mounds on cookie sheet. Make an indentation in the center of each mound to make it look like a cloud. The indentation should be deep enough to hold about ¼ cup of fruit.

Bake 2 hours or until meringues are dry and crisp. Turn off heat and leave clouds in oven at least 1 more hour (overnight if desired). Store in an airtight tin.

4 servings (makes 4 meringue shells)
1 serving = 1 meringue shell

CAL.	CHO*(g)*	PRO.*(g)*	TOTAL FAT*(g)*	SAT. FAT*(g)*	CHOL.*(mg)*	FIBER*(g)*	SODIUM*(mg)*
90	20	2	0	0	0	0	0

Food exchange per serving: 1 Other Carbohydrate
Low-sodium diets: An excellent choice.

Pudding in Cookie Flowers

These cookie shells can also be filled with fresh fruits or other fillings.

Cookies	Filling
¼ cup margarine	1 package sugar-free, fat-free
¼ cup sugar	vanilla or chocolate pudding
3 packets heat-stable sugar	(vanilla is in 0.9-ounce boxes,
substitute equivalent to 2	chocolate in 1.4-ounce boxes)
tablespoons sugar	1¾ cups skim milk
½ teaspoon pure vanilla extract	¼ cup fresh blueberries or
½ cup all-purpose flour	raspberries
2 egg whites	

Preheat oven to 350°F. To prepare cookies, cream together margarine, sugar, sugar substitute, and vanilla in a medium bowl. Add flour alternately with egg whites, mixing well after each addition.

Measure 1 heaping tablespoonful dough for each cookie. Place 3 inches apart on an ungreased nonstick cookie sheet, pressing cookie batter with back of spoon in circular motion to extend circle to 4 inches. Six cookies will fit on each pan. Have muffin pan available for shaping after baking. Bake cookies 8–10 minutes or until golden around edges.

Remove cookies immediately with a spatula. Gently press warm cookies into the muffin tin, giving each cookie a cup shape. Return to oven and bake 5 minutes more.

Allow cookie shells to cool. Remove from pan and store them in a tightly covered tin.

To prepare filling, prepare pudding with skim milk according to package directions. Refrigerate until set.

When ready to serve, fill each cookie cup with about ¼ cup pudding. Garnish each filled cup with a few fresh berries. Serve immediately.

8 servings (makes 8 cookie cups)
1 serving = 1 filled cookie cup

Pudding in Cookie Flower:

CAL.	CHO(g)	PRO.(g)	TOTAL FAT(g)	SAT. FAT(g)	CHOL.(mg)	FIBER(g)	SODIUM(mg)
145	19	4	6	1	0	0.5	260

Food exchanges per serving: 1 Starch plus 1 Fat *or* 1 Other Carbohydrate plus ½ Skim Milk plus 1 Fat
Low-sodium diets: Use unsalted margarine. If sodium is very restricted, fill cups with fresh fruit and omit pudding.

Cookie shell only:

CAL.	CHO(g)	PRO.(g)	TOTAL FAT(g)	SAT. FAT(g)	CHOL.(mg)	FIBER(g)	SODIUM(mg)
75	13	2	6	1	0	0	90

Food exchanges per serving: 1 Starch plus 1 Fat
Low-sodium diets: This recipe is excellent.

24

Beverages

Iced Mocha Latte

1 tablespoon instant coffee crystals
1 tablespoon Dutch-process cocoa
    powder
Sugar substitute equivalent to
    2 tablespoons sugar

⅓ cup strong hot coffee or espresso
2 cups ice cubes
1 cup evaporated skim milk

Dissolve instant coffee crystals, cocoa, and sugar substitute in hot coffee.

Put ice cubes and evaporated milk in a blender or food processor; process 20 seconds to crush ice. Add coffee mixture, and process 30 seconds more. Serve immediately.

5 servings (makes 5½ cups)
1 serving = 1 cup

CAL.	CHO(g)	PRO.(g)	TOTAL FAT(g)	SAT. FAT(g)	CHOL.(mg)	FIBER(g)	SODIUM(mg)
45	7	4	0	0	0	0	65

Food exchange per serving: ½ Skim Milk
Low-sodium diets: This recipe is excellent.

Cherry Shake

⅓ cup reduced-calorie cranberry
   juice cocktail
¾ cup ice cubes
1½ cups frozen pitted dark sweet
   cherries

½ cup evaporated skim milk
Sugar substitute equivalent to
   1 tablespoon sugar
½ teaspoon pure vanilla extract

*P*ut all ingredients in a blender or food processor. Process about 1 minute until ice cubes are crushed and mixture is thick and creamy.

Taste and add more sugar substitute if desired.

4 servings (makes 4 cups)
1 serving = 1 cup

CAL.	CHO(g)	PRO.(g)	TOTAL FAT(g)	SAT. FAT(g)	CHOL.(mg)	FIBER(g)	SODIUM(mg)
70	14	3	1	0	0	1	40

Food exchange per serving: 1 Fruit
Low-sodium diets: This recipe is excellent.

Orange Fizz

1 orange   Sugar substitute equivalent to
6 ice cubes   1 tablespoon sugar
1 teaspoon fresh lemon juice   1 10-ounce bottle club soda
½ teaspoon pure orange extract

Cut orange in half; cut one slice from center of orange to use as garnish.
Squeeze juice from orange halves.

Crush ice cubes and divide between 2 10-ounce glasses. Mix together
orange juice, lemon juice, and orange extract; dissolve sweetener in fruit
juices.

Pour ¼ cup of mixed juices into each glass. Pour half bottle club soda
into each glass. Stir briskly. Cut orange slice in half crosswise; fit onto edge
of glass. Serve immediately.

2 servings
1 serving = 1 12-ounce glass

CAL.	CHO*(g)*	PRO.*(g)*	TOTAL FAT*(g)*	SAT. FAT*(g)*	CHOL.*(mg)*	FIBER*(g)*	SODIUM*(mg)*
25	5	0	0	0	0	0	30

Food exchange per serving: ½ Fruit
Low-sodium diets: This recipe is excellent.

Foamy Orange Cup

This beverage is a first cousin to an Orange Julius, an old-fashioned fountain beverage.

¾ cup skim milk or low-fat (1½% milk fat) buttermilk
½ cup orange juice
Sugar substitute equivalent to 1 teaspoon sugar

¼ teaspoon pure vanilla extract
⅛ teaspoon pure almond extract
Dash salt
3 ice cubes, cracked into small pieces

*P*lace all ingredients in a blender or food processor; cover. Blend on low speed until ice cubes are crushed and the drink is foamy.

2 servings (makes 2 cups)
1 serving = 1 cup

CAL.	CHO(g)	PRO.(g)	TOTAL FAT(g)	SAT. FAT(g)	CHOL.(mg)	FIBER(g)	SODIUM(mg)
80	15	4	0	0	0	0	115

Food exchange per serving: 1 Fruit or 1 Skim Milk
Low-sodium diets: Omit salt.

Champagne Fooler

Bubble, bubble, no toil, no trouble!

*⅓ cup chilled unsweetened apple
juice or apple cider*

*¼ teaspoon fresh lemon juice
About ½ cup chilled club soda*

Chill a champagne glass or wineglass. Measure apple and lemon juices into a measuring cup. Add enough club soda to make a total of ¾ cup; stir gently to blend.

Pour into chilled champagne glass or wineglass. Serve immediately.

1 serving
1 serving = ¾ cup

CAL.	CHO(g)	PRO.(g)	TOTAL FAT(g)	SAT. FAT(g)	CHOL.(mg)	FIBER(g)	SODIUM(mg)
40	10	0	0	0	0	0	25

Food exchange per serving: 1 Fruit
Low-sodium diets: This recipe is excellent.

Appendix:
Sources of Information

People with diabetes as well as their families and friends can benefit from understanding the disease and its effects. The more you know, the more in control you will feel. With this confidence, you will find it easier to make wise decisions about food choices, exercise, and medication adjustments.

Remember that you are not alone. Many individuals and organizations are ready to help. Your primary sources of information are your doctor, registered dietitian, diabetes educator, and other members of your health care team. Your relationship with these health professionals becomes quite personal. It's important to be frank about your concerns and problems. Honesty is essential if you are to get the individualized care you need. If you are dissatisfied with the quality of your care, find other professionals to help you. Take charge! It's your life.

Two national organizations have referral services that can help you find a credentialed nutrition counselor. One of these is the National Center for Nutrition and Dietetics, the public education initiative of The American Dietetic Association and its Foundation (1-800-366-1655). The other is the American Association of Diabetes Educators (1-312-644-AADE).

Your local affiliate of the American Diabetes Association is another source of referrals to physicians and registered dietitians who specialize in diabetes care. Some major medical centers have diabetes centers that are wonderful sources of information and counseling. Ask the American Diabetes Association for the location of the nearest Diabetes Education and Training Center. Call for an appointment if you have recently diagnosed diabetes or problems in managing your condition.

The American Diabetes Association also offers a number of publications. When you join the national organization, you automatically become a member of a local affiliate. These organizations sponsor useful programs and support groups.

Your local library is yet another source of information. If you have a computer modem, you may want to join one of the on-line services, such as CompuServe, which has an active Diabetes Forum featuring literature as well as discussion groups.

Organizations

All of these organizations will send you information about their materials and/or programs for people with diabetes:

American Association of Diabetes Educators   (800) 832-6874
Suite 1240
444 N. Michigan Ave.
Chicago, IL 60611-3901
Referrals to certified diabetes educators in your local area

The American Diabetes Association   (800) 232-3472
1660 Duke St.
Alexandria, VA 22314

The American Dietetic Association   (800) 877-1600
National Center for Nutrition and Dietetics
216 W. Jackson Blvd.
Chicago, IL 60606-6995
Pretaped nutrition messages; registered dietitian available to answer questions; referral to a local registered dietitian for individual counseling

American Heart Association   (800) 242-8721
7272 Greenville Ave.
Dallas, TX 75231

Canadian Diabetes Association   (416) 214-1900
Suite 500
15 Toronto St.
Toronto, ON Canada M5C 2E3

International Diabetes Center   (612) 993-3393
3800 Park Nicollet Blvd.
Minneapolis, MN 55416
Excellent books, cookbooks, and information on many aspects of diabetes care

International Diabetic Athletes Association   (602) 433-2113
1647-B W. Bethany Home Rd.
Phoenix, AZ 85015

Joslin Diabetes Center   (617) 732-2400
1 Joslin Place
Boston, MA 02215
Ask for a list of current publications.

Juvenile Diabetes Foundation   (212) 889-7575
432 Park Avenue
New York, NY 10016
Ask for your local chapter's name and address.

National Diabetes Information Clearinghouse   (301) 654-3327
1 Information Way
Bethesda, MD 20892
Listings of material on specific diabetes-related topics

Periodicals for People with Diabetes

Diabetes Forecast   (800) 232-3472
*A monthly magazine for the members of the American Diabetes Association (a
benefit of membership and not available separately)*

Diabetes Self-Management   (212) 989-0200
150 W. 22nd St.
New York, NY 10011
*A bimonthly magazine featuring information on diabetes self-care, nutrition,
exercise, medical advances, and research*

The Diabetic Reader   **(800) 735-7726**
5623 Matilija Ave.
Van Nuys, CA 91401
A semiannual newsletter written by June Biermann and Barbara Toohey featuring book and audiotape reviews and excerpts and mail-order sources

Books for People with Diabetes

Franz, Marion J. *Exchanges for All Occasions: Meeting the Challenge of Diabetes*, 3rd ed. Minneapolis: Chronimed Publishing, 1993.

Franz, Marion J. *Fast Food Facts.* Minneapolis: Chronimed Publishing, 1994.

Franz, Marion J., et al. *Learning to Live Well with Diabetes.* Minneapolis: Chronimed Publishing, 1991.

Guthrie, Diana W., and Guthrie, Richard A. *The Diabetes Sourcebook.* Los Angeles: Lowell House, 1995.

Hollerorth, Hugo J., and Kaplan, Dora. *Everyone Likes to Eat*, 2nd ed. Boston: Joslin Publications, 1993. Activities, exercises, and information on managing a child's diabetes.

Pennington, J. A. T. *Bowes and Church's Food Values of Portions Commonly Used*, 16th ed. Philadelphia: J. B. Lippincott Company, 1994. This book lists food values in grams and milligrams if you want to compute your own recipes. It is used by professionals and is a comprehensive reference useful for counting grams of carbohydrate.

Polin, Ronnie S., and Giedt, Frances T. *The Joslin Diabetes Gourmet Cookbook.* New York: Bantam Books, 1993.

Powers, Margaret A. *Handbook of Diabetes Nutritional Management*, 2nd ed. Rockville, Maryland.: Aspen Publishers, Inc., 1995. An excellent reference for diabetes counselors.

Thom, Susan, and Betschart, Jean. *In Control: A Guide for Teens with Diabetes.* Minneapolis: Chronimed Publishing, 1995.

Warshaw, Hope. *Eating Out: Your Guide to More Enjoyable Dining.* New York: Diabetes Self-Management Books, 1990.

Warshaw, Hope. *The Healthy Eater's Guide to Family and Chain Restaurants.* Minneapolis: Chronimed Publishing, 1993.

Warshaw, Hope. *The Restaurant Companion: A Guide to Healthier Eating Out.* 2nd ed. Chicago: Surrey Books, 1995.

Videotapes

Know Your Diabetes, Know Yourself. Boston: Joslin Diabetes Center.

Living with Diabetes: A Winning Formula. Boston: Joslin Diabetes Center.

Glossary

Acesulfame K: A heat-stable artificial sweetener, 200 times sweeter than sucrose, that is not metabolized by the body and is excreted in the urine.

Alcohol: A substance produced when carbohydrates are fermented. Alcohol is an ingredient of beer, wine, liquors, and other beverages. Each gram of pure alcohol yields 7 calories. See Chapter 3, "The Food Exchange System."

Amino acids: The building units of proteins. There are 22 amino acids, 9 of which must be supplied by the diet; others can be made in the body.

Antioxidants: Substances that protect the cells in the body from damages and may prevent or delay the onset of some forms of cancer and heart diseases, and slow aging. *Vitamins* E, C, and A and the mineral selenium have antioxidant properties.

Aspartame: The chemical name of a sugar substitute derived from amino acids. Products containing NutraSweet®, such as Equal®, contain this sweetener. It is found in many sugar-free sodas, yogurts, and other products. See Chapter 4, "What You Need to Know About Carbohydrates."

Atherosclerosis: Deposits of fat and other substances in the walls of arteries that cause loss of elasticity and decreased blood flow. Severe atherosclerosis, sometimes called heart disease, can lead to heart attacks, circulatory problems, and strokes.

Blood glucose: Sugar in the blood. Blood glucose level can be determined by a simple test, using only a drop of blood from a fingerstick.

Calorie: A unit used to measure heat energy provided by food. Carbohydrates, proteins, fats, alcohol, and sugar alcohols provide calories. Vitamins, minerals, and dietary fiber do not provide calories.

Carbohydrates: Compounds that contain carbon, hydrogen, and oxygen and are found in sugars and starches. Carbohydrates are in foods from the Milk, Vegetable, Fruit, Starch, and Other Carbohydrates Exchange lists. Carbohydrates are the major source of energy for the body, yielding 4 calories per gram. The abbreviation for carbohydrate in our recipes is *CHO*. See Chapter 4, "What You Need to Know About Carbohydrates."

Cardiovascular: Referring to the heart and blood vessels.

Certified Diabetes Educator (C.D.E.): A health care professional who has mastered a core of knowledge and skill in the biological sciences and social sciences, communication and counseling, and education, and who has experience in the care of patients with diabetes. Various health care professionals—physicians, registered dietitians, nurses, pharmacists, social workers, podiatrists, and exercise physiologists—may have fulfilled the requirements to become certified diabetes educators.

Cholesterol: A waxy fatlike substance found in animals as a part of the brain, hormones, cells, bile, nerve tissue, and blood. When too much cholesterol is present, it deposits in artery walls, causing atherosclerosis. Cholesterol is made by the liver but is also found in foods of animal origin, particularly egg yolks and organ meats. It is found in some foods from the Milk, Meat, and Fat Exchange lists. Every recipe in this book has a cholesterol value listed as CHOL.

Diabetes mellitus: The failure of the body cells to use glucose from food due to an absolute (in Type I diabetes) or relative (in Type II diabetes) lack of insulin; often referred to simply as diabetes. The literal translation is "a flowing of honey."

Diabetologist: A doctor who specializes in the treatment of individuals with diabetes mellitus.

Dietitian: A specialist in applying the principles of nutrition and meal planning. A registered dietitian (R.D.) is recognized by the medical profession as the primary provider of medical nutrition therapy, including nutritional care, education, and counseling. The initials R.D. after a dietitian's name ensure that she or he has met the standards of The American Dietetic Association and has passed a national registration exam. Look for this credential when you seek advice on nutrition. Some states also have licensed dietitians (L.D.). This additional credential does not replace the R.D. A registered or licensed dietitian may also become a certified diabetes educator (C.D.E.).

Endocrinologist: A physician who specializes in the treatment of individuals with endocrine (hormonal) diseases, including diabetes.

Enrichment: The replacement of nutrients in a food that were lost in food processing. Enriched bread, for example, has added thiamin, riboflavin, niacin, and iron.

Exchanges: Foods with similar nutrient values grouped together on a list. Specified amounts of each food on the list have values of carbohydrate, protein, fat, and calories similar to other foods on the same list.

Fat: Oily substances found in meat, fish, poultry, eggs, butter, cheese, milk, and some starches and vegetables; a concentrated source of calories, yielding 9 calories per gram. May be *saturated* or *unsaturated.* See Chapter 5, "A New Look at Fats."

Fiber: Indigestible carbohydrates found in whole grains; dried beans, peas, and lentils; seeds; and fruits and vegetables. After digestion, fiber yields bulk but no calories. Fibers are classified as *soluble* or *insoluble.* Different types of fiber have different benefits to the body. See Chapter 4, "What You Need to Know About Carbohydrates."

Food habits: A person's pattern of choosing, preparing, and eating foods; a result of cultural, economic, family, and religious influences.

Fortification: The addition to a food of nutrients that are not naturally occurring in that food. Milk is almost always fortified with vitamins A and D. Many cereals, breakfast drinks, and processed foods are fortified.

Free Foods: Foods that contain few calories and carbohydrates. People with diabetes may use Free Foods in their diet without measuring portions or may use them in limited quantities without counting them as exchanges. Usually, Free Foods have fewer than 20 calories per serving. Free Foods that contain calories should be limited to three servings per day, because even small numbers of calories add up. Herbs, spices, and other ingredients that contain no calories may be used safely in any amount. See Free Foods list in Chapter 3, "The Food Exchange System."

Fructose: A type of simple sugar naturally found in fruits. See Chapter 4, "What You Need to Know About Carbohydrates."

Gastrointestinal: Referring to the digestive tract.

Glucagon: A hormone produced by the pancreas that raises blood glucose by breaking down glycogen produced by and stored in the liver; its activity opposes that of insulin. This hormone can be given by injection if the blood glucose level is so low that treatment must be administered by another person.

Gluconeogenesis: The conversion of amino acids to glucose by the liver, which thus raises blood glucose levels.

Glucose: A simple sugar that results from the digestion of carbohydrate-containing foods. All sugars and starches, and some protein and fat, are converted to glucose, which is the form of sugar used by the body for energy. See Chapter 4, "What You Need to Know About Carbohydrates."

Glycated hemoglobin: A test that provides the average of blood glucose levels during the preceding two to three months. When blood glucose is above normal, more glucose attaches to the hemoglobin in red blood cells. Because these cells remain altered for about 100 days, the amount of glucose in the hemoglobin can be measured. The level is used to evaluate adherence to the meal plan.

Glycogen: Form of carbohydrate stored in the liver as a reserve source of fuel. During fasting (including overnight and in the morning until you eat) or during an insulin reaction (hypoglycemia), glycogen breaks down to glucose and is released into the bloodstream to provide fuel for cells.

Gram: A unit of mass and weight in the metric system. A gram is approximately the weight of a paper clip. An ounce is about 28 grams. In recipe calculations and nutrient lists, *g* is the abbreviation for gram.

Healthy weight: The best weight a person can achieve and maintain over time. Healthy weights are individually determined based on genetics, frame size, body shape, medical risks, and other factors.

High-density lipoproteins (HDLs): The "good" type of cholesterol that protects against heart disease by returning excess cholesterol to the liver to be processed and excreted into the digestive tract as bile. HDL can be raised by increasing exercise.

Hormones: Chemical messengers that work in the bloodstream to regulate metabolic processes in each cell of the body. Insulin is a hormone.

Hydrogenation: The process of adding hydrogen to a liquid fat (oil); makes the fat more solid at room temperature and more saturated. This process is used to make margarine or shortening from oil.

Hyperglycemia: An abnormally high blood glucose level. It is treated with insulin and replacement of lost fluids. Hyperglycemia can lead to diabetic emergencies and/or long-term complications of diabetes mellitus.

Hypoglycemia: A low blood glucose level (usually below 70 milligrams per deciliter) that can lead to unconsciousness if untreated. Hypoglycemia can be caused by too much insulin, not enough food, a delayed meal, or extra activity. Common symptoms include confusion, tiredness, shakiness, dizziness, headaches, and/or emotional stress. Treatment requires quickly increasing blood glucose levels by eating rapidly absorbed sugars or injecting glucagon.

IDDM: Insulin-dependent diabetes mellitus (Type I diabetes). Individuals with IDDM are ketosis-prone and will develop ketoacidosis if they do not take insulin regularly. This type of diabetes was formerly called "juvenile-onset diabetes," because it is usually diagnosed in childhood or adolescence.

Insoluble fiber: Fiber that has poor water-holding capability; found in foods such as wheat bran and other whole grains. Insoluble fiber (cellulose) appears to speed the passage of foods through the stomach and intestines and aids elimination. This type of fiber probably does not significantly affect blood glucose levels or the risk of atherosclerosis.

Insulin: A hormone produced by the beta cells of the pancreas that helps the body use food. Insulin regulates glucose going from the blood into body cells. Commercially prepared insulin is an injectable substance used by people who do not make enough insulin of their own.

Ketoacidosis: A deficiency of available insulin. This imbalance results in an increase in ketones in the blood (hyperglycemia) and dehydration, causing the body's acid balance to shift to abnormal levels. Ketoacidosis is an emergency situation that may result in coma and death if untreated.

Ketone: An acid (such as acetone) formed in the body when fats are burned for energy because the cells do not have enough carbohydrate within them to use as fuel. Although blood glucose levels are high enough, insulin isn't available to allow glucose to enter the cells.

Lipids: Another word for *fats*. In addition to stored body fats, there are several types of lipids, such as cholesterol and triglycerides, that circulate in the bloodstream. See Chapter 5, "A New Look at Fats."

Lipoprotein: Complexes of fat joined with protein. Lipoproteins transport *cholesterol* in the bloodstream. May be high-density, low-density, or very low-density. See Chapter 5, "A New Look at Fats."

Low-density lipoproteins (LDLs) and Very-low density lipoproteins (VLDLs): The "bad" lipoproteins that transport cholesterol throughout the circulatory system. In excess, LDLs and VLDLs contribute to the formation of deposits on artery walls that can lead to heart attack and stroke.

Low-sodium diet: A modified diet that may be prescribed by a physician to treat high blood pressure or cardiovascular disease. A registered dietitian can mark this book to help you select recipes with limited amounts of sodium. On the exchange lists, foods high in sodium are marked with this symbol: 🧂. Follow the directions at the end of each recipe if you are on a low-sodium diet. This diet may also be called a low-salt or sodium-restricted diet.

Low-sodium foods: Foods that are processed or prepared without the addition of salt or other high-sodium ingredients. According to food label regulations, low-sodium means there is 140 milligrams of sodium or less per standard serving of that food. Reduced-sodium (unsalted) alternatives for high-sodium foods (soy sauce, canned vegetables, cereals, catsup, baking powder, cheese, etc.) may be available at your grocery store.

Meal plan: A specific plan prepared by a registered dietitian that reflects the nutrition prescription and the food habits of an individual. The guide shows the number of food exchanges or grams of carbohydrate per meal and snack. Some meal plans may monitor calories, fats, or other nutrients. See Chapter 1, "The Meal Plan."

Metabolism: The chemical and physical processes within all cells of the body that use energy (calories).

Milligram: A metric weight equal to 1/1,000 gram. In the recipe calculations, sodium and cholesterol are measured in milligrams, the abbreviation for which is *mg*.

Mineral: Chemically inorganic substances found in nature that are needed in small amounts to build and repair body tissue or to control metabolism. Calcium, iron, magnesium, phosphorus, potassium, sodium, and zinc are important minerals.

Monounsaturated fat: An unsaturated fat that may help lower "bad" LDL cholesterol levels without lowering "good" HDL cholesterol levels. Olive, canola, and peanut oils are good sources of monounsaturated fat. For information on the special role monounsaturated fat can play in the diet, see Chapter 5, "A New Look at Fats."

NIDDM: Non-insulin-dependent diabetes mellitus (Type II diabetes). Individuals with NIDDM may or may not take insulin for better control of their blood glucose levels; however, they are not ketosis-prone. NIDDM is the current terminology that has generally replaced "adult-onset (maturity-onset) diabetes." It is usually diagnosed after the age of 40.

Nutrients: Substances necessary to life that are found in and must be provided by food. Carbohydrates, proteins, fats, vitamins, minerals, and water are nutrients.

Nutrition: The process of taking in and utilizing food to nourish the body.

Omega-3 fatty acids: A type of polyunsaturated fat found in the oil of fish. These fatty acids have been shown to reduce levels of blood cholesterol. See Chapter 5, "A New Look at Fats."

Oral hypoglycemic agents: Drugs, taken by mouth, that lower blood sugar; sometimes called "antidiabetic pills."

Pancreas: A gland in the upper abdomen that secretes digestive enzymes into the intestine. The pancreas contains cells that produce many hormones, including insulin and glucagon, that are released directly into the bloodstream and regulate blood sugar levels.

Phytochemicals: Nonnutrient chemicals found in plants that may have disease-preventing potential or medicinal effects on the body. For example, indole-3-carbinol (found in cruciferous vegetables) and polyphenols (found in green tea) may protect against cancer. There may be hundreds, perhaps thousands of phytochemicals. Research is ongoing to identify these chemicals, and their specific effects.

Polyunsaturated fat: An unsaturated fat that may decrease both "good" HDL cholesterol and "bad" LDL cholesterol. It is found in fish and in vegetable oils such as corn, safflower, and sunflower.

Postprandial: After eating.

Preprandial: Before eating.

Protein: A major nutrient made up of amino acids that are necessary to build and repair tissue. Protein provides 4 calories per gram when burned for energy. It is found primarily in foods from the Milk and Meat Exchange lists. Small amounts are found in grains and some vegetables. The abbreviation for protein in our recipe calculations is *PRO.*

Animal protein is protein from animal sources—milk, meat, poultry, fish, eggs, and cheese. Animal proteins contain all nine essential amino acids that cannot be manufactured by the body.

Vegetable protein (plant protein) is protein from soybeans, nuts, dried peas and beans, seeds, oatmeal, wheat germ, and grains. These proteins usually contain some, but not all, of the essential amino acids. Combinations of vegetable proteins, however, can provide all essential amino acids. All essential amino acids must be present for the body to make proteins for cell maintenance, hormone formation, healing, and growth.

Saccharin: An artificial sweetener that provides no carbohydrate or calories. See Chapter 4, "What You Need to Know About Carbohydrates."

Salt: Sodium chloride, a compound containing about 40 percent sodium, that is used as a food flavoring and preservative.

Saturated fat: Fats that have no double bonds in their chemical structure are often firm at room temperature. Saturated fats tend to raise blood cholesterol levels. These fats are found in butter, stick margarine, lard, meat fat, eggs, solid shortening, palm oil, and coconut oil. All fats actually contain some saturated and some unsaturated fatty acids. When we categorize a fat as "saturated," it means that there are more of these types of fatty acids in the chemical structure of the food than "unsaturated" fatty acids.

Sodium: A mineral, needed by the body to maintain life, found mainly as a component of salt. Sodium-sensitive individuals need to limit the amount of sodium (and salt) they eat to prevent or control high blood pressure. Each recipe calculation includes a sodium value and instructions on how to reduce the sodium level if a low-sodium diet is prescribed.

Soluble fiber: Fiber that has high water-holding capability and turns to gel during digestion, thus slowing digestion and the rate of nutrient absorption from the stomach and intestine. This type of fiber is in oat bran, pectin (from fruits and vegetables), and various gums found in seeds and legumes, including dried beans, peas, and lentils. Soluble fiber may play a role in reducing the elevation of blood glucose after eating and in lowering the risk of atherosclerosis by reducing blood cholesterol levels.

Starch: One of the two major types of carbohydrate. Starch is a complex molecule of linked sugar units that do not taste sweet. Foods with starches are found on the Starch Exchange list.

Sugar: One of the two major types of carbohydrate. Foods with simple sugars are found on the Milk, Vegetable, and Fruit Exchange lists. Other simple sugars include table sugar and the sugar alcohols. See Chapter 4, "What You Need to Know About Carbohydrates."

Sugar alcohols: Isomalt, sorbitol, mannitol, and xylitol—chemical substances that taste sweet but are more slowly absorbed by the body than sugars. In excess, they have a laxative effect. Sugar alcohols are found in sugar-free gums and some sugar-free processed foods. Like sugar and other carbohydrates, most contain 4 calories per gram. See Chapter 4, "What You Need to Know About Carbohydrates."

Trans-fatty acids: A chemically modified fatty acid that can result when polyunsaturated oils are hydrogenated or partially hydrogenated. They are found in shortening, stick margarine, and some whipped toppings.

Triglycerides: The main storage form of fat (three fatty acids linked by a glycerol molecule) that circulates in the bloodstream. Excess weight and consuming too much fat, alcohol, or sugar may increase blood triglycerides to an unacceptably high level. See Chapter 5, "A New Look at Fats."

Unsaturated fats: Fats with specific chemical structures that are usually liquid at room temperature. Unsaturated fats tend to lower blood cholesterol levels. They may be *monounsaturated* or *polyunsaturated*, depending on their chemical structure. Examples of foods containing primarily unsaturated fats are vegetable oils such as corn, cottonseed, canola, sunflower, safflower, soybean, olive, and peanut and some fats in fish and chicken.

Urinalysis: Chemical analysis of the urine. Urine can be tested for the presence of glucose (sugar), an indication of diabetes mellitus. When blood sugar levels get very high, glucose can be found in the urine.

Vitamins: Organic substances found in food that are needed in very tiny amounts for normal body functions; include vitamins A, B complex, C, D, E, and K. Vitamins in foods or pills do not provide calories.

Index